The rapid growth of knowledge in molecular biology during the last decade has had far-reaching implications for the understanding, diagnosis and management of haematological malignant disease. The response of many conditions to treatment, and the ease with which patient material can be repeatedly sampled, have made this a fruitful area of study, and in parallel with the expanding contribution of molecular biology there has been growing awareness of the importance of epidemiology, techniques of drug administration, patient support and the evaluation of treatment results.

Haematological Oncology will serve as a regular forum for the evaluation and dissemination of this new information, and the topics selected for review range from basic science to clinical applications.

This series provides a comprehensive and up-to-date review of the current state of research and will be an important source of information and knowledge for oncologists, immunologists, postgraduate trainees and other clinical and laboratory workers in the field.

Cambridge Medical Reviews

Haematological Oncology   Volume 1

Cambridge Medical Reviews, a programme of review volumes for the clinical sciences, focuses attention on fields in which rapid and continuing advances in biomedical science have increased significantly our understanding and treatment of disease. Each review series is devoted to a single, clinical discipline. The purpose is to provide a regular evaluation and commentary on the growth of knowledge in that subject. Rigorous standards of selection and editing ensure a reliable and topical series of volumes which will meet the requirements of clinicians and research workers alike.

Haematological Oncology

Series editors

Adrian Newland
Department of Haematology, The London Hospital
Whitechapel, London, UK

James Armitage
Department of Medicine, University of Nebraska Medical Center
Omaha, Nebraska, USA

Alan Burnett
Department of Haematology, Glasgow Royal Infirmary
Glasgow, UK

Armand Keating
Autologous Bone Marrow Transplant Program
Toronto General Hospital
Ontario, Canada

Cambridge Medical Reviews

Haematological Oncology
Volume I

EDITORS

ADRIAN NEWLAND
Department of Haematology, The London Hospital
Whitechapel, London, UK

JAMES ARMITAGE
Department of Medicine, University of Nebraska Medical Center
Omaha, Nebraska, USA

ALAN BURNETT
Department of Haematology, Glasgow Royal Infirmary,
Glasgow, UK

ARMAND KEATING
Autologous Bone Marrow Transplant Program
Toronto General Hospital, Ontario, Canada

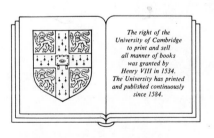

The right of the
University of Cambridge
to print and sell
all manner of books
was granted by
Henry VIII in 1534.
The University has printed
and published continuously
since 1584.

CAMBRIDGE UNIVERSITY PRESS

Cambridge
New York · Port Chester · Melbourne · Sydney

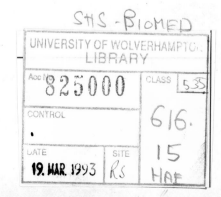

SHS - BIOMED

UNIVERSITY OF WOLVERHAMPTON
LIBRARY

Acc No 825000

CLASS 535

CONTROL

616.

DATE 19. MAR. 1993

SITE RS

15

HAE

Published by the Press Syndicate of the University of Cambridge
The Pitt Building, Trumpington Street, Cambridge CB2 1RP
40 West 20th Street, New York, NY 10011-4211, USA
10 Stamford Road, Oakleigh, Victoria 3166, Australia

First published 1991

Printed in Great Britain at the University Press, Cambridge

British Library cataloguing in publication data

Haematological oncology. Vol. 1
I. Newland, A.C. (Adrian Charles)
616.15

Library of Congress cataloguing in publication data available

ISBN 0 521 40193 3 hardback

WV

Contents

	page
Contributors	viii
Haemopoietic regulation by growth factors	1
V DEVALIA and D C LINCH	
Mechanisms of multi-drug resistance	29
D HOCHHAUSER and A L HARRIS	
Immunotoxins in haematological oncology	49
V S BYERS and R W BALDWIN	
Alpha interferon: uses and possible mechanisms of action	63
D W GALVANI and J C CAWLEY	
The genetics of the Philadelphia chromosome	79
R KURZROCK and M TALPAZ	
Treatment options for remission in acute myeloid leukaemia	111
A K BURNETT and B LÖWENBERG	
Gene rearrangements and minimal residual disease in lymphoproliferative disorders	145
F E COTTER	
Controversies in therapy for the low grade lymphomas	173
P McLAUGHLIN, F CABANILLAS and A C NEWLAND	
The management of high grade non-Hodgkin's lymphomas	195
J M VOSE and J O ARMITAGE	
CNS prophylaxis – who and how	209
O B EDEN	
Multiple myeloma: Host–tumour and tumour–host interactions	225
D E JOSHUA	
Index	241

Contributors

ARMITAGE, J O, University of Nebraska Medical Center, Department of Internal Medicine, Section of Oncology/Haematology, 600 South 42nd Street, Omaha, NE 68198-3330, USA

BALDWIN, R W, Cancer Research Campaign Laboratories, University of Nottingham, Nottingham NG7 2RD, UK

BURNETT, A K, Department of Haematology, Glasgow Royal Infirmary, Castle Street, Glasgow G4 0SF, UK

BYERS, V S, Cancer Research Campaign Laboratories, University of Nottingham, Nottingham NG7 2RD, UK

CABANILLAS, F, MD Anderson Cancer Center, 1515 Holcombe, Box 68, Houston, Texas 77030, USA

CAWLEY, J C, University Department of Haematology, Duncan Building, Royal Liverpool Hospital, Prescot Street, Liverpool L69 3BX, UK

COTTER, F E, ICRF Department of Medical Oncology, St Bartholomew's Hospital, London, EC1A 7BE, UK

DEVALIA, V, Department of Haematology, University College and Middlesex School of Medicine, London WC1E 6HX, UK

EDEN, O B, Department of Haematology, Royal Hospital for Sick Children, 17 Millerfield Place, Edinburgh EH9 1LF, UK

GALVANI, D W, University Department of Haematology, Duncan Building, Royal Liverpool Hospital, Prescot Street, Liverpool L69 3BX, UK

HARRIS, A L, Molecular Oncology Laboratory, Imperial Cancer Research Fund Laboratories, Institute of Molecular Medicine, University of Oxford, John Radcliffe Hospital, Headington, Oxford OX3 9DU, UK

HOCHHAUSER, D, Molecular Oncology Laboratory, Imperial Cancer Research Fund Laboratories, Institute of Molecular Medicine, University of Oxford, John Radcliffe Hospital, Headington, Oxford OX3 9DU, UK

JOSHUA, D E, Haematology Department, Royal Prince Alfred Hospital, Camperdown NSW 2050, Australia

KEATING, A, University of Toronto, Toronto General Hospital, Mulock Larkin Wing, 1-010, 200 Elizabeth Street, Toronto, Ontario, Canada M5G 2C4

KURZROCK, R, The Department of Clinical Immunology and

viii

Biological Therapy, Box 41, MD Anderson Cancer Center, 1515 Holcombe Blvd, Houston, Texas 77030, USA

LINCH, D C, Department of Haematology, University College and Middlesex School of Medicine, London WC1E 6HX, UK

LÖWENBERG, B, Dr Daniel den Hoed Cancer Centre and Erasmus University, Rotterdam, The Netherlands

McLAUGHLIN, P, MD Anderson Cancer Center, 1515 Holcombe, Box 68, Houston, Texas 77030, USA

NEWLAND, A C, Department of Haematology, The London Hospital Medical College, Turner Street, London E1 2AD, UK

TALPAZ, M, Department of Clinical Immunology and Biological Therapy, Box 41, MD Anderson Cancer Center, 1515 Holcombe Blvd, Houston, Texas 77030, USA

VOSE, J M, University of Nebraska Medical Center, Department of Internal Medicine, Section of Oncology/Haematology, 600 South 42nd Street, Omaham, NE 68198-3339, USA

Haemopoietic regulation by growth factors

V DEVALIA and D C LINCH

Introduction

In adult life, the cells that circulate in the blood are produced in the 'red bone marrow' restricted to the flat bones and proximal ends of the long bones. In the 1920s, Maximov and others proposed that all the blood cells were derived from a common haemopoietic stem cell. In 1961, Till and McCulloch[1] demonstrated that when a lethally irradiated mouse was rescued by a syngeneic bone marrow infusion, the injected cells, as well as repopulating the marrow, formed colonies within the spleen. These colonies were derived from single cells and contained cells of several myeloid lineages. Further work by Wu and colleagues[2] and Abramson[3] using chromosome markers in mouse bone marrow transplants suggested that all haemopoietic cells were derived from a common stem cell and this has been confirmed in elegant transplantation experiments using retroviral molecular markers.[4,5]

The most primitive haemopoietic cells can either undergo self-renewal or give rise to cells of the different lineages. As the cells differentiate within the bone marrow, there is progressive loss of lineage potential and the later progenitors can give rise to progeny of only one type. The stem cells are predominantly in a resting state but their recruitment into the proliferating pool, or the insertion of extra divisions in the differentiation pathway, would lead to an amplification of the mature cell pool.

The steady state level of peripheral blood cells is remarkably constant and yet the bone marrow can respond rapidly to stress by increasing output many fold, indicating that there is a complex and finely controlled regulatory mechanism.

In 1906, Carnot and Deflandre[6] suggested that erythropoiesis was regulated by a factor present in the plasma which later became known as erythropoietin.[7]

In the 1960s, Pluznik and Sachs[8] and Bradley and Metcalf[9] developed in vitro colony assays for mouse haemopoietic cells, and these were later adapted

All correspondence to: Professor David C Linch, Department of Haematology, University College and Middlesex School of Medicine, London WC1E 6HX.

Cambridge Medical Reviews: Haematological Oncology Volume 1
© Cambridge University Press 1991

for use in man.[10,11] As well as providing further information on the structural organization of the haemopoietic system, these culture systems provided assays for regulatory molecules. The colony stimulating factors (CSFs) were first identified in a variety of tissue fluids and cell culture supernatant, and in 1983 Nicola and colleagues[12] reported the purification to homogeneity of G-CSF.

The application of recombinant DNA technology has allowed molecular cloning of genes for these substances and production of synthetic material.[13,14] A substantial number of factors have been characterized in this way and named according to the lineage stimulated in vitro, or designated as interleukins. The term haemopoietic growth factors (HGFs) is used here to include the CSFs, the interleukins directly involved in myeloid proliferation, and erythropoietin.

The bone marrow micro-environment is extremely complex. Whereas only late progenitor cells can be propagated in semi-solid culture, primitive stem cells can be maintained in long-term liquid culture systems, which require the establishment of a feeder layer comprising fibroblastoid cells, adipocytes and other cell types.[15] The precise role of the stromal cells is not clear. With the exception of M-CSF it has been difficult to demonstrate that the stromal layer produces HGFs, and it is possible that, in the appropriate micro-environment, HGF independent proliferation can occur. It has been shown, however, that the stromal matrix can bind some HGFs with high affinity,[16,17] and the alternative possibility is that the stromal cells produce low amounts of HGFs which are presented with high efficiency over a short range to adherent stem cells and progenitor cells.

The HGFs are all glycoproteins possessing biological activity at picomolar concentrations. GM-CSF, G-CSF, IL-3 and IL-6 are single subunit proteins whereas M-CSF and IL-5 are composed of two identical disulphide-linked subunits. Although the factors have some overlap of biological activity and specificity, there is very little sequence homology between them. Interspecies sequence conservation and biological activity is also variable, for example, comparison of human and murine amino acid sequence for M-CSF, G-CSF and IL-5 show approximately 75% homology with some cross-species biological activity; GM-CSF and IL-6 approximately 50%; and IL-3 approximately 28% with little cross species biological activity.

The carbohydrate moieties on the growth factors do not seem to be directly necessary for biological activity, and may act to enhance the solubility, stability, and resistance to proteolysis.

Cloning of the HGFs and chromosomal location

Three major strategies have been used to clone the genes encoding for the HGFs (see Table 1). First, the relevant factor may be purified from biological fluids or tissue culture supernatant, the protein sequenced and relevant

Table 1. *Chromosomal localization and molecular size of the principal human haemopoietic growth factors*

Growth factor	Cromosomal location	Mol. wt. (kD)	Cloning ref
Erythropoietin	7q	34–39	18, 19
G-CSF	17q	18	20
M-CSF	5q	40–50, 70–90	21
IL-5	5q	29–66	22
GM-CSF	5q	14–35	23, 24, 25
IL-3	5q	14–28	26
IL-6	7q	23–32	27
IL-1α	2q	12–19	28

oligonucleotides made to probe a cDNA library. Murine GM-CSF, human G-CSF, and IL-6 cDNAs were identified using this approach. Secondly, a cDNA library can be expressed in a eukaryotic system and the protein product screened for by the use of antibodies or bioassay. The identities of cDNAs coding for murine and human IL-3, human GM-CSF, and murine IL-5 were thus established. Thirdly, when the relevant gene has been cloned in another species by the above methods, it can be used as a probe to cross-hybridize with the human cDNA library. Success with this strategy relies on the presence of a sufficient degree of homology of the gene between the two species, exemplified by the murine IL-3 probe failing to hybridize with the human gene (45% homology) whereas use of a gibbon IL-3 gene probe (99.5% homology) was successful. Having cloned the genes, their chromosomal location can be determined by in situ hybridization techniques. The HGF genes are present in single copies and show a striking clustering in both the murine and human genomes. The genes for murine GM-CSF and IL-3 are located close together as chromosome 11, which also contains the G-CSF and IL-5 genes as well as the gene for the M-CSF receptor (c-*fms*).[29] Part of the murine chromosome 11 is homologous to the long arm of human chromosome 5, which also shows a similar topography of human GM-CSF, IL-3, M-CSF, IL-5 genes, as well as the M-CSF receptor gene, which have all been mapped to this region of chromosome 5.[30] Interestingly, this region is deleted in a certain group of patients who suffer from a type of myelodysplastic syndrome, the 5q-syndrome, and is also a common cytogenetic abnormality in myeloid malignancies. It is difficult to define any direct correlation between the clinical entities and the possible loss of one or more growth factors or receptor gene(s). Although the genes for GM-CSF and IL-3 are very closely linked (about 10 kb apart) they are independently controlled since many cell types synthesize GM-CSF, but only activated T-cells produce IL-3. The human gene for G-CSF is located on chromosome 17 at locus q21–q22[31] and this region too is homologous to the corresponding region of murine chromosome 11. In close proximity to the gene for G-CSF is the gene for myeloperoxidase, an enzyme found in the primary granules of neutrophils. Although human promyelocytic leukaemias are associated with a translocation between chromosome 15 and 17, the G-CSF gene does not appear to be altered by this translocation. Human IL-6 is found on chromosome 7, as is the gene for erythropoietin.[32]

Production of HGFs

The haemopoietic growth factors are produced by a wide range of activated cell types (Table 2).[33] Such cells are found in sites of inflammation and the HGFs may have a role in the mediation of the inflammatory response. Although the production of factors at local sites of inflammation may partly explain the attendant bone marrow response, the resting control of steady state haemopoiesis is not explained in this way and the internal marrow processes by which circulating blood cell numbers remain so constant in health remains obscure.

It is noteworthy that several sources of haemopoietic growth factors are themselves mature haemopoietic cells, and such cells also modulate the production of these growth factors by endothelial cells and fibroblasts. It is thus possible that a major insult to the bone marrow would not only reduce the progenitor cell pool but would also impair the homeostatic response mechanisms.

Analysis of the genes of HGFs has revealed interesting findings, with particular reference to control of transcription and hence gene expression. A common structural element at their 5′ ends in the GM-CSF, IL-3, G-CSF, IL-5, and IL-6 genes, called CK1, is found at a position 73–183 nucleotides upstream of the TATA box. In the GM-CSF and IL-3 genes, another conserved region called CK2 is found just 3′ to the CK1. Despite the demonstration of nuclear binding proteins in gel-retardation studies for these sites, only limited specificity in their tissue expression has been shown.[34] In addition, in stimulated T-cells, DNase I footprinting studies of the human GM-CSF gene have identified the importance of a different nuclear-protein binding region[35] distinct from CK1 and CK2. The role of these regions in gene expression therefore remains to be determined. Initiation of transcription at different sites has also been described for a number of the growth factor genes, including GM-CSF, IL-3, and IL-6, resulting in production of different size transcripts and altered protein molecules. The less common initiation site seems to lie up to 10 kb upstream to the more common site, resulting in production of an altered protein with a hydrophilic domain N-terminal to the hydrophobic leader sequence. Alternative splicing of primary mRNA transcripts may also give rise to different sizes of translatable message, and has been shown for some haemopoietic growth factors. For example, the

Table 2. *Main cellular sources and functions in vitro of the principal haemopoietic growth factors*

Growth factor	Cellular source	In vitro effects	
		Immature cells	*Mature cells*
Erythropoietin	Renal peritubular cells Liver, bone marrow macrophage	Erythroid proliferation Megakaryocyte proliferation	Nil
G-CSF	Monocyte, endothelial cell	Granulocyte proliferation Synergistic factor for growth of early stages of other lineages	Enhancement of neutrophil function and survival
M-CSF	Monocyte, endothelial cell, fibroblast	Monocytic proliferation Synergistic factor for growth of other lineages	Enhancement of monocyte function and differentiation to macrophages
IL-5	T cells	Eosinophil proliferation	Enhancement of eosinophil function
GM-CSF	Monocyte, endothelial cell, fibroblast	Multilineage proliferation	Enhancement of survival and function of neutrophils, monocytes, and eosinophils
IL-3	T cells Neuronal cells (murine)	Multilineage proliferation including mast cell series and lymphoid cells	Enhancement of monocyte and basophil function
IL-6	Monocyte Numerous other cell types	Synergistic factor for early cells	Multiple activities on numerous cell types
IL-1α	Monocyte Numerous other cell types	Synergistic factor for early cells	Multiple activities on numerous cell types

expression of M-CSF gene exhibits alternative splicing resulting in either 4 kb or 1.6 kb mRNA, with differential expression in different cells.[36] However, the functional significance of the altered proteins resulting from alternate initiation and alternative splicing is unknown. An A/U rich sequence in the 3' untranslated region, which is conserved in the mRNAs for GM-CSF, IL-3, G-CSF, and several lymphokines and oncogenes[37,38] seems to impart nuclease sensitivity to the mRNA since insertion of this region from GM-CSF mRNA into the beta globin mRNA resulted in a decrease in the latter's stability.[39] The induction of HGF expression by some activated cells appears to be due to the induction of a ribonuclease inhibitor.[40]

Haemopoietic growth factor receptors

Growth factors exert their biological activity upon binding to their receptors on target cells, and therefore considerable effort is centred on characterization of biochemical and functional properties of the receptors. Apart from affinity studies using radioactively labelled ligand, and molecular weight analysis from cross-linking experiments, investigation of the receptors is hampered by the unavailability of purified receptor preparations since they are expressed at low numbers on responsive cells. In general, between 10 and 1000 copies are present per positive bone marrow cell[41,42], for example, 200–800 for human GM-CSFR. Additional information has therefore been obtained following cloning of a number of receptors in the past 5 years using expression cloning systems of cDNA libraries made from tissue (placenta in the case of human GM-CSF) or cell lines (mouse myeloid leukaemia NFS-60 for G-CSF) expressing the respective receptor (see Table 3).

Sequence analysis of the receptor cDNAs is consistent with a transmembrane protein comprising an extracellular and intracellular component linked by a single intramembranous segment which remains virtually constant in size between receptors. The variation in size of the receptors is due to variation in the extracellular and intracellular regions. Comparison of the receptor cDNA sequences with database gene sequences has revealed interesting features. On the basis of sequence homologies, the receptors can be grouped into families exhibiting common structural characteristics. The human M-CSF receptor, human IL-6 receptor, and murine IL-1 receptor have sequences characteristic of the immunoglobulin supergene family in the extracellular region, ie one or more immunoglobulin-like domains.[51] The M-CSF receptor has a clearly defined sequence motif characteristic of a tyrosine kinase[52] and has been shown to be part of a group of families of receptors with tyrosine kinase activity.[53] Receptors for GM-CSF, G-CSF, erythropoietin, IL-3, IL-4, and IL-6 all have significant sequence homologies between each other and also to the IL-2 beta chain, IL7, prolactin, and growth factor receptors.[54] Idzerda[55] et al have suggested these be referred to as the haemopoietin receptor superfamily (HRS superfamily). Further cDNA

Table 3. *Characteristics of haemopoietic growth factor receptors*

	Molecular wt(kD)		Affinity K_D (pM)	Source of cDNA	cDNA analysis				Homology	ref
	Predicted from cDNA (non-glycosylated)	Observed mol. wt (glycosylated)			Total number of amino acids	Extra-cellular	Trans-membranous	Cytoplasmic		
Human M-CSFR	105	150	100–400	placenta	972	512	25	435	IGS and tyrosine kinase receptor family	43
Human GM-CSFR	45	84	2000–8000 (low) 40–46 (high)	placenta	400	297	27	54	HRS	44
Human IL-6R	26	–	1000 (low) 10 (high)	YT cells	468	359	27	82	HRS and IGS	45
Murine G-CSFR	90.8	95–125	290	NFS-60	812	601	24	187	HRS	46
Murine Epo-R	55	85–100	210 (low) 30 (high)	MEL	507	224	22	234	HRS	47
Murine IL-4R	85	138–145	1400–3600 1500–1700[a]	CTLL-2	785 230[a]	208	24	553	HRS	48
Murine IL-3R	94.7	140	17 900	MC 9	878	417	26	413	HRS	49
Murine IL-1R	62	80	3000–4000	EL4 6.1 C10	576	319	40	217	IGS	50

[a]soluble receptor.
IGS = Immunoglobulin gene superfamily.
HRS = Haematopoietin receptor superfamily

analysis of the haematopoietin receptor family by Patthy[56] has shown the presence of the type III domain in the C-terminal part of the extracellular portion of members of the family. This domain was initially described in fibronectin[57] and later in several other proteins. In view of its demonstrated interaction with the fibronectin receptor,[58] it suggests a possible role in receptor–ligand interactions in members of this family. The presence of a sequence motif within the type III domain which is unique to the HRS family, the WS × WSE box, raises the possibility that it may serve as a recognition site for some common or homologous constituent of the receptor–ligand complexes. Within this group, separate cDNAs encoding a soluble form of the receptor, in addition to the membrane-bound form, have been found for IL-4 and IL-7 which may play a part in an, as yet, unknown regulatory role.

The gene encoding for M-CSF receptor is on the long arm of chromosome 5[30] and the 'low affinity' GM-CSF receptor is encoded on the pseudo-autosomal region of the sex chromosomes.[59]

Several growth factor receptors have been reported to have varying high and low affinity of binding to ligand which has been difficult to explain apart from the IL-2 receptor. IL-2 binds to two distinct receptor molecules, with a low affinity to IL-2 alpha receptor and a higher affinity to IL-2 beta receptor.[60] When both alpha and beta receptors are co-expressed, the binding affinity is increased still further, suggesting that interaction between the two separate components is responsible for converting a low affinity receptor into a high affinity one. This seems to occur despite a much smaller intra-cytoplasmic segment in the alpha receptor, and therefore the significant inter-action presumably occurs at the level of the extracellular ligand binding segment. Support for this is provided in the case of the IL-7 receptor. When a cDNA construct lacking almost all of the cytoplasmic portion was expressed in a cell line,[61] comparison of its binding affinity with that of the full-length receptor showed no difference in binding. Both low and high affinity binding was demonstrated in the deficient construct. This suggests that the cytoplasmic domain of the receptor is not involved in the formation of high affinity sites. Therefore, although only one receptor component has been positively identified to date with respect to other receptors expressing varying affinity, for example, GM-CSF and IL-7, the modulation of the affinity may be due to other membrane component(s).

The specificity of binding of a growth factor receptor with its ligand is extremely high, and yet the binding of one type of colony-stimulating factor to its receptor can affect the binding of other receptors to their respective ligands. This phenomenon was investigated initially in the murine system where binding of various growth factors to their receptors, and cross-competition of binding to a particular receptor between growth factors, was determined at 4 °C and 37 °C in mouse bone marrow progenitor cells.[62] There was no cross-competition of binding of ligand at 4°C, but a hierarchical binding was observed at 37°C with IL-3 inhibiting binding of GM-CSF, M-CSF, and G-CSF; GM-CSF inhibiting binding of G-CSF and M-CSF; G-CSF inhibiting binding of M-CSF and M-CSF inhibiting binding of GM-CSF. Since receptor internalization and down-regulation is known to occur at 37°C and not at 4°C, this suggested that the cross-competition was a consequence of a similar down-regulation of receptors by heterologous ligands, termed *trans*-modulation.[41]

In contrast to the murine system, recent ligand binding in human cells shows that cross-competition between growth factors undeniably occurs at 4°C in addition to 37°C. Park et al[63] showed that GM-CSF partially inhibited the binding of IL-3 to human monocytes, and both IL-3 and GM-CSF showed partial competition for binding to KG-1 cells. Similar competition has also been demonstrated in human eosinophils,[64] and cell lines and primary leukaemia cells.[65] This direct competition between growth factors occurring at 4°C is therefore unlikely to be due to the transmodulation of receptors as described for murine CSFs. It has been suggested that this may be due to a subset of receptors which bind to both ligands, to a close association of the receptors on the membrane or to the use of a shared receptor component.[66]

In the myeloid leukaemic cell line where IL-3 blocks binding of GM-CSF and vice versa,[67] chemical crosslinking of radiolabelled ligands shows that GM-CSF and IL-3 bind to distinct molecules indicating that there is not a subset of receptors binding both ligands, and, if there is a common auxiliary component to the IL-3 and GM-CSF receptors, it is not covalently linked. A recent report from Taga and colleagues shows that the IL-6 receptor can associate with a membrane protein (gp 130) in a non-covalent manner after binding ligand and that the signal transduction occurs through gp 130 rather than through the IL-6 binding protein.[68]

Biological activity of the HGFs

The HGFs can be considered as three families of factors with overlapping activities. First, there are the late-acting factors which are relatively lineage restricted and stimulate the terminal divisions and differentiation of a specific cell lineage. Secondly, there are the multi-CSFs, the paradigm example of which is interleukin 3 (IL-3). The activity of this factor is largely limited to cells at an intermediate stage of differentiation, although the earlier cells of many haemopoietic lineages express receptors and respond to this factor.[67] Granulocyte-macrophage colony-stimulating factor (GM-CSF) does not fit readily into either of the above two categories. It shares many of the multi-CSF activities with IL-3, although probably acting on a slightly 'later' cell. In addition, as its name implies, it also stimulates the terminal divisions of the granulocyte and monocyte series, and modulates the function of mature granulocytes and monocytes analogous to the other 'late acting factors'.[70]

Thirdly, there are the factors such as IL-1 (also called haemopoietin 1) and IL-6 which affect very primitive haemopoietic cells. These cells are difficult to study by virtue of their rarity and their requirement for the marrow micro-environment[15] so that the precise effects of IL-1 and IL-6 are not fully clear. It appears that these factors render the most primitive cells sensitive to the 'multi CSFs' and later acting factors, by stimulating division and maturation of these early cells, by upregulating the receptors for the multi-CSFs and later acting factors independent of cell division, or by inducing the transition of primitive cells from G0 to G1 and thus rendering them more sensitive to the effects of other factors. In vitro, IL-1 alone does not cause colony growth but, combined with other factors, it permits the growth of very large colonies from primitive cells.[71] For this reason, it is often referred to as a synergistic factor.

It must be acknowledged that this type of subdivision of the HGFs is an over simplification as there is good evidence that G-CSF has 'synergistic activity' as well as affecting the late stages of granulocytic proliferation and differentiation.[72] It is interesting that leukaemia inhibitory factor (LIF) (also known as HILDA) also possesses synergistic activity.[73–75]

As one moves from the late-acting factors to the early-acting factors there is increasing promiscuity of target cell reactivity so that, whereas the effects of G-CSF are largely restricted to cells of the granulocyte lineage, IL-1 and IL-6 have multiple activities including effects on lymphocytes and hepato-cytes and the induction of fever.[76,77] This has obvious implications for clinical exploitation.

The mechanism of action of the HGFs is not clear, and, as well as stimulat-ing proliferation and differentiation, they maintain the survival of the primi-tive cells. Studies with murine growth factor-dependent cell lines and erythroid progenitor cells indicate that HGF deprivation results in early cell death by the active process of apoptosis.[78,79] This implies that there is con-stant cell death of early haemopoietic cells within the bone marrow analogous to thymocyte death in the thymus. This may appear 'wasteful' but could result in a system able to respond rapidly to stress and a rise in HGFs within the marrow environment.

As well as the effects on primitive cells, the HGFs have a range of effects on the survival and function of mature myeloid cells. Thus both neutrophils and eosinophils undergo rapid morphological changes when exposed to GM-CSF; neutrophils assuming an elongated polarised shape and eosinophils becoming triangular. These changes are reflected in altered forward angle light scatter measured by flow cytometry.[80] In vitro studies of neutrophil mobility have yielded conflicting results probably because of different experimental systems. In agarose gel, GM-CSF treated neutrophils show reduced migra-tion[81] whilst in Boyden chambers GM-CSF acts as a potent chemotactic factor.[82] In vivo studies using skin windows in patients receiving rhGM-CSF have shown reduced migration of neutrophils compared to baseline and non-rhGM-CSF treated controls.[83,84]

GM-CSF causes an increase in neutrophil surface membrane expression of cellular adhesion molecules (CAMs) both in vitro[85] and during in vivo use in humans.[86,87] This may contribute to the transient margination and pulmonary sequestration of neutrophils and monocytes that is observed when GM-CSF administration is commenced.[88] Although antibodies to neutrophil CAMs inhibit GM-CSF induced adherence to cultured endothelial cells in vitro, changes in expression of neutrophil CAMs cannot be the sole explanation for GM-CSF induced margination/demargination as CAM levels remain high long after demargination has occurred.[87] Neutrophil CAMs are stored in the membranes of specific granules and are translocated to the cell surface following activation by chemotactic factors and other agonists.[89] This fact and the observation that plasma levels of the granule components lactoferrin and transcobalamins 1 and 3 rise during GM-CSF therapy[90] strongly suggest that GM-CSF causes release of neutrophil secondary granules.

Various in vitro assays of neutrophil function show enhancement after exposure to GM-CSF. These include: superoxide production in response to f met leu phe (fmlp) and Fc receptor cross-linking, phagocytosis of opsonized yeast and antibody-dependent cytotoxicity (ADCC).[80,91–94] Eosinophils and monocytes show similarly enhanced function.

Both the killing of intracellular parasites[95] and tumour cell targets[96] by monocytes are increased, the latter by induction of TNF production.[97] Murine antigen presenting cell function is augmented by GM-CSF, an effect that is associated with increased expression of Ia antigens.[98]

G-CSF has similar priming properties for neutrophil function although when studied in whole blood it is a much weaker effector molecule than GM-CSF.[99] IL-3 primes monocytes, eosinophils, and basophils but probably not neutrophils although there is controversy as to whether neutrophils do express IL-3 receptors. M-CSF activates monocytes and macrophages and, in man, M-CSF has more potent effects on mature cells than on monocyte progenitor cells. The priming effects of the HGFs underline their potentially important role as inflammatory mediators.

Signal transduction

Factor-dependent cell lines, enriched marrow progenitors, and mature end cells have all been used for studying HGF signal transduction. It cannot be assumed that a given ligand–receptor interaction leads to the same biochemical sequence of events in different cell types at different stages of differentiation, and the use of these different target cells compounds the problems of interpreting the available data.

The M-CSF receptor possesses tyrosine kinase activity[100–102] with considerable homology to the platelet-derived growth factor (PDGF) receptor.[53] It is likely that the tyrosine phosphorylation induced by receptor occupancy contributes to a series of metabolic events in the cell ultimately resulting in activation and proliferation. It is worth noting that the phosphorylation and dephosphorylation of enzymes is one of the major regulatory mechanisms in intermediate metabolism[103,104] although the important substrates phosphorylated by the M-CSFR have not yet been characterized.

M-CSF is thought to activate the receptor tyrosine kinase by inducing receptor dimers or higher order aggregates analogous to the activation of the PDGF receptor.[105] The aggregation facilitates phosphorylation of the receptor which has been shown to occur in *trans*[106] although true autophosphorylation may also occur. Receptor phosphorylation may modulate its interaction with potential substrates which in turn may be phosphorylated. One such molecule is the phosphatidyl inositol 3 kinase (Pts Ins 3 kinase) which becomes associated with the M-CSF R following ligand binding. Pts Ins 3 kinase phosphorylates the inositol ring of Pts Ins at the D3 position and may also phosphorylate Pts Ins 4 Phosphate and Pts Ins 4, 5, *bis* P. Studies with site-directed mutants of the M-CSF R indicate that the association of the M-CSR R and Pts Ins 3 kinase is dependent on the tyrosine phosphorylation of the M-CSF rather than the direct kinase activity of M-CSFR. This illustrates how one receptor type (tyrosine kinase) can recruit enzymes involved in other potential signal transduction pathways such that several distinct secondary messenger events could occur simultaneously. By analogy with cells transformed by 'v fms' it is also likely that M-CSF binding to M-CSF R phosphorylates and activates the c-*raf* oncogene product, which is a serine kinase.[107]

Within 10 minutes of M-CSF administration to murine macrophages, there is activation of the Na+/H+ pump, an event common to many HGFs,[108] but it is not clear whether the resulting cytoplasmic alkalinization is a central event in signal transduction or a phenomenon secondary to cell activation.

Following the binding of M-CSF to its receptor, the surface receptor is rapidly down modulated by internalization. Alternatively, activation of protein kinase C (PKC) by phorbol esters down regulates surface M-CSF R expression by activation of a protease which cleaves off the extracellular domain of the receptor.[109] Recent studies suggest that M-CSF itself directly activates PKC.[110]

None of the other HGF receptors has a tyrosine kinase domain. There is evidence for erythropoietin, GM-CSF,[111] and IL-3[112] that signalling is mediated by a G protein, in that the response to these factors can be blocked by pertussis toxin which ADP ribosylates and thus inhibits many such G proteins. The situation is complex, however, a pertussis toxin has also been reported to inhibit M-CSF induced bone marrow proliferation.[112] G proteins are a family of regulatory molecules, and the range of enzyme systems that can be activated by these molecules has only recently been appreciated.

The interaction of IL-3 with its receptor has been reported to cause activation and translocation of the serine/threonine kinase protein kinase C.[113] This occurs without generation of IL-3 or changes in intracellular calcium[114-116] and may be due to the generation of diacyl glycerol from phosphatidyl choline analogous to the events that occur with IL-I-mediated stimulation.[117] In several factor-dependent cell lines, the requirement for IL-3 can be reduced or abrogated by phorbol myristate acetate (PMA) which directly activates PKC, adding support to the idea that PKC may have a pivotal role in IL-3 induced proliferation.[118]

A number of rapid phosphorylations have been described occurring within seconds of IL-3 binding. Some occur on serine residues and are also produced by 12 orthotetradecanoylphorbol 13 acetate (TPA), whereas others occur on tyrosine and would thus appear to be non-PKC dependent. IL-3 binding to factor-dependent cell line and immature primary cells also causes cytoplasmic alkalinization and increased ATP levels and glucose uptake but such events may be non-specific housekeeping events subsequent to activation. Carrol and colleagues have shown that the c raf protein is phosphorylated and simultaneously activated which is an important potential mechanism of growth regulation.[119] Down regulation of the IL-3 response has not been studied in detail but Murthy et al have reported that binding of IL-3 to its receptor results in proteolytic cleavage of the receptor from a 140 kD to a 70 kD molecule.[120]

The mechanism of activation of GM-CSF is obscure. Although it has been reported that GM-CSF causes a rapid rise in intracellular calcium in myeloid blast cells,[121] we have found no such changes. Similarly, we and others[122] have observed no rise in intracellular calcium $[Ca^{2+}]_i$, in neutrophils exposed to GM-CSF. In both neutrophils and GM-CSF dependent cell lines, GM-CSF induces a number of rapid phosphorylation events.[119,123,124] In the murine GM-CSF responsive cell line, B6SUta GM-CSF induces tyrosine phosphorylation of a 90 kD protein and serine phosphorylation of a cytoplasmic and membrane 68 kD protein: only the membrane 68 kD protein is phosphorylated on addition of TPA. The importance of PKC in GM-CSF signal transduction is also called into doubt by the facts that GM-CSF does not cause translocation of PKC from cytosol to membrane in neutrophils,[122] and the kinase inhibitors H7 and H8 at concentrations which will block TPA induced neutrophil responses will actually enhance rather than inhibit the response to GM-CSF.[91] As with IL-3 and M-CSF, GM-CSF has also been reported to cause phosphorylation and activation of the c-*raf* gene product.[119] In neutrophils, GM-CSF causes priming and in some instances this is brought about by upregulation of receptors such as the f met leu phe receptor.[125] This is not the complete story however, as GM-CSF also primes the superoxide response to crosslinking of the Fcδ RII with no change in surface receptor expression.[92] Furthermore, in whole blood systems, GM-CSF has been reported to augment the stimulatory effects of phorbol esters which bypass classical receptor pathways.[93] Following binding of GM-CSF to its receptor, the complex is rapidly internalized by endocytosis and then recycled or resynthesized after about 6 hours.[126,127] This internalization appears to down regulate the response as H7 and H8 inhibit internalization and also augment the effects of GM-CSF. Whether internalization of the receptor is consequent upon direct phosphorylation of the receptor is not known.

Studies with a murine erythroid cell line have suggested that erythropoietin causes cells to pass from the G to the S phase of the cell cycle, and that further progression through the cycle is independent of erythropoietin[128] although earlier studies had implicated erythropoietin activity at other phases of the cell cycle.

Conflicting evidence on the mechanism of erythropoietin-mediated signal transduction has been reported. Miller and colleagues reported that erythopoietin caused a rapid rise in intracellular $[Ca^{2+}]$[129] in human erythroblasts but this was not found in studies of murine erythroid colony-forming cells[130] or in human fetal liver proerythroblasts.[131] Bonanou-Tzedaki found that erythropoietin caused an increase in adenylate cyclase activity in rabbit erythroblasts[132] but erythropoietin-dependent rises in cyclic AMP have not been found in other systems. In a study of a murine erythropoietin-dependent cell line, Tsuda et al[133] in fact showed that the proliferative effects of erythropoietin were markedly down regulated by agents that elevated cyclic AMP levels. Other studies have implicated arachadonic acid metabolites[134] and a calcium-ATP ase[135] in erythropoietin signal transduction.

Choi and colleagues have described rapid erythropoietin-induced phosphorylation changes, in particular the serine dephosphorylation of a 43 kD membrane protein.[136] Although the significance of this event is not known, it is of interest that HGF signal transduction may involve phosphatase as well as kinase activation.

In summary, little is yet known about HGF signalling, but the recent cloning of the receptor molecules will hopefully allow more detailed structure and functional analyses to be performed in the near future.

Negative regulators of haemopoiesis

Haemopoiesis appears to be regulated by a balance between the haemopoietic growth factors and a number of inhibitory molecules. These are outlined in Table 4 and this topic was recently reviewed by Axelrad.[150]

With the exception of lactoferrin, which inhibits the production of HGFs by accessory cells,[149,151] the negative regulators act rapidly and reversibly to

Table 4. *Haemopoietic negative regulators*

Name	Hamopoietic target cells	Native mol. wt.	Ref.
Transforming growth factor-β (TGF-β)	Stem cells Progenitor cells	25 000	137
Macrophage inflammatory protein-1α (MIP-1α)	Stem cells	–	138, 139
La Jolla negative regulator (Inhibin)	Progenitor cells	32 000	140
Villejuif negative regulator (SDKP)	Stem cells	487	141
Toronto negative regulatory protein (NRP)	Progenitor cells	79 000	142
Vienna–Bergen hæmoregulatory peptide (HP and HP5b) (EEDCK)	Stem cells Progenitor cells	590	143
Lund negative regulator (LAI)	Progenitor cells	500 000	144
Acidic isoferritins	Progenitor cells	–	145
Prostaglandins	Progenitor cells	–	146
Tumour necrosis factor	Progenitor cells	18 000	147
Gamma interferon	Progenitor cells	–	148
Lactoferrin	Accessory	–	149

either arrest cells during S phase or to prevent them entering S phase (G0 or G1 arrest). The mechanisms by which the negative regulators exert their action is as yet unknown.

The gene for transforming growth factor beta (TGF beta) was the first of the negative regulatory genes to be cloned.[152] TGF beta is a potent non-lineage specific inhibitor of haemopoietic stem cell and early progenitor cell proliferation when added in vitro, whereas unipotential more mature progenitors are insensitive to its action. TGF beta is produced by many cell types and has effects on multiple other cell types, being inhibitory in some cells and stimulatory in others (eg fibroblasts and epithelial cells). This inevitably raises doubts about the physiological relevance of such a promiscuous factor. When blocking anti-TGF beta antibodies are added to human long-term marrow cultures, however, there is an increase in the number of primitive BFU-E in cell cycle indicating that in this culture system, at least, TGF beta is produced and keeps the early cells in a quiescent state.[153] The stem cell inhibitor originally described by Lord et al[138] has recently been shown to be macrophage inflammatory protein-lα (MIP 1α).[139] This factor inhibits stem cells but not GM-CFC.[154] It appears that MIP-1α is produced by macrophage-like cells in quiescent marrow but not in regenerating bone marrow, supporting the idea that this is an important physiological regulator.

The Lund negative regulator, also called 'leukaemia associated inhibitor', is notable in that, as well as being produced by a range of normal cells, it is also produced constitutively by myeloid leukaemic cells. It inhibits normal progenitor cells but not leukaemic cell growth, raising the possibility that escape from inhibitory signals is an important mechanism of leukaemogenesis.

Prostaglandins E and TNF α inhibit progenitor cell growth in vitro.[155] Gamma interferon has little inhibitory activity alone but synergizes markedly with TNF α.[156] The physiological role of these molecules is not clear but it has been suggested that they play a role in immune-mediated cytopaenias and in aplastic anaemia.

Clinical use of HGFs

Erythropoietin, G-CSF, GM-CSF, IL-1, IL-3 and IL-4, have all entered into clinical trials. It is not the intention of this review to analyse the results of these trials in any detail but merely to point out that the clinical experience supports the models of haemopoiesis derived from in vitro studies. Thus, when erythropoietin is given to patients with chronic renal failure (erythropoietin deficient), there is correction of the anaemia with a very small rise in platelet counts and no significant change in the white cell count.[157–159] G-CSF administration causes a neutrophilia which can exceed $100 \times 10^9/l$[160,161] whereas GM-CSF causes a neutrophilia accompanied by a monocytosis and eosinophilia.[162–164] IL-3 has been reported to cause a rise in reticulocytes, leucocytes including basophils, and platelets in accordance with its multilineage activity in vitro.[165]

Both G-CSF and GM-CSF are effective in reducing the period of neutropaenia following conventional chemotherapy and autologous bone marrow transplantation.[163,164] To what extent the improvement in blood counts will translate into clinical benefits such as reduced infections and shorter periods in hospital is not yet clear but randomized trials are in progress. It might be anticipated that, in patients receiving transplants, in whom the stem cell and progenitor cell numbers are likely to be less than with conventional therapy, GM-CSF might be more effective than G-CSF because of the former's apparent activity on more primitive cells in vitro. This does not appear to be the case. Furthermore, one study has suggested that, if a bone marrow transplant contains a small number of progenitor cells, such as may happen with pharmacological purging, then GM-CSF does not accelerate haemopoietic recovery.[166] Only preliminary data is available with IL-3, but the early results suggest that it may induce earlier recovery of red cells and platelets as well as phagocytes.[167]

Finally, the in vivo experience of administering HGFs to man has confirmed the in vitro findings that GM-CSF, G-CSF and M-CSF all augment some of the functional attributes of mature phagocytes.[168]

It is possible that the negative regulators of haemopoiesis may find valuable clinical application. If normal stem cells are kept out of cell cycle whilst tumour stem cells are unaffected, then escalation of cycle-specific agents may be possible without undue myelosuppression. This strategy may also be possible in some cases of myeloid leukaemia if the leukaemic stem cells are resistant to the particular inhibitor. This approach may, however, be hampered by the apparent lack of specificity of the negative regulators.

Conclusions

The understanding of haemopoietic regulation has been facilitated by the development of in vitro culture systems and more recently by the cloning of most of the haemopoietic growth factors and their receptors. It is also clear that there is a dynamic balance between these stimulatory factors and a range of inhibitory molecules. The analysis of ligand receptor interactions and the association of the receptors with other molecules and their substrate will help unravel the mechanisms of signal transduction and growth control. It is to be hoped that such studies will provide clues to the pathogenesis of leukaemia. At a more practical level, the availability of recombinant HGFs is already finding clinical application although the precise indications for their use have yet to be determined.

References

(1) Till J E, McCulloch E A. A direct measurement of the radiation sensitivity of normal mouse bone marrow cells. *Radiat Res* 1961; 14: 213–22.

(2) Wu AM, Till JE, Siminovitch L, McCulloch EA. Cytological evidence for a relationship between normal haematopoietic colony forming cells and cells of the lymphoid system. *J Exp Med* 1963; 127: 453–63.

(3) Abramson S, Miller RG, Phillips RA. The identification in adult bone marrow of pluripotent and restricted stem cells of the myeloid and lymphoid systems. *J Exp Med* 1977; 145: 1567–79.

(4) Keller G, Paige C, Gilboa E, Wagner EF. Expression of a foreign gene in myeloid and lymphoid cells derived from multipotent hematopoietic precursors. *Nature* 1985; 318: 149–54.

(5) Jordan CT, Lemischka IR. Clonal and systemic analysis of long-term hematopoiesis in the mouse. *Gene Dev* 1990; 4: 220–32.

(6) Carnot P, Deflandre G. Sur l'activité hémopoiétique du sérum au cours de la régéneration du sarig. *Compte Rendu de l'Académie des Sciences*, Paris. 1906; 143, 384.

(7) Reissman KR. Studies on the mechanisms of erythropoietic stimulation in parabiotic rats during hypoxia. *Blood* 1950; 5: 372.

(8) Pluznik DH, Sachs L. The cloning of normal mast cells in cell culture. *J Cell Comp Physiol* 1965; 66: 319–24.

(9) Bradley TR, Metcalf D. The growth of mouse bone marrow cells in-vitro. *J Cell Comp Physiol* 1966; 66: 283–300.

(10) Pike B, Robinson WA. Human bone marrow growth in agar gel. *J Cell Physiol* 1970; 76: 77–84.

(11) Iscove NN, Sieber F, Winterhalter KH. Erythroid colony formation in cultures of mouse and human bone marow: analysis of the requirement for erythropoietin by gel filtration and affinity chromatography on agarose Con A. *J Cell Physiol* 1974; 83: 309–20.

(12) Nicola NA, Metcalf D, Matsumoto M, Johnson GR. Purification of a factor inducing differentiation in murine myelomonocytic leukaemia cells: identification as granulocyte colony-stimulating factor (G-CSF). *J Biol Chem* 1983; 258: 9077.

(13) Metcalf D. The molecular biology of the granulocyte-macrophage colony stimulating factors. *Blood* 1986; 67: 257–67.

(14) Clark SC, Kamen R. The human haematopoietic colony stimulating factors. *Science* 1987; 236: 1229–37.

(15) Dexter TM, Allen TD, Lajtha LG. Conditions controlling the growth of haemopoietic stem cells in-vitro. *J Cell Physiol* 1977; 91: 336–44.

(16) Gordon MY, Riley GP, Watt SM, Greaves MF. Compartmentalisation of a haemopoietic growth factor (GM-CSF) by glycosaminoglycans in the bone marrow microenvironment. *Nature* 1987; 326: 403–5.

(17) Roberts R, Gallagher J, Spooncer E, Allen TD, Bloomfield F, Dexter TM. Heparan sulphate bound growth factors: a mechanism for stromal cell mediated haemopoiesis. *Nature* 1988; 332: 376–8.

(18) Jacobs K, Shoemaker C, Rudersdorf R et al. Isolation and characterisation of genomic and cDNA clones of human erythropoietin. *Nature* 1985; 33: 806–10.

(19) Lin F-K, Suggs S, Lin C-H et al. Cloning and expression of the human erythropoietin gene. *Proc Natl Acad Sci USA* 1985; 82: 580–4.

(20) Nagata S, Tsuchiya M, Asano S et al. Molecular cloning and expression of a cDNA for human granulocyte colony-stimulating factor. *Nature* 1986; 319: 415–18.

(21) Wong GS, Temple PA, Leary AC et al. Human CSF-1: molecular cloning and expression of 4kb cDNA encoding the human urinary protein. *Science* 1987; 235: 1504–8.

(22) Campbell HD, Tucker WQJ, Hort Y et al. Molecular cloning, nucleotide sequence, and expression of the gene encoding human eosinophil differentiation factor (interleukin-5). *Proc Natl Acad Sci USA* 1987; 84: 6629–33.

(23) Wong GC, Witek J, Temple PA et al. Human GM-CSF: molecular cloning of the complementary DNA and purification of the natural and recombinant proteins. *Science* 1985; 228: 810.

(24) Lee F, Yokata T, Otsuka T et al. Isolation of cDNA for a human granulocyte-macrophage colony stimulating factor by functional expression in mammalian cells. *Proc Natl Acad Sci USA* 1985; 82: 4360.

(25) Cantrell MA, Anderson D, Cerretti DP et al. Cloning, sequence and expression

of a human granulocyte-macrophage colony stimulating factor. *Proc Natl Acad Sci USA* 1985; 82: 6250–4.

(26) Yang YC, Ciarletta AB, Temple PA et al. Human IL-3 (multi-CSF): identification by expression cloning of a novel hemopoietic growth factor related to murine IL-3. *Cell* 1986; 47: 3–10.

(27) Hirato T, Yatsuka K, Harada H, Taga T, Watanabe Y, Matsuda T. Complementary DNA for a novel human interleukin (BSF-2) that induces lymphocytes to produce immunoglobulin. *Nature* 1986; 324: 73.

(28) Mochizuki DY, Eisenman JR, Conlon PJ, Larsen AD, Tushinski RJ. Interleukin 1 regulates hemopoietic activity, a role previously ascribed in hemopoietin 1. *Proc Natl Acad Sci USA* 1987; 84: 5267.

(29) Buchberg AM, Bedigian HG, Taylor BA et al. Localization of Evi-2 to chromosome 11: linkage to other proto-oncogene and growth factor loci using interspecific backcross mice. *Oncogene Research* 1988; 149–65.

(30) Le Beau MM, Pettenati MJ, Lemons RS et al. Assignment of the GM-CSF, CSF-1 and fms genes to human chromosome 5 provides evidence for linkage of a family of genes regulating hemopoiesis and for their involvement in the deletion 5q in myeloid disorders. *Cold Spring Harbor Symp Quant Biol* 1986; LI: 899.

(31) Simmers RN, Weber LM, Shannon MF et al. Localization of the G-CSF gene on chromosome 17 proximal to the breakpoint in the t(15:17) in acute promyelocytic leukaemia. *Blood* 1987; 70: 330.

(32) Powell JA, Berkner KL, Lebo RV et al. Human erythropoietin gene: high level expression in stably transfected mammalian cells and chromosomal localisation. *Proc Natl Acad Sci USA* 1986; 83: 6465–9.

(33) Quesenberry P, Souza L, Krantz S. Growth factors: In: Education session booklet, *American Society of Haematology Annual Meeting* 1989. 98–113.

(34) Shannon MF, Gamble JR, Vadas MA. Nuclear proteins interacting with the promoter region of the human granulocyte/macrophage colony-stimulating factor gene. *Proc Natl Acad Sci USA* 1988; 85: 674–8.

(35) Nimer SD, Morita EA, Martis MJ, Wachsman W, Gasson JC. Characterization of the human granulocyte-macrophage colony-'stimulating' factor promoter region by genetic analysis: correlation with DNase I footprinting. *Mol Cell Biol* 1988; 8: 1979–84.

(36) Rajavashisth TB, Eng R, Shadduck RK et al. Cloning and tissue-specific expression of mouse macrophage colony-stimulating factor mRNA. *Proc Natl Acad Sci USA* 1987; 84: 1157–61.

(37) Caput D, Beutler B, Hartog K, Thayer R, Brown-Shimer S, Cerami A. Identification of a common nucleotide sequence in the 3'-untranslated region of mRNA molecules specifying inflammatory mediators. *Proc Natl Acad Sci USA* 1986; 83: 1670–4.

(38) Wreschner DH, Rechavi A. Differential mRNA stability to reticulocyte ribonucleases correlates with 3' non-coding (U)n A sequences. *Eur J Biochem* 1988; 172: 333–40.

(39) Shaw G, Kamen R. A conserved AU sequence from the 3' untranslated region of GM-CSF mRNA mediates selective mRNA degradation. *Cell* 1986; 46: 659–67.

(40) Bagby GC, Shaw G, Brown MA et al. Interleukin-1 induces granulocyte-

macrophage colony stimulating factor mRNA accumulation in human stromal cells by inducing ribonuclease inhibitory activity. *Blood* 1988; 2 (suppl 1): 347.

(41) Nicola NA. Why do hemopoietic growth factor receptors interact with each other? *Immunol Today* 1987; 8: 134–40.

(42) Nicola NA. Haemopoietic growth factors and their receptors. *Ann Rev Biochem* 1989; 58: 45–77.

(43) Coussens L, Van Beveren C, Smith D et al. Structural alteration of viral homologue of receptor proto-oncogene *fms* at carboxyl terminus. *Nature* 1986; 320: 277–80.

(44) Gearing DP, King JA, Gough NM, Nicola NA. Expression cloning of a receptor for human granulocyte-macrophage colony-stimulating factor. *EMBO J* 1989; 8: 3667–76.

(45) Yamasaki K, Taga T, Hirata Y et al. Cloning and expression of the human Interleukin-6 (BSF-2/IFNb2) receptor. *Science* 1988; 214: 825–8.

(46) Fukunaga R, Ishizaka-Ikeda E, Seto Y, Nagata S. Expression cloning of a receptor for murine granulocyte colony-stimulating factor. *Cell* 1990; 61: 314–50.

(47) D'Andrea AD, Lodish HF, Wong GG. Expression cloning of the murine erythropoietin receptor. *Cell* 1989; 57: 277–85.

(48) Mosley B, Beckmann P, March CJ, Cosman D et al. The murine interleukin-4 receptor: molecular cloning and characterization of secreted and membrane bound forms. *Cell* 1989; 59: 335–48.

(49) Itoh N, Yonehara S, Schreurs J et al. Cloning of an interleukin-3 receptor gene: a member of a distinct receptor gene family. *Science* 1990; 247: 324–7.

(50) Sims JE, March CJ, Cosman D et al. cDNA expression cloning of the IL-1 receptor, a member of the immunoglobulin superfamily. *Science* 1988; 241: 585–9.

(51) Williams AF. A year in the life of the immunoglobulin superfamily. *Immunol Today* 1987; 8: 298–303.

(52) Hanks SK, Quinn AM, Hunter T. The protein kinase family: conserved features and deduced phylogeny of the catalytic domains. *Science* 1988; 241: 42–52.

(53) Ullrich A, Schlessinger J. Signal transduction by receptors with tyrosine kinase activity. *Cell* 1990; 61: 203–12.

(54) Bazan JF. A novel family of growth factor receptors: a common binding domain in the growth hormone, prolactin, erythropoietin, and IL-6 receptors. *Biochem Biophys Res Commun* 1989; 164: 788–95.

(55) Idzerda RL, March CJ, Mosley B et al. Human interleukin-4 receptor confers biological responsiveness and defines a novel receptor superfamily. *J Exp Med* 1990, in press.

(56) Patthy L. Homology of a domain of the growth hormone/prolactin receptor family with type III modules of fibronectin. *Cell* 1990; 61: 13–14.

(57) Skorstengaard K, Jensen MS, Sdahl P, Petersen TE, Magnusson S. Complete primary structure of bovine plasma fibronectin. *Eur J Biochem* 1986; 161: 441–53.

(58) Ruoslahti E. Fibronectin and its receptors. *Ann Rev Biochem* 1988; 57: 375–413.

(59) Gough NM, Gearing DP, Nicola NA et al. Localization of the human GM-CSF receptor gene to the X-Y pseudoautosomal region. *Nature* 1990; 345: 734–6.

(60) Hatakeyama M, Tsudo M, Minamoto S et al. Interleukin-2 receptor B chain gene: generation of three receptor forms by cloned human alpha and beta chain cDNAs. *Science* 1989; 244: 551–6.

(61) Goodwin RG, Friend D, Ziegler SJ et al. Cloning of the human and murine interleukin-7 receptors: demonstration of a soluble form and homology to a new receptor superfamily. *Cell* 1990; 60: 941–51.

(62) Walker F, Nicola NA, Metcalf D, Burgess AW. Hierarchical down-modulation of haemopoietic growth factor receptors. *Cell* 1985; 43: 269–76.

(63) Park LS, Friend D, Price V et al. Heterogeneity in human interleukin-3 receptors. A subclass that binds human granulocyte/macrophage colony simulating factor. *J Biol Chem* 1989; 10: 5420–7.

(64) Lopez AF, Eglinton JM, Gillkis D, Park LS, Clark S, Vadas MA. Reciprocal inhibition of binding between interleukin 3 and granulocyte-macrophage colony-stimulating factor to human eosinophils. *Proc Natl Acad Sci USA* 1989; 86: 7022–6.

(65) Park LS, Waldron PE, Friend D et al. Interleukin-3, GM-CSF, and G-CSF receptor expression on cell lines and primary leukaemia cells: receptor hetero-geneity and relationship to growth factor responsiveness. *Blood* 1989; 74: 56–65.

(66) Elliot MJ, Vadas MA, Eglinton JM et al. Recombinant interleukin-3 and granulocyte-macrophage colony-stimulating factor show common biological effects and binding characteristics on human monocytes. *Blood* 1989; 74: 2349–59.

(67) Gesner T, Mufson RA, Turner KJ, Clark SC. Identification through chemical cross-linking of distinct granulocyte-macrophage colony-stimulating factor and interleukin-3 receptors on myeloid leukemic cells, KG-1. *Blood* 1989; 8: 2652–6.

(68) Taga T, Hibi M, Hirata Y et al. Interleukin-6 triggers the association of its receptor with a possible signal transducer, gp 130. *Cell* 1989; 58: 573–81.

(69) Bor DJ, Wagemaker G, Lowenberg B. Stimulatory spectrum of human recom-binant multi CSF (IL-3). *Blood* 1988; 1: 1609.

(70) Sieff CA, Emerson SG, Donahue RE et al. Human recombinant granulocyte-macrophage colony-stimulating factor: a human multilineage hemopoietin. *Science* 1985; 230: 1171.

(71) Stanley ER, Bartocci A, Patinkin D, Rosendaal M, Bradley TR. Regulation of very primitive multipotent haemopoietic cells by haemopoietin 1. *Cell* 1986; 45: 667.

(72) Ikebudni K, Clark SC, Ihle JN, Souza LM, Ogawa M. Granulocyte colony-stimulating factor enhances interleukin-3 dependent proliferation of multipotential hemopoietic progenitors. *Proc Natl Acad Sci USA* 1988; 85: 3445.

(73) Moreau J-F, Donaldson DD, Bennett Frances, Witek-Giannotti J, Clark SC, Wong GG. Leukaemia inhibitory factor is identical to the myeloid growth factor human interleukin for DA cells. *Nature* 1988; 336: 690–2.

(74) Williams RL, Hilton DJ, Peare S et al. Myeloid leukaemia inhibitory factor

V Devalia and D C Linch

maintains the developmental potential of embryonic stem cells. *Nature* 1988; 336: 684–7.

(75) Leary AG, Wong GG, Clark SC, Smith AG, Ogawa M. Leukaemia inhibitory factor differentiation-inhibiting activity/human interleukin for DA cells augments proliferation of human haematopoietic stem cells. *Blood* 1990; 75: 1960–4.

(76) Durum SK, Schmidt JA, Oppenheim JJA. Interleukin 1: an immunological perspective. *Ann Rev Immunol* 1985; 3: 263.

(77) Wong GC, Clark SC. Multiple actions of interleukin 6 within a cytokine network. *Immunol Today* 1988; 9: 137.

(78) Williams GT, Smith CA, Spooncer E, Dexter TM, Taylor DR. Haemopoietic colony stimulating factors promote cell survival by suppressing apoptosis. *Nature* 1990; 343: 76–9.

(79) Koury MJ, Bohdurant MC. Erythropoietin retards DNA breakdown and prevents programmed death in erythroid progenitor cells. *Science* 1990; 248: 378–81.

(80) Lopez AF, Williamson J, Gamble JR et al. Recombinant human granulocyte-macrophage colony stimulating factor stimulates in vitro mature human neutrophil and eosinophil function, surface receptor expression and survival. *J Clin Invest* 1986; 8: 1220–8.

(81) Gasson JC, Weishart RH, Kaufaman SE et al. Purified human granulocyte-macrophage colony-stimulating factor: direct action on neutrophils. *Science* 1984; 226: 1339–42.

(82) Wang JM, Cotella S, Allavena P, Mantovani A. Chemotactic activity of human recombinant granulocyte-macrophage colony-stimulating factor. *Immunology* 1987; 60: 439.

(83) Addison IE, Johnson B, Devereux S, Goldstone AH, Linch DC. Granulocyte-macrophage colony stimulating factor may inhibit neutrophil migration in-vivo. *Clin Exp Immunol* 1989; 76: 149–53.

(84) Peters WP, Stuart A, Affronti ML, Kim CS, Coleman RE. Neutrophil migration is defective during recombinant human granulocyte-macrophage colony-stimulating factor infusions after autologous bone marrow transplantation in humans. *Blood* 1988; 72: 1310–15.

(85) Arnaout MA, Wang EA, Clark SC, Sieff CA. Human recombinant granulocyte-macrophage colony-stimulating factor increases cell to cell adhesion and surface expression of adhesion promoting glycoproteins on mature granulocytes. *J Clin Invest* 1986; 8: 597–601.

(86) Socinski MA, Canistra SA, Sullivan R et al. Granulocyte-macrophage colony-stimulating factor induces the expression of the CD 11b surface adhesion molecule on human granulocytes in-vivo. *Blood* 1988; 72: 691–7.

(87) Devereux S, Bull HA, Campos-Costa D, Saib R, Linch DC. Granulocyte-macrophage colony stimulating factor induced changes in cellular adhesion molecule expression and adhesion to endothelium: in vitro and in-vivo studies in man. *Br J Haematol* 1989; 71: 323.

(88) Devereux S, Linch DC, Campos-Costa D, Spittle MF, Jelliffe AM. Transient leucopenia induced by granulocyte-macrophage colony stimulating factor (letter). *Lancet* 1987; ii: 1523.

(89) Bainton DF, Miller LJ, Kishimoto TK, Springer TA. Leukocyte adhesion

receptors are stored in peroxidase negative granules of human neutrophils. *J Exp Med* 1987; 166: 1641–53.

(90) Devereux S, Porter JB, Hoyes KP, Abeysighe RD, Saib R, Linch DC. Secretion of neutrophil secondary granules occurs during granulocyte-macrophage colony stimulating factor induced margination. *Br J Haematol* 1990; 74: 17–23.

(91) Khwaja A, Roberts PJ, Jones HM, Yong K, Linch DC. The isoquinolinesulphonamide protein kinase C inhibitors H7 and H8 enhance the effects of granulocyte-macrophage colony stimulators factor (GM-CSF) on neutrophil function and inhibit GM-CSF receptor internalization. *Blood* 1990; 76: 1–8.

(92) Roberts PJ, Devereux S, Pikington GR, Linch DC. FcδR11 mediated superoxide production by phagocytes is augmented by GM-CSF without a change in FcδR11 expression. *J Leuk Biol* 1990; 48: 247–57.

(93) Jaswan MS, Khwaja A, Roberts PJ, Jones HM, Linch DC. The effects of rhGM-CSF on the neutrophil respirator burst when studied in whole blood. *Br J Haem* 1990; 75: 181–7.

(94) Weisbart RH, Golde DW, Clark SC, Wong GC, Gasson JC. Human granulocyte-macrophage colony-stimulating factor is a neutrophil activator. *Nature* 985; 314: 361–3.

(95) Handman E, Burgess AW. Stimulation by granulocyte-macrophage colony stimulating factor of *Leishmania tropica* killing by macrophages. *J Immunol* 1979; 122: 1134.

(96) Grabstein KH, Urdal DL, Tushinski RJ et al. Induction of tumoricidal activity by granulocyte-macrophage colony-stimulating factor. *Science* 1986; 232: 506–8.

(97) Cannistra SA, Vellenga E, Groshek P, Rambaldi A, Griffin JD. Human granulocyte-monocyte colony-stimulating factor and interleukin 3 stimulate monocyte cytotoxicity through a tumour necrosis factor dependent mechanism. *Blood* 1988; 1: 672–6.

(98) Morrissey PJ, Bressler L, Park LS, Alpert A, Gillis S. Granulocyte-macrophage colony-stimulating factor augments the primary antibody response by enhancing the function of antigen presenting cells. *J Immunol* 1987; 139: 113–19.

(99) Khwaja A, Linch DC. Cytokine interactions on neutrophil priming. (Submitted)

(100) Roussel MF, Dull TJ, Rettenmier CW, Ralph P, Ullrich A, Sherr CJ. Transforming potential of the c-fms proto-oncogene (CSF-1 receptor). *Nature* 1987; 325: 549–52.

(101) Downing JR, Rettenmier CW, Sherr CJ. Ligand-induced tyrosine kinase activity of the colony-stimulating factor 1 receptor in a murine macrophage cell line. *Mol and Cell Biol* 1988; 8: 1795–9.

(102) Sengupta A, Liu WK, Yeung YG, Yeung DCY, Frackelton AR, Stanley E R. Identification and subcellular localisation of proteins that are rapidly phosphorylated in tyrosine in response to colony-stimulating factor. *Proc Natl Acad Sci USA* 1988; 85: 8062–6.

(103) Lord JM, Bunce CM, Brown G. The role of protein phosphorylation in the control of cell growth and differentiation. *Br J Cancer* 1988; 58: 549–55.

(104) Cohen P. The structure and regulation of protein phosphatases. *Ann Rev Biochem* 1989; 58: 433–508.

(105) Heldin CH, Ernuld A, Rorsman C, Ronnstrand L. Dimerization of beta-type

platelet-derived growth factor receptors occurs after ligand binding and is closely associated with receptor kinase activation. *J Biol Chem* 1989; 264: 8905–12.

(106) Shurtleff SA, Downing JR, Rode CO, Hawkins SA, Roussel MF, Sherr CJ. Structural features of the colony-stimulating factor 1 receptor that affect its association with phosphatidyl inositol 3-kinase. *EMBO J* 1990; 9: 2415–21.

(107) Morrison DK, Kaplan DR, Escobedo JA, Rapp UR, Roberts TM, Williams LJ. Direct activation of the serine/threonine kinase activity of *raf*-1 through tyrosine phosphorylation by the PDGF beta-receptor. *Cell* 1989; 58: 649.

(108) Cook N, Dexter TM, Lord BI, Cragoe EJ, Whetton AD. Identification of a common signal associated with cellular proliferation stimulated by four haemopoietic growth factors in a highly enriched population of granulocyte/ macrophage colony-forming cells. *EMBO J* 1989; 8: 2967–74.

(109) Downing JR, Roussel MF, Sherr CJ. Ligand and protein kinase C downmodulate colony-stimulating factor 1 receptor by independent mechanisms. *Mol and Cell Biol* 1989; 9: 2890–6.

(110) Imamura K, Dianoux A, Nakamuna T, Kufe D. Colony-stimulating factor 1 activates protein kinase C in human monocytes. *EMBO J* 1990; 9: 2423–39.

(111) Gomez-Cambronemo J, Yamazaki M, Metwally F et al. Granulocyte-macrophage colony-stimulating factor and human neutrophils: role of guanine nucleotide regulatory proteins. *Proc Natl Acad Sci USA* 1989; 86: 3569–73.

(112) He Y, Hewlett E, Temeless D, Quesenberry P. Inhibition of interleukin 3 and colony-stimulating factor 1-stimulated marrow cell proliferation by pertussis toxin. *Blood* 1988; 5: 1187–95.

(113) Farrar WL, Thomas TP, Anderson WB. Altered cytosol/membrane enzyme redistribution on interleukin-3 activation of protein kinase C. *Nature* 1985; 315: 235–7.

(114) Whetton AD, Monk PN, Consalvery SD, Downes CP. The haemopoietic growth factors interleukin-3 and colony stimulating factor-1 stimulate proliferation but do not induce inositol lipid breakdown in murine bone-marrow-derived macrophages. *EMBO J* 1986; 5: 3281–6.

(115) Whetton AD, Monk PB, Consalvery SD, Huang SJ, Dexter TM, Downes CP. Interleukin 3 stimulates proliferation via protein kinase C activation without increasing inositol lipid turnover. *PNAS* 1988; 85: 3284–8.

(116) Whetton AD, Vallance SJ, Monk PN, Cragoe EJ, Dexter TM, Heyworth CM. Interleukin-3-stimulated haemopoietic stem cell proliferation. Evidence for activation of protein kinase C and Na+/H+ exchange without inositol lipid hydrolysis. *Biochem J* 1988; 256: 585–92.

(117) Rosoff PM, Savage N, Dhavello CA. Interleukin-1 stimulates diacylglycerol production in T lymphocytes by a novel mechanism. *Cell* 1988; 54: 73–87.

(118) Whetton AD, Heyworth CM, Dexter TM. Phorbol esters activate protein kinase C and glucose transport and can replace the requirement for growth factor in interleukin-3-dependent multipotent stem cells. *J Cell Sci* 1986; 84: 93–104.

(119) Carroll M, Rapp UR, Clarke-Lewis I, May WS. IL-3 and GM-CSF induced phosphorylation and activation of the c-raf protein. A model for cytoplasmic growth factor signal transduction [Abstract] *Blood* 1989; 74 (Suppl 1) 195a.

(120) Murthy SC, Mui ALF, Krystal G. Characterization of interleukin 3 receptor. *Exp Haematol* 1990; 18: 11–17.

(121) Strauss L, Meade-Cobun K, Englee M, Civin C, Tucker R. Conditioned medium (5637) stimulates increased intracellular free calcium in normal human marrow. My-10-positive blast cells [Abstract] *Blood* 1986; 68 (Suppl 1) 181a.

(122) Sullivan R, Griffin JD, Simons ER et al. Effects of recombinant human granulocyte and macrophage colony stimulating factors on signal transduction pathways in human granulocytes. *J Biol Chem* 1987; 139: 3422–30.

(123) Sorensen PHB, Mui ALF, Murthy SC, Krystal G. Interleukin-3, GM-CSF, and TPA induce distinct phosphorylation events in an interleukin 3-dependent multipotential cell line. *Blood* 1989; 2: 406–18.

(124) Evans JPM, Mire-Sluis AR, Hoffbrand AV, Wickremasinghe RG. Binding of G-CSF, GM-CSF, Tumor Necrosis Factor-α, and Gamma-Interferon to cell surface receptors on human myeloid leukemia cells triggers rapid tyrosine and serine phosphorylation of a 75-kd protein. *Blood* 1990; 75: 88–95.

(125) Weisbart RH, Kwan L, Golde DW, Gasson JC. Human GM-CSF primes neutrophils for enhanced oxidative metabolism in response to the major physiological chemoattractants. *Blood* 1987; 69: 18–21.

(126) Walker F, Burgess AW. Internalisation and recycling of the granulocyte-macrophage colony-stimulating factor (GM-CSF) receptor on a murine myelomonocytic leukaemia. *J Cell Physiol* 1986; 130: 255–61.

(127) Cannistra SA, Groshek P, Garlick R, Miller J, Griffin JD. Regulation of surface expression of the granulocyte-macrophage colony stimulating factor receptor in normal human myeloid cells. *Proc Natl Acad Sci USA* 1990; 87: 93–7.

(128) Tsuda H, Sawada T, Kawakita M, Takatsuki K. Mode of action of Erythropoietin (Epo) in an epo-dependent murine cell line. 11. Cell cycle dependency of epo action. *Exp Haematol* 1989; 17: 218–22.

(129) Miller BA, Scaduto RC, Tillotson DC, Botti JJ, Cheung JY. Erythropoietin stimulates a rise in intracellular free calcium concentration in single early human erythroid precursors. *J Clin Invest* 1988; 82: 309.

(130) Imagawa S, Smith BR, Palmer-Crocker R, Bunn HF. The effect of recombinant erythropoietin on intracellular free calcium in erythropoietin-responsive cells. *Blood* 1989; 3: 452–7.

(131) Linch DC, Jones HM, Tidman N, Roberts PJ. The effects of erythropoietin on primitive human erythroid cells. [Abstract] *Blood* 1989; 70 (Suppl 1): 177a.

(132) Bonanou-Tzedaki SA, Sctchenska MS, Arnstein HRV. Stimulation of the adenylate cyclase activity of rabbit bone marrow immature erythroblasts by erythropoietin and haemin. *Eur J Biochem* 1986; 155: 363–70.

(133) Tsuda H, Smada T, Sakaguchi M, Kawakita M, Takatsulci K. Mode of action of erythropoietin (epo) in an epo-dependent murine cell line. 1. Involvement of adenosine 3′, 5′-cyclic monophosphate not as a second messenger but as a regulator of cell growth. *Exp Haematol* 1989; 17: 211–17.

(134) Beckman BS, Mason-Garcia M, Nystuen L, King L, Fisher JW. The action of erythropoietin is mediated by lipoxygenase metabolites in murine fetal cells. *Biochem Biophys Res Comm* 1987; 47: 392–8.

(135) Beckman BS, Seferynska I. Possible involvement of phospholipase activation in erythroid progenitor cell proliferation. *Exp Haematol* 1989; 17: 309–12.

(136) Choi HS, Wojchowski DM, Sythkowski AJ. Erythropoietin rapidly alters phosphorylation of pp43 on erythroid membrane protein. *J Biol Chem* 1987; 262: 2933–6.

(137) Roberts AB, Sporn MB. Transforming growth factor-beta. *Adv Cancer Res* 1988; 51: 107.

(138) Lord BI, Mori KJ, Wright EG, Lajtha LG. An inhibitor of stem cell proliferation in normal bone marrow. *Br J Haematol* 1976; 34: 441.

(139) Graham GJ, Wright EG, Hewick R et al. Identification and characterization of an inhibitor of haemopoietic stem cell proliferation. *Nature* 1990; 344: 442–4.

(140) Yu J, Shao L-E, Lemas V, Yu A, Vaughan J, Rivier J, Vale W. Importance of FSH-releasing protein and inhibitin in erythrodifferentiation. *Nature* 1987; 330: 765.

(141) Lenfant M, Wdzieczak-Bakala J, Guittet E, Prome J-C, Sotty D, Frindel E. Inhibitor of hematopoietic pluripotent stem cell proliferation: purification and determination of its structure. *Proc Natl Acad Sci USA* 1989; 86: 779.

(142) Del Rizzo DF, Eskinazi D, Axelrad AA. Negative regulation of DNA synthesis in early erythropoietic progenitor cells (BFU-E) by a protein purified from medium of a C57BL/6 mouse marrow cell line. *Proc Natl Acad Sci USA* 1988; 85: 4320.

(143) Paukovits WR, Laerum OD, Paukovits JB, Guigon M, Schanche J-S. Regulatory peptides inhibiting granulopoiesis. In: Najman A, Guigon M, Gorin N-C, Mary J-Y, eds. *The inhibitors of haematopoiesis*. Paris: Colloque INSERM/ John Libbey Eurotext. 1987; 162: 31.

(144) Olofsson TBJ. Leukaemia associated inhibitor (LAI): biological characterization and purification of the active subunit. In: Najman A, Guigon M, Gorin N-C, Mary J-Y, eds. *The inhibitors of haematopoiesis*. Paris: Colloque INSERM/ John Libbey Eurotext. 1987; 162: 177.

(145) Broxmeyer HE, Juliano L, Lu L, Platzer E, Dupont B. HLA-DR Human histocompatibility leukocyte antigens-restricted lymphocyte-monocyte interactions in the release from monocytes of acidic Isoferritins that suppress haematopoietic progenitor cells. *J Clin Invest* 1984; 73: 939–53.

(146) Pelus LM, Broxmeyer HE, Moore MAS. Regulation of human myelopoiesis by prostaglandin E and lactoferrin. *Cell Tissue Kinetics* 1981; 14: 515.

(147) Degliantoni G, Murphy M, Kobayashi M, Francis MK, Perussia B, Trinchieri A. Natural Killer (NK) cell derived haematopoietic colony inhibiting activity and NK cytotoxic factor. Relationship with tumour necrosis factor and synergism with immune interferon. *J Exp Med* 1985; 162: 1512–30.

(148) Broxmeyer HE, Lu L, Platzer E, Feit C, Juliano L, Rubin BY. Comparative analysis of the influences of human gamma, alpha, and beta interferons on human multipotential (CFU-GEMM), erythroid (BFU-E) and granulocyte-macrophage (CFU-GM) progenitor cells. *J Immunol* 1983; 131: 1300–5.

(149) Broxmeyer HE, Smithyman A, Eger R, Meyers A, De Sousa M. Identification of lactoferrin as the granulocyte-derived inhibitor of colony-stimulating activity production. *J Exp Med* 1978; 148: 1052–67.

(150) Axelrad AA. Some hemopoietic negative regulators. *Exp Haematol* 1990; 18: 143–50.

(151) Bagby GC, Vasiliki DR, Bennett RM, Vanderbark AA, Garewal H S. Interac-

tion of lactoferrin, monocytes, and T lymphocyte subsets in the regulation of steady-state granulopoiesis in vitro. *J Clin Invest* 1981; 68: 56–63.

(152) Derynck R, Jarrett JA, Chen EY et al. Human transforming growth factor – beta complementary DNA sequence and expression in normal and transformed cells. *Nature* 1985; 316: 701–5.

(153) Del Rizzo DF, Eskinazi D, Axelrad AA. Interleukin 3 opposes the action of negative regulatory protein (NRP) and of transforming growth factor beta (TGF beta) in their inhibition of DNA synthesis of the erythroid stem cell BFU-E. *Exp Haematol* 1990; 18: 138–42.

(154) Tejero C, Testa NG, Lord BI. The cellular specificity of haemopoietic stem cell proliferation regulators. *Br J Cancer* 1984; 50: 335–41.

(155) Pelus LM, Gentile PS. In vivo modulation of myelopoiesis by Prostaglandin E2III. Induction of suppressor cells in marrow and spleen capable of mediating inhibition of CFU-GM proliferation. *Blood* 1988; 1: 1633–40.

(156) Pelus LM, Ottoman O, Nocka K. Interferons α, beta and gamma induce tumour necrosis factor (TNF) release by marrow adherent cells which synergizes with prostaglandin E2 to inhibit human CFU-AM [Abstract] *Blood* 1986.

(157) Winearls CG, Oliver DO, Pippard MJ, Reid C, Downing MR, Cotes PM. Effect of human erythropoietin derived from recombinant DNA on the anaemia of patients maintained by chronic haemodialysis. *Lancet* 1986; ii: 1175–8.

(158) Eschbach JW, Egrie JC, Downing MR, Browne JK, Adamson JW. Correction of anaemia of end stage renal disease with recombinant human erythropoietin: results of a combined phase 1 and 2 clinical trial. *New Eng J Med* 1987; 316: 73–8.

(159) Moia M, Mannucci PM, Vizzotto L, Casati S, Cattaneo M, Ponticelli C. Improvement in the haemostatic defect of uraemia after treatment with recombinant human erythropoietin. *Lancet* 1987; ii: 1227–9.

(160) Bronchud MH, Scarffe JH, Thatcher N et al. Phase I/II study of recombinant human granulocyte stimulating factor in patients receiving intensive chemotherapy for small cell lung cancer. *Br J Cancer* 1987; 56: 809.

(161) Morstyn G, Cambell L, Souza LM et al. Effect of granulocyte colony stimulating factor on neutropaenia reduced by cytotoxic chemotherapy. *Lancet* 1988; i: 667.

(162) Antman LK, Griffin J, Elias A et al. Use of rGM-CSF to ameliorate chemotherapy induced myelosuppression in sarcoma patients. *Blood* 1987; 70 (Suppl.) 373.

(163) Brandt SJ, Peters WP, Atwater et al. Effect of recombinant human granulocyte-macrophage colony-stimulating factor on haemopoietic reconstitution following high dose chemotherapy and autologous bone marrow transplantation. *N Eng J Med* 1988; 318: 869.

(164) Devereux S, Linch DC, Patterson KP, Gribben JG, McMillan A, Goldstone AHG. GM-CSF accelerates neutrophil recovery after autologous bone marrow transplantation for Hodgkins disease. *Bone Marrow Transpl* 1989; 4: 49–54.

(165) Ganser A, Lindemann A, Seipelt G et al. Effect of recombinant human interleukin-3 (rhIL-3) in patients with bone marrow failure – a phase I/II trial [Abstract] *Blood* 1989; 74 (Suppl 1): 50a.

(166) Blazar BR, Kersey JH, McGlave PB et al. In vivo administration of GM-CSF in acute lymphoblastic leukaemia patients receiving purged autografts. *Blood* 1989; 73: 849–57.

(167) Kurzrock R, Talpaz M, Salewski E, Gutterman JU. Phase 1 study of recombinant human interleukin-3 in patients with bone marrow failure [Abstract] *Blood* 1989; 74 (Suppl 1): 154a.

(168) Baldwin GC, Gasson JC, Quan SG et al. GM-CSF enhances neutrophil function in acquired immunodeficiency syndrome patients. *Proc Natl Acad Sci USA* 1988; 85: 2763–6.

Mechanisms of multi-drug resistance

D HOCHHAUSER and A L HARRIS

Introduction

The failure of chemotherapy to cure more than a minority of tumours is predominantly due to drug resistance. Resistance may be inherent or acquired: either as a stable change within the cell or induced following drug administration. Currently, although a majority of childhood tumours are curable, only a minority of adult tumours (eg Hodgkin's and non-Hodgkin's lymphoma, acute leukaemia, teratoma) respond fully although significant prolongation of survival has been shown for small cell lung cancer, ovarian cancer and breast cancer, the latter when used as adjuvant.

Multi-drug resistance (MDR) is the phenomenon whereby exposure to one drug induces cross-resistance to a variety of agents to which the cell has not been exposed. Several mechanisms may mediate MDR, primarily expression of the MDR gene, topoisomerases and glutathione transferases.

Most of the drugs used in haematological malignancies have been implicated in multi-drug resistance which may constitute a major factor in relapse. This review will concentrate on recent advances in the understanding of this phenomenon.

The hallmark of MDR is the expression of P-glycoprotein (PGP), a 170 kD protein with 12 hydrophobic domains and a tandemly duplicated ATP binding domain.[1-4] PGP acts as a transmembrane exporter of drugs but the normal substrates have yet to be identified.

Homologies of PGP

Clear homologies exist between PGP and several bacterial transport proteins, in particular with conservation of the ATP binding domains.[5] These proteins transport individual peptide and carbohydrate species into bacterial cells. In bacteria, the hydrophilic and hydrophobic domains associate as independent integral membrane proteins rather than linked within a single polypeptide

All correspondence to: D Hochhauser, Molecular Oncology Laboratory, Imperial Cancer Research Fund Laboratories, Institute of Molecular Medicine, University of Oxford, John Radcliffe Hospital, Headington, Oxford OX3 9DU, UK.

Cambridge Medical Reviews: Haematological Oncology Volume 1

chain, and are energized by hydrolysis of ATP. The transport protein Hly B exports α haemolysin protein from haemolytic bacteria. Its carboxy terminal contains the ATP binding site and is identical to P-glycoprotein in 50% of its amino acids, as well as having extensive homology of the amino terminal portion. P-glycoprotein may be considered a duplication of the Hly B structure.

In eukaryotes, the only defined normal role for an MDR homologous gene has been found with the STE6 gene of *Saccharomyces cerevisiae*.[6] The product of this locus actively transports the α factor mating pheromone (MAT). It is not essential for cell viability and does not confer a drug-resistant phenotype.

Chromosomal location and genomic organization of MDR
In man, the MDR1 gene is located on chromosome 7q 21–31 and contains an open reading frame of 1280 amino acids. There are 2 known human and 3 rodent MDR genes with control of expression of both human genes occurring at the levels of gene copy number, transcription, translation and post-translationally[1,7] (see Table 1).

Molecular and genetic studies
The major evidence for PGP involvement in drug resistance has come through gene transfection studies. In man, only the MDR1 gene has been shown to mediate MDR phenotype by transfection; MDR3 fails to confer any resistance. In rodents, both PGP1 and PGP2 may mediate resistance. For example, expression of a full-length MDR1 cDNA in NIH3T3 cells conferred resistance to colchicine, doxorubicin and vinblastine.[8] There may also be involvement of an MDR homologue in mediating chloroquine resistance in *Plasmodium falciparum* though the association remains to be clarified.[9]

Regulation of MDR
A variety of physical and chemical agents affect expression of MDR1, predominantly through increased transcription. The renal carcinoma cell line HDP 46 demonstrated an 8-fold increase in MDR1 RNA levels in response to heat shock, ethanol, sodium arsenite and cadmium, consistent with a role for PGP as a stress-inducible gene product following environmental insults.[10] These effects are not found in all cell types.

Furthermore, the differentiating agents dimethyl sulphoxide (DMSO) and sodium butyrate increased PGP expression in a variety of colon carcinoma cell lines as measured by Northern blots and immunoblotting.[11] However, in one line (SW 620), increased expression was not accompanied by increased doxorubicin or vinblastine resistance. The regulation of MDR1 by gene amplification was suggested initially by the presence of double minutes and homogeneously staining regions.[12] Several genes co-amplify with MDR1 including sorcin, an acidic 22 kD protein homologous to calpain, which binds

Table 1. *Multi-drug resistance genes family*

	Class 1		Class 2
Human	*MDR* 1		*MDR 2* (3)
Hamster	*pgp* 1	*pgp* 2	*pgp* 3
Mouse	*mdr* 3	*mdr* 1	*mdr* 2
	(*mdr* 1a)	(*mdr* 1b)	

calcium. It is possible that differential amplification of sorcin and other gene products may be partially responsible for the differential drug sensitivities found in different MDR expressing resistant cell lines, but no correlations have been found with resistance patterns.

Work in rodents has identified differential overexpression of MDR isotypes as a source of variable resistance patterns.[13,14] There are different RNA species detectable in resistant cell lines isolated after exposure to increasing concentrations of colchicine, vinblastine and taxol. The expression of different MDR genes encoding separate PGP isoforms may be a mechanism for generating diversity of response. Expression of these genes may occur through different pathways as MDR1a (MDR3) is primarily transcriptionally activated with MDR1b (MDR1) levels paralleling gene amplification. Furthermore, transfection experiments using mouse MDR1 and MDR3 confer overlapping but distinct drug specificities. In the former case, preferential resistance to colchicine and adriamycin is conferred, whilst the latter gave preferential resistance to actinomycin D. Such phenomena have not been demonstrated in man where only one MDR gene confers resistance.

Protein modification

Post-translational modification of MDR is also significant. In man, a 140 kD precursor protein is gradually converted to a 170 kD form over 2 to 4 hours. There are 10 potential *N*-glycosylation sites on PGP but only 3 appear on the external surface of the plasma membrane. Glycosylation-deficient mutants of MDR cells show no change in resistance profiles compared with parental cells, and the further finding that tunicamycin (a glycosylation inhibitor) does not affect resistance indicates that this may be of questionable significance.

The PGP expressed in the mouse line J774-2 has been shown to be a substrate for cyclic AMP-dependent protein kinase A with phosphorylation of serine and threonine residues having been demonstrated in vitro. PGP seems to be phosphorylated in its basal state by protein kinase C and this may be important in affecting drug transport. Drug accumulation assays of a multi-drug-resistant human carcinoma line showed that PMA treatment significantly reduced [³H]-vinblastine accumulation induced by verapamil and that basal phosphorylation of PGP was increased 2-fold by phorbol ester treatment. However, it has also been demonstrated that staurosporine and H7, which are inhibitors of protein kinase C and cAMP-dependent protein kinase activity, do not affect overall PGP phosphorylation. Studies of vincristine resistant HL 60 cells demonstrated another membrane associated protein kinase (PK 1) which also phosphorylates PGP on serine and threonine residues and may regulate levels of multi-drug resistance.[15,16]

Mutation of MDR I

Mutations within the MDR1 gene may alter patterns of cross-resistance. In KB cells, a glycine to valine mutation at codon 185 resulted in a changed preferential resistance pattern from vinblastine to colchicine.[17] Analysis of nucleotide sequences using the polymerase chain reaction demonstrated the colchicine specific sequences to be present within KB cellular DNA prior to selection. Transfections of wild-type and colchicine-resistant cDNAs conferred the appropriate preferential resistance indicating a key role for amino acid 185 in PGP drug interaction. This amino acid is located within the first hydrophobic region on the cytoplasmic side of the membrane and may be part of a drug binding site. However, a recent study on KB lines transfected with both cDNAs also showed that the 'mutant' PGP led to a significant increase in etoposide (VP16) resistance as well as to increased resistance to vincristine, actinomycin D and taxol; reversal of resistance was achieved with 1μM verapamil.[18] Interestingly, studies using photoactive drug analogues showed that, against expectations, the mutant line binds *less* colchicine and more vinblastine than the wild type. This suggests that altered resistance may not be due to initial association of PGP with drug but by a subsequent dissociation of drug from PGP. This argues against an effect solely on the drug binding site and in favour of two critical points in PGP-mediated translocation of drug: one in the drug binding site and another involved in intracellular drug localization and transport.

RNA stabilization

Recent evidence on the MDR1 gene in regenerating rat liver reveals another possible level of control with mRNA degradation being controlled by sequences in the non-coding region.[19] Following hepatectomy, a 2-fold increase in MDR transcription was demonstrated by nuclear run-on experiments, whereas gene expression was increased 22-fold. Analysis of the 3' encoding sequences of MDR reveals an AU rich sequence associated with unstable mRNA messages.

Summary of mechanisms of regulation

Expression of MDR is regulated by amplification, transcription and translation. The relative contributions of each may vary throughout the selection process. In a multi-drug resistant ovarian carcinoma cell line, overexpression of MDR1 mRNA was found without evidence of amplification at low levels of drug resistance.[20] At intermediate drug concentrations, amplification became increasingly significant while, at high drug level, PGP increased without further changes in mRNA or gene copy number, consistent with translational modification or mutation. Apart from indicating that MDR may be mediated at different levels of protein in the same tumour under different selection pressures, this study also indicates that measurement of MDR1 mRNA alone may give a misleading impression of the amount of functional PGP present.

Tissue distribution of PGP

Studies on tissue distribution of PGP and MDR expression have involved immunohistochemistry with mouse and human monoclonal antibodies, ribonuclease protection assays and in situ mRNA hybridization. Specific monoclonals have been developed to distinguish between the various PGP isoforms.[21,22] Nevertheless, problems of non-specific hybridization continue to confuse results. The widely used C219 recognizes highly conserved amino acid sequences found in all PGP isoforms characterized to date, including MDR3; it also cross-hybridizes to a small percentage of skeletal muscle fibres. Similarly, MRK 16 recognizes external regions of the molecule but gives occasional staining of smooth muscle cells in the walls of the stomach and intestine. Recently, it was found that treatment of cells with neuraminidase, thus affecting sialylation patterns, greatly increased the amount of detectable fluorescence by the antibody MRK 16 in samples of lymphocytes from CLL patients.[23]

Generally, the highest levels of PGP have been found in kidney (lumina of the proximal tubules), adrenal cortex (zona fasciculata and reticulata), stomach, duodenum, colon and placenta. Expression occurs primarily in specialized epithelial cells with secretory or excretory functions on the luminal surfaces as well as in placental trophoblasts.[24]

Strong expression was also found in endothelial cells of capillary blood vessels at blood–tissue barrier sites, primarily capillaries of the central nervous system and testes as well as the dermis.[25] These observations have significance in the light of the fact that the brain and testis constitute sanctuary sites in which relapse following systemic chemotherapy in conditions such as acute lymphoblastic leukaemia occurs presumably because of failure of drug penetration. Location of PGP in these cells is primarily on the luminal surface consistent with the role of PGP in secretion of an, as yet, unknown substrate.

Clinical significance – expression in tumours
Solid tumours

Studies of the significance of MDR in human tumours have recently become available. The most extensive study reported on levels of MDR1 mRNA in over 400 human cancers.[26] Quantification of mRNA was measured using slot blot analysis comparing tumour samples to known drug sensitive (KB-3-1) and resistant (KB-8-5) cells. Expression was defined as common if MDR1 mRNA was detectable in over 50% of cancers in each group. The overall findings have been that there is an inverse correlation of levels of MDR expression with chemosensitivity of the tumour type, though numerous exceptions have been found. Thus, for example, breast and ovarian cancers had lower levels of MDR and less frequent expression than colon and renal cell carcinomas. However, sarcomas and non-small cell lung cancers had low levels of MDR and low frequency despite showing a resistant phenotype. This may reflect sensitivity of the assay and our ignorance of the level at which MDR expression becomes significant within the clinical context as well as the use of other resistance pathways.

Studies on other tumour types have also appeared. The earliest report of PGP elevation in a human malignancy was in 5 cases of relapsed ovarian cancer where cells showed raised MDR expression compared with normal ovarian tissue which did not express MDR.[27] One of these patients showed increased MDR expression following failure of therapy. Clinical significance has also been assessed in a retrospective immunohistochemical study of rhabdomyosarcoma and undifferentiated sarcoma in which all 9 PGP positive patients relapsed and, of 21 PGP negative patients, 20 showed durable complete response.[28]

A study of various lung cancers and non-tumorous lung tissue showed no significant differences in MDR with minimal changes following therapy.[29] Once again, completely opposing results have been found from a study of 212 untreated primary lung neoplasms using the monoclonal antibodies H1B612 which gave the frequency of MDR as 76.3% of non-small cell lung cancers compared with 57% of small cell lung cancer.[30] These are the findings which would be expected to correlate with the known drug responsiveness of these tumour types. However, it should be noted that positivity in this study was confirmed if only a single positive cell was detected. Furthermore, stromal cell contamination may be particularly problematic in analysis of lung tumour material.

A recent study attempted to analyse MDR1 RNA levels quantitatively using the polymerase chain reaction (PCR) on RNA derived from cell lines, tumours and normal tissue.[31] In 26 of 28 normal tissue samples, MDR1 expression was detected with highest levels in adrenal, kidney, colon and liver, in keeping with previous studies. However, 25% of all tumours and tumour-derived cell lines were negative for MDR1 expression. Results on tumour samples largely confirmed and expanded previous findings with osteosarcoma, chondrosarcoma and soft tissue sarcomas having low to moderate MDR mRNA and the sensitive Ewing's sarcoma having no detectable expression. Both non-small cell lung cancer and small cell lung cancer had similar MDR1 expression implicating other resistance pathways in the former tumours.

The increased MDR1 mRNA in normal tissues compared with tumour samples is explained by the authors on the basis of potential clonal expansion of an MDR1 negative cell compared with heterogeneous normal cell populations. It emphasizes that the term 'drug resistance' is misleading to the extent that most normal tissues are drug resistant and it is, in fact, the chemosensitivity of tumours that represents an abnormal state of affairs.

Haematological malignancies

A variety of studies on human leukaemias have recently appeared and, despite contradictory findings, there does appear to be a correlation between MDR and chemosensitivity.[32–35] In a study of 9 newly diagnosed patients with ALL, 8 had low levels of MDR RNA at the time of diagnosis. The one patient with elevated MDR RNA failed to achieve remission. In the same study, 14 of 19 relapsed patients had elevated MDR expression. Similarly, in another small study of 15 patients with acute non-lymphoblastic leukaemia, 3 out of 10 with elevated MDR1 levels relapsed after a short interval. In contrast, 4 out of 5 with minimal or absent MDR expression achieved remission. An immunohistochemical study of CML patients in blast crisis showed that, initially, PGP negative tumours became positive following chemotherapy when measured at relapse.[36]

Studies of MDR expression in leukaemias and other tumours could potentially allow prediction of subgroups likely to respond to particular drug regimens.[37,38] A recent study of 74 patients with AML found the highest MDR RNA levels in leukaemic cells of patients with a history of toxic exposure or preleukaemia syndrome.[34] Patients with high MDR1 transcript levels were difficult to induce into remission and, when occurring, the remissions were short. Nevertheless, another analysis of 19 patients with adult leukaemia (14 AML and 5 ALL) involving analyses using MRK 16 antibodies and gene-specific probes differed considerably.[35] Unusually, no PGP expression was found in any sample treated, whether using immunohistochemistry or Northern blotting. Cases were studied at presentation and relapse. It should be noted that this result is contrary to other recently published studies.

A study of 26 patients with myeloma, lymphoma and breast cancer showed highly significant correlations between positive PGP staining and in vitro resistance to doxorubicin.[38] All 12 patients with PGP positive levels showed in vitro resistance as well as 3 out of 14 PGP negative subjects. No clinical data are available on these patients to determine in vivo significance.

As previously mentioned, cross-reactivity of several of the monoclonals may render interpretation difficult. Thus, a study of 15 non-Hodgkin's lymphomas showed that minimal PGP staining obtained using C219 and MRK 16 antibodies was due to strong background staining of macrophages which are positive for PGP rather than for tumour expression.[39]

Conclusion

To conclude, the majority of studies thus far have included too few patients to allow clinical significance of MDR expression to be fully clarified. On-going longitudinal studies will help to clarify whether identifying subgroups of tumour patients expressing MDR helps to predict response to chemotherapy and might therefore be appropriate for the use of MDR modulators. It is clear that, for haematological neoplasms, MDR expression is insufficient to fully explain patterns of resistance, particularly as it does not confer antimetabolite or steroid resistance.

Problems are still significant with regard to correlative analysis of PGP and in vivo resistance profiles. Assays may be insufficiently sensitive to detect significant PGP expression; this may be particularly important in mRNA measurement where degradation of biopsy samples may occur. Similarly, as previously mentioned, there have been difficulties in developing specific monoclonal probes. Recently, expression of MDR3 has been demonstrated in the absence of MDR1 as shown by RNAse protection assays and dot–blot analysis in B-cell prolymphocytic leukaemia.[40] In one study, daunorubicin accumulation could be reversed by cyclosporine and, to a lesser extent, by verapamil. This does suggest that MDR3 may encode a functional drug pump in these patients. Problems of non-specific staining may be overcome by using panels of several different monoclonal probes for PGP.

Reversal of MDR

A variety of pharmacological agents reverse MDR and this has been extensively reviewed.[41] These range from the calcium blockers, particularly verapamil and nifedipine to tamoxifen, phenothiazines and cyclosporin, among others. The concentrations of some drugs required to reverse MDR in vitro would produce toxicity in vivo and this has been a major limitation to effective clinical use of, for example, verapamil. Some of these agents probably act by binding to PGP and thereby cause intracellular accumulation of drug. Others, including phenothiazines, may act by binding calmodulin or do not affect efflux but cause redistribution within the cell. Normal basal to apical flux of vinblastine in multidrug-resistant epithelial cells is reversed by verapamil with enhanced phosphorylation of PGP, but verapamil has also been noted to potentiate bleomycin, cisplatin and 5-fluorouracil toxicity which are not associated with the MDR phenotype.

The most extensive studies on MDR reversal occurred with verapamil. For example, a study of calcium antagonists in multi-drug resistant primary human renal cell carcinomas demonstrated significant enhancement of a vinblastine cytotoxicity with verapamil, but high concentrations (1 μM) were required and this failed to abolish the tumour resistance completely.[42] Recent studies on the use of verapamil in multiple myeloma have shown a significant improvement in remission rate and are encouraging.[43] This detailed study involved analysis of PGP in 8 patients with multiple myeloma and non-Hodgkin's lymphoma with progressive disease despite having received regimes containing vincristine and doxorubicin. In 3 out of 8 patients, addition of verapamil to the VAD + dexamethasone regime led to response; these patients were PGP positive. Verapamil increased intracellular accumulation of doxorubicin and vincristine in vitro for both a PGP myeloma cell line and tumour cells from 2 PGP positive patients. Effective verapamil concentrations caused transient hypotension and arrhythmias. However, in 3 patients, despite expression of PGP, there was only minimal response implicating other mechanisms than MDR in modulating resistance. Responses were in the range of 4 to 6 months' duration. It is possible that using combinations of different MDR antagonists together at lower levels such as tamoxifen with verapamil may overcome MDR without the undue toxicity seen with the higher levels of each drug. Alternatively, chemotherapeutic drug analogues not binding to PGP, eg the adriamycin derivative, aclacinomycin, could be used. Further studies on whether higher doses of drugs can cure previously unresponsive tumours may be facilitated by studies of transgenic mice expressing high levels of PGP in bone marrow.[44]

Although expression of P-glycoprotein thus far appears to be the most significant cause of the multi-drug resistance phenotype, increasing attention has recently been paid to the so-called atypical multi-drug resistance (atMDR). This has always been applied to circumstances where the multi-drug resistance phenotype has occurred without over-expression of the MDR gene. The commonest pattern appears to be of drugs which act on cellular topoisomerase II as a target.

Topoisomerase II

Topoisomerase II (topo II), the eukaryotic homologue of bacterial DNA gyrase, is a 170 kD homodimeric protein which plays a role in DNA replication, chromosome scaffold formation, chromosomal segregation, and possibly recombination and gene transcription.[45,46] In *Saccharomyces cerevisiae*, topo II null mutations are lethal because of the inability to separate chromosomes at mitosis. The enzyme acts by producing DNA single and double strand breaks and it attaches covalently to the 5' ends of the break. Double strand breaks are staggered by 4 base pairs on opposite strands and the protein attaches as a dimer. Subsequently, strand passage occurs with changes in both supercoiling and DNA relaxation. In proliferating cells, the functional topo II is probably that which is incorporated into the salt insoluble nuclear matrix. In *Drosophila*, topo II is enriched at the sites of attachment of chromatin loops to the nuclear matrix.

Topoisomerase II as a drug target

Several classes of drugs are termed topoisomerase inhibitors though they do not inhibit the initial stages of topoisomerase action. These drugs include intercalating agents such as acridines (*m*AMSA), anthracyclines (adriamycin, daunomycin) anthracene-diones (mitoxantrone) and ellipticines. There is also an important group of non-intercalating agents which appear to bind directly to topo II, most notably teniposide (VP26) and etoposide (VP16). These drugs bind to topo II forming a cleavable complex; so called because denaturation of the trapped protein with SDS or alkali reveals the DNA strand breaks with protein covalently linked to the 5-phosphoryl end of each broken strand.

Since each complex requires two proteins, an increase in the amount of topoisomerase will correlate with increased strand breakage and potential toxicity. It has been shown, for example, that CHO cell lines hypersensitive to etoposide over-expressed topoisomerase II.[47] Although the exact mode of cell death is unclear, presumably the cleavable complex prevents chromosome segregation as well as DNA synthesis. Almost all topoisomerase inhibiting drugs increase the number of topo II-associated DNA strand breaks although this does not always correlate with cytotoxicity because the drugs may have other modes of action. Recent evidence suggests that the common mode of action of the structurally disparate anti-topo II drugs is their inhibition of the enzyme's ability to relegate its cleaved DNA intermediate.[48] Thus, rather than forming the initial cleavable complex, these drugs act by stabilizing the ternary complex and preventing the final relegation step.

Regulation of topo II

Topo II is expressed primarily during the proliferative phases of growth and is down regulated at plateau phase. The amount of topo II increases at the onset of DNA replication, continues to increase through S and G2 phases, peaks in the late G2 to M phase and then drops after mitosis. At confluence, topo II is switched off in untransformed, but not in transformed, cells.

The regulation of topo II during the cell cycle may be relevant as to which phase is most sensitive to topo II inhibitors.[49] Following serum stimulation of BALB-c 3T3 cells, actively proliferating cells showed much greater sensitivity to etoposide than quiescent cells. The increase in drug sensitivity began during S phase and reached a peak just before mitosis with a maximal 2.5-fold increase in drug sensitivity. However, although the maximal number of topo II-associated strand breaks occurred during G2, cytotoxicity was maximal during S phase, suggesting that interactions with other mechanisms lead to cell death.

Modulation of topo II activity during the cell cycle involves phosphorylation.[50] This has been demonstrated for casein kinase and protein kinase C, and these changes may be crucial in switching on the activity of topoisomerase. Phosphorylation has been shown to lead to a 3-fold increase in enzyme activity, and dephosphorylation inactivates the enzyme. Studies of [^{32}P]-incorporation into DNA topo II in vivo in chicken lymphoblastoid cells showed phosphorylation highest at G2 and M, suggesting that phosphorylation may be involved in enzyme activation for sister chromatid disjunction. Glucose deprivation, hypoxia and the stress response to heavy metals have been shown to downregulate the amount of topo II while epidermal growth factor (EGF) is an upregulator.[51] The latter effect may be simply due to causing increased cell proliferation.

Topoisomerase II and drug resistance

There has been demonstration of so-called atypical multi-drug-resistant phenotype in numerous cell lines. Characteristically, there is cross-resistance to the full range of anti-topo II drugs though not to the vinca alkaloids.

These mechanisms may include:

Point mutations and abnormally functioning topoisomerases An HL60 human leukaemia cell line showed 100-fold resistance to *m*AMSA in contrast to a 2- to 3-fold increase in etoposide resistance.[52] Cleavage of DNA produced by *m*AMSA or etoposide had an absolute requirement for ATP in contrast to the situation in wild-type cells. A new restriction enzyme polymorphism was found in the resistant forms. This correlated with a mutation in the ATP binding site. A mutation has been found to induce *m*AMSA resistance in the bacteriophage T4 DNA topoisomerase.[53,54]

The extent to which down regulation of the total amount of topo II is a significant resistance mechanism remains unclear, although reduced levels of topo II shown in some studies could be due to decreased half-life of the mutant protein. However, in a VP16-resistant mouse breast cancer cell line, quantitative analysis of drug-stimulated cleavage activity showed one-fifth of the wild-type topo II activity as measured by cleavable complex formation while mRNA slot blot analyses showed significant reductions within resistant cells.[55]

Several studies have demonstrated abnormal functional forms of topo II in resistant cells with different drug cleavage patterns.[56]

In a study of teniposide-resistant human CEM lines, the amount of topo II bound to the nuclear matrix decreased due to a mutant enzyme which differs in salt stability thereby affecting attachment to the nuclear matrix.[57] It is probable that the functional topo II is that which is associated with the matrix, and with newly replicated DNA.

Methylation Several studies have demonstrated hypermethylated sites. This could be of significance in regulating the transcription of non-mutant alleles.[58]

Glucose deprivation and hypoxia These factors may be relevant within the tumour mass and contribute towards decreased topoisomerase expression.

Cytosolic factors A PGP negative human fibrosarcoma cell line was found to express 150-fold etoposide cross resistance compared to the wild-type cells. The amount of topoisomerase II as measured by immunoactivity was only 3- to 10-fold lower in the resistant lines (DR4).[59]

Nuclear topoisomerase II function as measured by cleavage and decatenation assays was identical in both cell types. However, whole cell extracts of the resistant line showed significantly reduced VP16 induced DNA breaks implicating cellular mechanisms. A variety of antioxidant enzyme activities were increased in the resistant cells, including glucose-6-phosphate dehydrogenase, glutathione peroxidase and catalase. These enzymes may inactivate the free radical drug metabolites but their exact role in mediating resistance remains unclear.

Upregulation of topoisomerase I This has been shown in several cases. Topoisomerase I, an enzyme which produces single strand breaks in DNA and is involved in transcription, may increase as a compensatory effect with topo II downregulation (as occurs in *S. cerevisiae*) and may be able to carry out the functions of topo II at least partially when it is downregulated.

Switch to a novel form of topo II (β) Purification of a topoisomerase II from *m*AMSA resistant P388 leukaemia cells indicated another form of topo II of 180 kD differing in several respects from the previously known 170 kD form. Partial cloning of the gene shows that it may lack the leucine zipper motif which is probably important in dimerization of the 170 kD form and that it differs in expression throughout the cell cycle (topo II β levels peak during G1 and fall during the rest of the cell cycle), and in drug sensitivity.[60,61]

The 170 kD topo II (topo IIα) is expressed in rapidly proliferating cells, and its ratio increases compared to the 180 kD form (topo IIβ) in *ras*-transfected NIH3T3 cells.[62] At plateau phase, the decrease in topo II in *ras* transformed cells was approximately 40% compared to 70% in normal cells. In both *ras* transformed and control lines the percentage of 180 kD protein increased as cells drew closer to plateau phase. Although the amount of

170 kD protein correlated with mRNA levels, the mRNA levels of the 180 kD form decreased by 45–60% following *ras* transformation while the amount of 180 kD enzyme differed only slightly. This suggests alterations in regulation between topo IIα and β and that topo II activity is less dependent on growth state in *ras*-transformed cells.

As the 170 kD protein is preferentially sensitive to teniposide and merbarone, this could account for drug effectiveness against tumours which possess a higher percentage of topo IIα, ie transformed cells as opposed to normal cells. Similarly, switch of expression from topo IIα to topo IIβ could lead to an 8-fold degree of resistance with equivalent protein expression.

Tissue distribution of topoisomerase II
Studies of topo II activity in normal tissues showed the highest levels in spleen and thymus.[63] Expression within tumours was highest in breast cancer and leiomyosarcoma. However, levels within these tumours were in the same range as normal tissues; possibly normal tissue topo II is relatively teniposide resistant. These results were surprising since one would expect the highest topo II levels to be in proliferating cells. Further studies on tissue levels are needed using antibodies and activity assays.

Clinical implications
Further studies are required to elucidate the clinical significance of altered topo II as well as possible methods of circumvention. It may be possible to reduce topo II resistance by molecular design. Mechanisms of resistance to the topo II inhibitor *m*AMSA include altered transport and MDR. By altering substituents on the anilino-acridine nucleus, resistance to both mechanisms was overcome.[64] Up-regulation of topo I could be significant as inhibitors, notably camptothecin, could be used and cells exhibiting this mechanism of resistance may be hypersensitive to topo I inhibitors. Nevertheless, evidence indicates that combined use of topo I and topo II inhibitors may, in fact, decrease cytotoxicity. This could be due to the inhibitory effects of camptothecin on cellular transcription. Another route could be through the development of competitive topoisomerase inhibitors rather than through the current stoichiometric agents, ie competition with topo II for binding to DNA would be more effective in low topo II expressers. There is possibly a link between MDR and topo II regulation with possible inverse correlation of these. A study of MDR induction showed simultaneous topo II reduction though this may simply be due to a generally inhibitory effect of the drugs on cellular metabolism rather than to a specific action on topo II regulation.[65]

Glutathione transferases
The involvement of glutathione and glutathione transferases (GST) in the multi-drug resistant phenotype has been difficult to clarify. Glutathione

transferases are enzymes involved in detoxification, distributed in all organs but primarily in the liver and kidney. Their mode of action is by conjugation of glutathione (a tripeptide present in all organs in millimolar amounts) via the sulphur atom of its cystine residue to various electrophiles. GSTs may also act as intracellular binding proteins (eg for bilirubin and steroids) and may constitute up to 10% of the total cellular protein in the liver. In man, GST exists in cytosolic and microsomal forms. There are 3 major classes of cytosolic GST: π, α, μ. Several comprehensive recent reviews deal with classification of the GSTs and their involvement in drug resistance.[66-69]

GST expression in drug resistance

Several anticancer drugs may be inactivated by GST catalysis, eg melphalan, chlorambucil and cyclophosphamide. There have been numerous reports correlating increases in GST isozymes, particularly the π family, with the onset of drug resistance. There may be increased amounts of enzymes involved in glutathione synthesis and also glutathione peroxidase. GSTπ has also been thought to be significant as it constitutes the predominant isozyme found in human cancers with 2- to 4-fold increases in RNA levels in tumours of the colon, bladder, ovary and stomach relative to normal tissues, and it has been found to be overexpressed in several multi-drug resistant lines, particularly in adriamycin resistant lines. Studies in ovarian cancer patients show expression of α and π isozymes following treatment. However, studies have also shown little difference between GST in tumour tissue and normal cells. In a study of patients with CLL, no correlation was found between chlorambucil resistance and GST expression which also did not vary significantly between control and CLL lymphocytes.[70]

Transfection studies

Transfection of GSTπ cDNA into *ras*-transformed NIH3T3 cells led to elevated GSTπ enzyme levels but, although there was a moderate 1.8- to 3-fold increase in resistance to adriamycin and ethacrynic acid (a substrate of GSTπ), there was no change in resistance to *cis* platinum, chlorambucil and melphalan.[71] In another study, a doxorubicin resistant line of human breast cancer MCF7 with both GSTπ and MDR expression was analysed. The MDR and GSTπ cDNAs from these cells were cloned and transfected but, although MDR conferred a resistance, phenotype GSTπ gave only moderate resistance to ethacrynic acid. The transfection of GTSπ, together with MDR, showed no significant additive effect.

Glutathione depletion

In view of the large amount of intracellular glutathione, it may be that non-enzymatic reaction of glutathione with electrophiles could be relevant.

Several studies have shown that glutathione depletion with buthionine sulphoximine (BSO), a blocker of glutathione synthesis, potentiates melphalan toxicity in numerous cell lines.

It has not been shown so far that GST activity changes amount to more than associated stress responses following treatment with alkylating agents rather than definitive resistance mechanisms. However, the increased protection against adriamycin, although small, has consistently been found to be correlated with GSTπ. It is of interest that transformation with vH-*ras* and v-*raf* oncogenes induces resistance to a number of cytotoxic agents and induces both PGP and GSTπ in NIH3T3 cells.[72] Definitive evidence with regard to gene transfection experiments awaits cloning the GST isozymes into a variety of cell types and the testing of different drug classes. Evidence so far suggests that resistance induced would be less than 3-fold. However, coordinate changes reducing ability to regenerate or transport glutathione may interact synergistically with other resistance pathways. Studies are in progress involving the clinical use of BSO and ethacrynic acid which deplete glutathione.

The role of other pathways in the mediation of multi-drug resistance remains to be clarified. Although the platinum drugs and alkylating agents are not implicated with MDR expression, over-expression of metallothioneins occurs following chronic exposure to heavy metals and confers resistance to *cis*diaminedichloroplatinum, melphalan and chlorambucil.[73] Transfection of vectors expressing metallothionein conferred the same resistance profile.

Conclusion

Multiple mechanisms may be responsible for multi-drug resistance. Furthermore, individual drugs may have several modes of action which could affect resistance. For example, adriamycin is demonstrated to be located within multiple cellular organelles suggesting several targets of action apart from the cell membrane. Even within the cell surface, other mechanisms may be significant. An interesting recent study produced an adriamycin-resistant MCF-7 breast carcinoma line by exposing to drug in the presence of verapamil.[74] PGP expression was not elevated but a novel uncharacterized 95 kD surface membrane protein was expressed. There was also a decrease in topo II activity which may have contributed to the resistance profile. Nevertheless, the presence of this protein in clinical samples of breast cancer refractory to ADR suggests actions on membrane mechanisms other than PGP. Clarification of the various resistance pathways will enable the development of newer strategies for their circumvention as well as allowing more accurate predictive analyses of effective treatment regimens.

References

(1) Endicott JA, Ling V. The biochemistry of P-glycoprotein mediated multidrug resistance. *Ann Rev Biochem* 1989; 58: 136–71.

(2) Deuchars KL, Ling V. P-glycoprotein and multidrug resistance in cancer chemotherapy. *Semin Oncol* 1989; 16(2): 156–65.

(3) Kane SE, Pastan I, Gottesman MM. Genetic basis of multidrug resistance of tumor cells. *J Bioenerg Biomem* 1990; 22(4): 593–618.

(4) van der Bliek AM, Borst P. Multidrug resistance. *Adv Cancer Res* 1989; 52: 165–203.

(5) Juranka PE, Zastawny RL, Ling V. P-glycoprotein: multidrug resistance and a superfamily of membrane associated transport proteins. *FASEB J* 1989; 3: 2583–92.

(6) McGrath JP, Varshavsky A. The yeast STE6 gene encodes a homologue of the mammalian multidrug resistant P-glycoprotein. *Nature* 1989; 340: 400–4.

(7) Ueda K, Pastan I, Gottesman MM. Isolation and sequence of the promoter region of the human multidrug resistance (P-glycoprotein) gene. *J Biol Chem* 1987; 262(36): 17432–6.

(8) Gros P, Ben-Nariah Y, Croop JM, Housman DE. Isolation and expression of a complementary DNA that confers multidrug resistance. *Nature* 1986; 323: 728–31.

(9) Foote SJ, Thompson JK, Cowman AF, Kemp I. Amplification of the multidrug resistance gene in some chloroquine-resistant isolates of *P. falciparum*. *Cell* 1989; 57: 921–30.

(10) Chin KV, Tanaka S, Darlington G, Pastan I, Gottesman MM. Heat shock and arsenite increase expression of the multidrug resistance (MDR1) gene in human renal cell carcinoma cells. *J Biol Chem* 1990; 265(1): 221–6.

(11) Mickley LA, Bates SE, Rikhert ND et al. Modulation of the expression of a multidrug resistance gene (MDR1/P-glycoprotein) by differentiating agents. *J Biol Chem* 1989; 264(30): 18031–40.

(12) Scotto KW, Biedler JL, Melera PW. Amplification and expression of genes associated with multidrug resistance in mammalian cells. *Science* 1986; 232: 751–5.

(13) Devault A, Gros P. Two members of the mouse MDR gene family confer multidrug resistance with overlapping but distinct drug specificities. *Mol Cell Biol* 1990; 10(4): 1652–63.

(14) Hsu SI, Lothstein L, Horwitz SB. Differential overexpression of 3 MDR gene family members in multidrug resistance J774.2 mouse cells. *J Biol Chem* 1989; 264(20): 12053–62.

(15) Chambers TC, McAvoy EM, Jacobs JW, Eilon G. Protein kinase C phosphorylates P-glycoprotein in multidrug resistant human KB carcinoma cells. *J Biol Chem* 1990; 265(13): 7679–86.

(16) Staats J, Marquardt D, Center MS. Characterisation of a membrane-associated protein kinase of multidrug-resistant HL60 cells which phosphorylates P-glycoprotein. *J Biol Chem* 1990; 265(7): 4084–90.

(17) Choi K, Chen C-J, Kriegler M, Roninson IB. An altered pattern of cross resistance in multidrug resistant cells results from spontaneous mutations in the MDR1 (P-glycoprotein) gene. *Cell* 1988; 53: 519–29.

(18) Safa AR, Stern RK, Choi K, Agresti M, Tamai I, Mehta ND, Roninson IB. Molecular basis of preferential resistance to colchicine in multidrug-resistant human cells conferred by GLY185 → VAL-185 substitution in P-glycoprotein. *Proc Natl Acad Sci USA* 1990; 87: 7225–9.

(19) Marino PA, Gottesman MM, Pastan I. MDR gene regulation in rat liver. *Cell Growth & Differentiation* 1990; 1: 57–62.

(20) Bradley B, Naik M, Ling V. P-glycoprotein expression in multidrug-resistant human ovarian carcinoma cell lines. *Cancer Res* 1989; 49: 2790–6.

(21) Weinstein RS, Kuszak JR, Kluskensl F, Coon JS. P-glycoprotein in pathology: the multidrug resistance gene family in humans. *Human Pathol* 1990; 21(1): 34–48.

(22) Georges E, Bradley G, Gariepy J, Ling V. Detection of P-glycoprotein isoforms by gene-specific monoclonal antibodies. *Proc Natl Acad Sci USA* 1990; 87: 152–6.

(23) Cumber PM, Jacobs A, Hoy T, Whittaker JA, Tsuruo T, Padua A. Expression of the multiple drug resistance gene (MDR-1) and epitope masking in chronic lymphatic leukemia. *Br J Haematol* 1990; 76: 226–30.

(24) Fojo AJ, Ueda K, Slamon DJ, Poplack DG, Gottesman MM, Pastan I. Expression of a multidrug resistance gene in human tumours and tissues. *Proc Natl Acad Sci USA* 1987; 84: 265–9.

(25) Cordon-Caroo C, O'Brien JP, Casals D et al. Multidrug resistance gene (P-glycoprotein) is expressed by endothelial cells at blood–brain barrier sites. *Proc Natl Acad Sci USA* 1989; 86: 695–8.

(26) Goldstein LJ, Galski H, Fojo A et al. Expression of a multidrug resistance gene in human cancers. *J Natl Cancer Inst* 1989; 81(2): 116–24.

(27) Bell DR, Gerlach JH, Kartner N, Buick RN, Ling V. Detection of P-glycoprotein in ovarian cancer: a molecular marker associated with multidrug resistance. *J Clin Oncol* 1985; 3(3): 311–15.

(28) Chan HSL, Thorner PS, Haddad G, Ling V. Immunohistochemical detection of P-glycoprotein: prognostic correlation in soft tissue sarcoma of childhood. *J Clin Oncol* 1990; 81(4): 689–704.

(29) Lai S-L, Goldstein LJ, Gottesman MM et al. MDR1 gene expression in lung cancer. *J Natl Cancer Inst* 1989; 81(15): 1144–50.

(30) Radosevich JA, Robinson PG, Rittmann-Grauer LS et al. Immunohistochemical analysis of pulmonary and pleural tumours with the monoclonal antibody of HYB-612 directed against the multidrug resistance (MDR-1) gene product P-glycoprotein. *Tumour Biol* 1989; 10: 252–7.

(31) Noonan KE, Beck C, Holzmayer TA et al. Quantitative analysis of MDR1 (multidrug resistance) gene expression in human tumours by polymerase chain reaction. *Proc Natl Acad Sci USA* 1990; 87: 7160–4.

(32) Rothenberg ML, Mickley, LA, Cole DE et al. Expression of the MDR1/P170 gene in patients with acute lymphoblastic leukaemia. *Blood* 1989; 74(4): 1388–95.

(33) Sato H, Gottesman MM, Goldstein LJ, Pastan I, Blouk AM, Sandberg AA, Preisler H D. Expression of the multidrug resistance gene in myeloid leukaemias. *Leukaemia Res* 1990; 14: 11–12.

(34) Sato H, Preisler H, Day R et al. MDR1 transcript levels as an indication of resistant disease in acute myelogenous leukaemia. *Br J Haematol* 1990; 75: 340–5.

(35) Ito Y, Tanimoto M, Kumazawa T et al. Increased P-glycoprotein expression and multidrug resistant gene (MDR1) amplification are infrequently found in fresh acute leukaemia cells. *Cancer* 1989; 63(8): 1534–8.

(36) Kuwazuru Y, Yoshimura A, Hanada S et al. Expression of the multidrug transporter, P-glycoprotein in chronic myelogenous leukaemia cells in blast crisis. *Br J Haematol* 1990; 74: 24–9.

(37) Dalton WS, Grogan TM, Rybski JA et al. Immunohistochemical detection and quantitation of P-glycoprotein in multiple drug resistant human myeloma cells. *Blood* 1989; 73(3): 747–52.

(38) Salmon SE, Grogan TM, Miller T, Scherer R, Dalton WS. Prediction of doxorubicin resistance in vitro in myeloma, lymphoma and breast cancer by P-glycoprotein staining. *J Natl Cancer Inst* 1989; 81(9): 696–701.

(39) Schlaifer D, Laurent G, Chittal S et al. Immunohistochemical detection of multidrug resistance associated P-glycoprotein in tumour and stromal cells of human cancers. *Br J Cancer* 1990; 62: 177–82.

(40) Herweijer H, Sonnenveld P, Baas F, Nooter K. Expression of MDR1 and MDR3 multidrug-resistance genes in human acute and chronic leukemias and association with stimulation of drug accumulation by cyclosporine. *J Natl Cancer Inst* 1990; 82(13): 1133–40.

(41) Stewart DJ, Evans WK. Non-chemotherapeutic agents that potentiate chemotherapy efficiency. *Cancer Treat Rev* 1989; 16: 1–40.

(42) Mickisch GH, Kossig J, Keilhauer G, Schlick E, Tschada RK, Alken PM. Effects of calcium antagonists in multidrug resistant primary human renal cell carcinomas. *Cancer Res* 1990; 50: 3670–4.

(43) Dalton WS, Grogan JM, Meltzer PS et al. Drug resistance in multiple myeloma and non-Hodgkin's lymphoma: detection of P-glycoprotein and potential circumvention by addition of verapamil in chemotherapy. *J Clin Oncol* 1989; 7: 415–24.

(44) Galski H, Sullivan M, Willingham MC, Khew-Voon C, Gottesman MM, Pastan I, Merlino K T. Expression of a human multidrug resistance cDNA (MDR1) in the bone marrow of transgenic mice: resistance to daunomycin-induced leukaemia. *Mol Cell Biol* 1989; 9(10): 4357–63.

(45) Wang JC. DNA topoisomerases. *Ann Rev Biochem* 1985; 54: 6654–97.

(46) Liu LF. DNA topoisomerase poisons as antitumour drugs. *Ann Rev Biochem* 1989; 58: 351–75.

(47) Davies SM, Robson CN, Davies SL, Hickson ID. Nuclear topoisomerase II levels correlate with the sensitivity of mammalian cells to intercalating agents and epipodophyllotoxins. *J Biol Chem* 1988; 263(33): 17724–9.

(48) Robinson MJ, Osheroff N. Stabilisation of the topoisomerase II-DNA cleavage complex by antineoplastic drugs: inhibition of enzyme-mediated DNA relegation by 4′(9′ acridinylamino) methanesulfon-*m*-anisidide. *Biochemistry* 1990; 29: 2511–15.

(49) Chow K-C, Ross WE. Topoisomerase-specific drug sensitivity in relation to cell cycle progression. *Mol Cell Biol* 1987; 7(9): 3119–23.

(50) Heck MMS, Hittelman WN, Earnshaw WL. In vivo phosphorylation of the 170 kD form of eukaryotic DNA topoisomerase II. *J Biol Chem* 1989; 264(26): 15161–4.

(51) Shen J-W, Subjeck JR, Lock RB, Ross WE. Depletion of topoisomerase II in isolated nuclei during a glucose-regulated stress response. *Mol Cell Biol* 1989; 9(8): 3284–91.

(52) Zwelling LA, Hinds M, Chan D et al. Characterisation of an amsacrine resistant line of human leukaemia cells. *J Biol Chem* 1989; 264(28): 16411–20.

(53) Huff AC, Leatherwood JK, Kreuzer KN. Bacteriophage T4 DNA topoisomerase is the target of antitumor agent 4' (9-acridinylamino) methanesolfon-*m*-anisidide (*m*-AMSA) in T4-infected *Escherichia coli*. *Proc Natl Acad Sci USA* 1989; 8: 1307–11.

(54) Huff AC, Ward RE, Kreuzer KN. Mutational alteration of the breakage/ resealing subunit of bacteriophage T4 topoisomerase confers resistance to anti-tumour agent *m*-AMSA. *Mol Gen Genet* 1990; 221: 27–32.

(55) Hong JH, Okada K, Kusano T et al. Reduced DNA topoisomerase II in VP-16 resistant mouse breast cancer cell line. *Biomed J Pharmacother* 1990; 44: 41–5.

(56) Pommier Y, Kerrigan D, Schwartz R et al. Altered DNA topoisomerase II activity in Chinese hamster cells resistant to topoisomerase II inhibitors. *Cancer Res* 1976; 46: 3075–81.

(57) Fernandes DJ, Danks MK, Beck WT. Decreased nuclear matrix DNA topoisomerase II in human leukaemia cells resistant to VM-26 and *m*-AMSA. *Biochemistry* 1990; 29: 4235–41.

(58) Tan KB, Mattern MR, Eng W-K, McCabe FL, Johnson RK. Non-productive rearrangement of DNA topoisomerase I and II genes: correlation with resistance to topoisomerase inhibitors. *J Natl Cancer Inst* 1989; 81: 1732–5.

(59) Zwelling LA, Slovak ML, Doroshow JH et al. HT1080/DR4: a P-glycoprotein-negative human fibrosarcoma cell line exhibiting resistance to topoisomerase II-reactive drugs despite the presence of a drug-sensitive topoisomerase II. *J Natl Cancer Inst* 1990; 82(19): 1553–60.

(60) Drake FH, Hofmann GA, Bartus HF et al. Biochemical and pharmacological properties of P170 and P180 forms of topoisomerase II. *Biochemistry* 1989; 28: 8154–60.

(61) Chung TDY, Drake FH, Tan KB, Per SR, Crooke ST, Mirabelli EK. Charac-terisation and immunological identification of cDNA clones encoding 2 human DNA topoisomerase II isozymes. *Proc Natl Acad Sci USA* 1989; 86: 9431–5.

(62) Woessner RD, Chung TDY, Hofmann GA, Mattern MR, Mirabelli CK, Drake F H, Johnson R K. Differences between normal and *ras* transformed NIH-3T3 cells in expression of the 170 kD and 180 kD forms of topoisomerase II. *Cancer Res* 1990; 50: 2901–8.

(63) Holden JA, Rolfson DH, Wittner CT. Human DNA topoisomerase II: evalua-tion of enzyme activity in normal and neoplastic tissues. *Biochemistry* 1990; 29: 2127–34.

(64) Finlay GJ, Baguley BC, Snow K, Judd WJ. Multiple patterns of resistance of human leukemia cell sublines to amsacrine analogues. *J Natl Cancer Inst* 1990; 82(8): 662–7.

(65) Chin K-V, Chauhan SS, Pastan I, Gottesman MM. Regulation of MDR RNA levels in response to cytotoxic drugs in rodent cells. *Cell Growth and Differenti-ation* 1990; 1: 361–5.

(66) Pickett CB, Lu AY. Glutathione S-transferases: gene structure, regulation and biological function. *Ann Rev Biochem* 1989; 58: 743–64.

(67) Morrow CS, Cowan KH. Glutathione S-transferases and drug resistance. *Cancer Cells* 1990; 2(1): 15–22.

(68) Cowan RH. The role of glutathione-S-transferase in drug resistance. *Proc Am Assn Cancer Res* 1989; 30: 674.

(69) Waxman DJ. Glutathione S-transferases: role in alkylating agent resistance and possible target for modulation chemotherapy – a review. *Cancer Res* 1990; 50: 6449–554.

(70) Schisselbauer JC, Silber R, Papadopoulos E, Abrams R, Lacreta FP, Tew KD. Characterisation of glutathione-S-transferase in lymphocytes from chronic lymphocytic leukaemia patients. *Cancer Res* 1990; 50: 3562–8.

(71) Nakagawa K, Saijo N, Tsuchida S et al. Glutathione S-transferase pi as a determinant of drug resistance in transfectant cell lines. *J Biol Chem* 1990; 265(8): 4296–301.

(72) Shklar MD. Increased resistance to *cis*-diaminedichloroplatinum in NIH3T3 cells transformed by *ras* oncogenes. *Cancer Res* 1988; 48: 793–7.

(73) Kelley SL, Basu A, Teicher BA, Hacker MP, Hamer DH, Lazo JS. Overexpression of metallothionein confers resistance to anticancer drugs. *Science* 1989; 241: 1813–15.

(74) Chen YN, Mickley LA, Schwartz AM, Acton EM, Hwang J, Fojo AT. Characterisation of adriamycin-resistant human breast cancer cells which display overexpression of a novel resistance related membrane protein. *J Biol Chem* 1990; 265(17): 10073–80.

Immunotoxins in haematological oncology

V S BYERS and R W BALDWIN

Introduction

Monoclonal antibodies defining human leukocyte surface antigens are being considered for targeted therapy of haematological malignancies. Treatment with unmodified antibody in order to activate host effector mechanisms including complement and cell-mediated cytotoxicity has been reported, but the clinical outcome has been widely variable ranging from prolonged remission to no effect.[1-3] An alternative approach is to employ the antibody for targeting therapeutic agents, particularly cytotoxic drugs. In this approach, a number of factors have to be considered including the choice of monoclonal antibody and cytotoxic agent, and the method of conjugating these two moieties to produce a cytotoxic immunoconjugate. The choice of cytotoxic agent is based upon a number of features such as its cytotoxic potency and the possibility of drug resistance being induced. From these considerations, antibody delivery of toxin molecules derived from plant and bacterial sources has been proposed. These are enzymes that, following entry into the cytosol of a cell, catalytically inactivate essential components required for protein synthesis.[4,5] One group of plant toxins, of which ricin is a typical example, act directly on ribosomes and so are referred to as ribosome-inhibiting proteins (RIP).[6] Diphtheria toxin and exotoxin A (*Pseudomonas aeruginosa*) inactivate an enzyme (elongation factor 2) required for the translocation of peptide chains in ribosomes.[7]

These toxins possess high enzymatic activity and a single molecule reaching the cytosol should be sufficient to produce cytotoxicity. For this to take place, the immunotoxin must first bind through the antibody moiety to the cell surface antigen. The cell-bound immunotoxin has then to be endocytosed, trafficked through intracellular organelles and the toxin component released into the cytosol (Fig. 1). Binding of immunotoxin to cell surface antigens is influenced by the affinity of the antibody component. The intracellular routing of the conjugate depends on a number of factors such as the

All correspondence to: Professor R W Baldwin, Cancer Research Campaign Laboratories, University of Nottingham, Nottingham NG7 2RD

Cambridge Medical Reviews: Haematological Oncology Volume 1

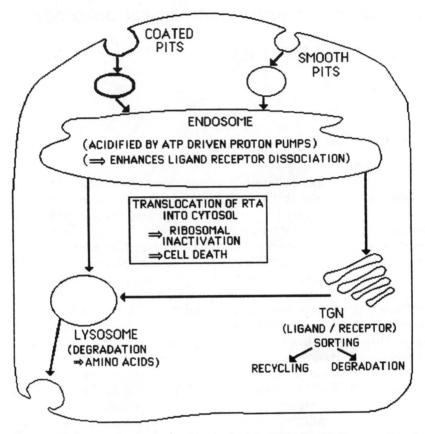

Fig. 1. Pathways of endocytosis of immunotoxins following binding to cell surface antigens.

rate of endocytosis of the cell surface receptor and its uptake into cell compartments such as endosomes for processing, or lysosomes for degradation. These intracellular processes are only poorly understood,[8] but, in practical terms, it is likely that a proportion of endocytosed immunotoxin will be lost from the system. Thus it will be necessary for a finite number of immunotoxin molecules to be internalized in order to ensure that sufficient toxin reaches the cytosol.

Design of immunotoxins
Ricin
Ricin isolated from the seeds of *Ricinus communis* plant has been used for the construction of a number of immunotoxins.[9,10] This toxin in its mature form

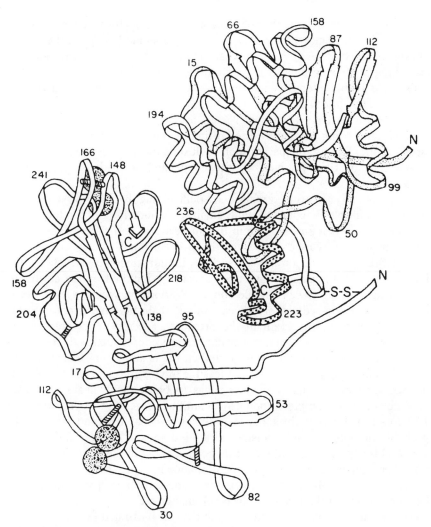

Fig. 2.   Ribbon representation of the ricin backbone.
Upper right: ricin A chain
Lower left: ricin B chain

is composed of two polypeptide chains A and B of approximately comparable
molecular size (30 kD) joined together through a disulphide bond (Fig. 2). In
the natural interaction, the toxin binds through a site on the B chain to
galactose-containing cell receptors.[11] The other role of the B chain is in
transporting endocytosed toxin into the cytoplasm of the cell. Following entry
into the cytoplasm through a series of endosome vesicles and trafficking
through the Golgi network, the ricin A chain (RTA) inhibits protein synthesis

51

by catalytically inactivating the 60S ribosomal subunit. This is achieved by an *N*-glycosidic cleavage which releases a specific adenine base from the sugar phosphate of 28S RNA.[12,13] The mechanism of ricin toxin entry into a cell and trafficking to the ribosomes is not well understood, but the overall cytotoxic response is highly effective such that one RTA-ribosome interaction is sufficient to result in cell death.

Immunotoxins have been constructed by conjugation of whole ricin to antibody, this being effected by directly linking the two proteins or by using a 'spacer-arm'. The use of spacers such as flexible polypeptides reduces steric interference or ricin B chain by the conjugated antibody so increasing potency.[14]

Immunotoxins constructed with intact ricin are highly cytotoxic since they retain the multiple functions of the B chain so augmenting cell binding. The B chain also plays a positive role in the intracellular trafficking of the toxin following its endocytosis. But, since the B chain binds non-specifically to carbohydrate structures on the cell surface, immunotoxins constructed with intact ricin lack the desired target-cell specificity imposed by the antibody component binding to cell surface antigen. Various manoeuvres have been utilized in order to reduce, or prevent, this B chain binding. Incubation of target cells and immunotoxin in the presence of excess concentrations of galactose or lactose has been used for in vitro procedures such as depletion of tumour cells from bone marrow prior to their use in autologous bone marrow transplantation. This approach is not feasible in vivo and methods have been devised for constructing conjugates so as to block the B chain galactose binding site. For example, a monoclonal antibody reacting with murine Thy 1 : 1 conjugated to ricin through a short linker was unable to bind to galactose probably through antibody causing steric hindrance of the B chain binding site.[15] This approach has subsequently been adopted in the construction of a thioether linked ricin-containing immunotoxin and fractionation into 'blocked' and 'non-blocked' components,[16] and a blocked ricin conjugate is being evaluated in the treatment of B cell malignancies.[17]

The potential of blocked ricin immunotoxins is illustrated further by comparison of immunotoxins constructed with a monoclonal antibody (M-T151) recognizing the CD4 antigen.[18] An immunotoxin constructed by linking intact ricin to antibody, so that the galactose binding sites of the B chain subunit were 'blocked', was cytotoxic in vitro for human T lymphoblastoid cells (CEM). Compared to an immunoconjugate prepared with ricin A chain, the 'blocked' ricin conjugate was some 100-fold more cytotoxic.

The in vivo toxicity of intact ricin-containing immunotoxins is a major obstacle for their use and methods continue to be explored for blocking the B chain carbohydrate binding sites. For example, treatment of ricin with ethylammonium nitrate has been claimed to inactivate the B chain carbohydrate binding activity, and the procedure has been used in constructing immunotoxins active against human monocytes.[19]

Ricin A chain immunotoxins

Immunotoxins constructed with ricin A chain (RTA) are specifically cytotoxic for target cells expressing the antigen recognized by the antibody component, although this is achieved at the expense of cytotoxic potential compared to whole ricin. In this approach, the A and B polypeptides of ricin are separated following reductive cleavage of the disulphide bond linking the two chains of the toxin, and the RTA conjugated to antibody. The choice of linker between antibody and RTA is a compromise since it must be sufficiently stable so as to preserve immunotoxin in the circulation, whilst readily undergoing cleavage intracellularly so as to release the RTA moiety. Many immunotoxins have been constructed using the heterobifunctional reagent N-succinimidyl-3(2-pyridyldithio) propionate (SPDP) as coupling agent,[9] but, in view of stability problems, other coupling reagents have been devised. These include iminothiolane and 4-succinimidyloxycarbonyl-α methyl α (2 pyridyldithio) toluene or SMPT[9,20] which result in the synthesis of more stable immunoconjugates.

Immunoconjugates constructed by conjugation of RTA with antibodies reacting with CD structures (Table 1) are cytotoxic in vitro for normal and neoplastic cells. These include immunotoxins T101-RTA and H65-RTA[21–23] reacting with the CD5 cell surface molecule, 67 kD glycoprotein expressed on the majority of human peripheral T lymphocytes. Immunotoxin 4A2-RTA is also cytotoxic for T cells reacting with the CD7 cell surface molecule (gp40).[24] Immunotoxins cytotoxic for B lymphocytes have been produced with several monoclonal antibodies reacting with CD19 (gp95) and CD22 (gp135) membrane components.[25,26] These immunotoxins have been constructed in various ways using intact antibodies as well as F(ab′)2 and Fab′ fragments. Also, native ricin A chain and deglycosylated RTA have been conjugated as the cytotoxic moiety. Deglycosylated RTA (dgA) is prepared by modification of the carbohydrate component of ricin by oxidation with metaperiodate--cyanoborohydride prior to separation of the ricin A and B chains. This modifies the mannose and fucose residues of the RTA which are involved in its uptake in vivo by non-parenchymal hepatic (Kupffer) cells.[27] As a result of this chemical modification, immunotoxins constructed with deglycosylated RTA have extended blood survival.

Clinical studies

Immunotoxins constructed with antibodies reacting with human leukocyte surface molecules are cytotoxic in vitro for normal and neoplastic cells. In addition, immunotoxins constructed with antibodies recognizing 'leukaemia

V S Byers and R W Baldwin

Table 1. *Ricin A chain immunotoxins for targeting to human leucocyte cell surface structures*

Binding structure	Target cell	Monoclonal antibody	Toxin	Ref.
CD2	T	9.6/35.1	RTA	41
CD3	T	64.1	RTA	41, 42
CD4	T	M.T151	RTA	42
CD5	T	T101	RTA	21, 22, 43
	B subset	H65	RTA	23, 42
CD7	T	4A2	RTA	24
CD19	B	HD37		
		HD37 (Fab')2	dgA	
CD22	B	HDG, RFB4	RTA)	
		UV 22.1 UV22.2	dgA	25, 26
		(also Fab'2) and		
		Fab fragments		

associated' antigens are cytotoxic and suppress growth of tumour xenografts. For example, RTA immunotoxins constructed with monoclonal antibodies reacting with leukaemia-associated antigens TALLA and GP37 have therapeutic activity against B and T cell leukaemia xenografts in athymic mice.[28,29] Clinical studies have now been initiated to examine the therapeutic applications of these immunotoxins in haematological malignancies. This includes the use of anti-T cell immunotoxins for the treatment of graft versus host disease following allogeneic bone marrow transplantation. These immunotoxins are also being evaluated in the treatment of T cell leukaemias and lymphomas. Immunotoxins reacting with B cell antigens are similarly being evaluated in the treatment of B cell malignancies including non-Hodgkin's lymphoma and lymphoblastic leukaemias.

Immunotoxins in the treatment of graft versus host disease arising following bone marrow transplantation

Bone marrow transplantation (BMT) from HLA-identical siblings has improved long-term survival in patients with haematological malignancies as well as genetic disorders and marrow failure. Graft versus host disease (GVHD), arising from transfer of donor T lymphocytes, is a major complication of BMT. The overall incidence of moderate to severe acute GVHD in recipients of bone marrow from an HLA-identical sibling has been reported to be 45 to 50%.[30] Immunosuppressive agents including corticosteroids, cyclosporin A and anti-thymocyte globulin (ATG) have been used as initial therapy of acute GVHD with partial or complete overall responses in some 40

54

to 60% of patients.[31] However, acute GVHD remains an important cause of mortality following allogeneic BMT.

Monoclonal antibodies reacting with human T cell antigens offer a new modality for therapy of acute GVHD. Several trials have utilized unmodified antibodies for treatment, the objective being to activate host responses such as complement or cell dependent cytotoxicity responses. Responses to treatment with unmodified antibodies have been of short duration and incomplete. In addition, therapy with murine monoclonal antibody reacting with the CD_3 antigen on T cells was associated with a high incidence of B cell lymphoproliferative disorders.[32]

Immunotoxin H65-RTA in the treatment of acute graft versus host disease

Immunotoxins constructed by conjugation of ricin A chain to anti-T cell monoclonal antibodies represent an alternative approach to antibody targeted treatment of acute GVHD.[23,33] The monoclonal antibody selected for immunoconjugate synthesis (H65) reacts with the CD5 differentiation antigen (67 kD glycoprotein) present on the surface of almost all peripheral T lymphocytes as well as thymocytes and a subset of B lymphocytes.[34] The antibody does not react with a wide range of normal tissues when examined by immunoperoxidase staining. This is important since antibodies selected as carriers for cytotoxic agents must have little, or no, reactivity with normal tissues so as to minimize non-specific toxicity. Since ricin A chain is only active intracellularly, it is also essential for the antibody used in constructing the immunotoxin to be efficiently endocytosed following binding to the target cell antigen. This was shown to be the case with antibody H65 in studying the endocytosis or radioiodine-labelled antibody and immunotoxin.[35] Finally, the immunotoxin was cytotoxic for cells expressing the CD5 marker.[23] For example, treatment of human bone marrow preparations with immunotoxin H65-RTA produced up to 98% depletion of T lymphocytes without decreasing the committed haematopoietic progenitor cells.

Patients with moderate to severe acute GVHD following an allogeneic bone marrow transplant as treatment mainly for leukaemia or lymphoma have been treated with immunotoxin H65-RTA.[33] Thirty-four patients received up to 14 daily intravenous doses of the immunotoxin. Side effects were identified as being constitutional symptoms such as fatigue and myalgias as well as hypoalbuminaemia with weight gain but without pulmonary oedema. Similar side effects have been noted with other RTA-containing immunotoxins in treating patients with malignant melanoma and colorectal cancer.[36,37] Immunotoxin treatment was associated with a rapid decrease in peripheral blood T lymphocyte levels which persisted for greater than one month after therapy. With a follow-up of 7–60 days after immunotoxin treatment, 16 of 32 evaluable patients had complete or partial overall responses without recurrence of

GVHD. Skin disease was the most responsive (73%) with gastrointestinal tract (45%) and liver (28%) being less responsive. Survival in responding patients was significantly prolonged at all times compared to those with no response.

BMT is a technique which is well suited for prophylactic therapy, since there is a 15–25 day period after the transplant before GVHD is expected to begin. Relatively low risk donor–recipient pairs are HLA matched siblings, in which the recipient is less than 20 years of age, and in these populations the incidence of GVHD is about 50%. Higher risk patients are those older than 30, or those receiving transplants from donors who are related but partially HLA mismatched, or HLA matched but unrelated (and thus mismatched at minor HLS loci). Clinical trials are ongoing in all three of these high risk populations, in which H65-RTA is given shortly after transplantation through day 10 post BMT, in an attempt to reduce incidence of severe GVHD. The first study is complete, in which patients received BMT from partially matched related donors starting 7–10 days post-BMT. Those patients with one and two antigen mismatches fared significantly better than controls, with severe GVHD developing in 4/21 patients, receiving immunotoxin as compared to 9/12 in controls. Similar results are being seen in other high risk populations, and it is anticipated that this agent will allow expansion of the procedure to other high risk patients (Henslee-Downey et al, in preparation).

Immunotoxin H65-RTA in cutaneous T Cell lymphoma (CTCL)

Immunotoxin H65-RTA has been used in a phase I/II study on the treatment of patients with cutaneous T cell lymphoma and Sezary syndrome.[38] Eleven patients were treated with escalating doses from 0.2 mg to 0.5 mg/kg/day for 10 days with re-treatment at the same doses at 35 day intervals. Side effects, as in the trial on patients with GVHD, included reversible myalgias, fatigue, chills, dyspnea and hypoalbuminemia with weight gain. Three patients showed a partial response by day 35; one of these had a greater than 80% reduction in Sezary cells after the first course with complete clearance during the second cycle of treatment. Although patients developed antibodies to the immunotoxin, this did not preclude re-treatment. A fourth patient attained a complete response after the second cycle of treatment in spite of the presence of anti-immunotoxin antibodies.

Anti-CD19 antibody-'blocked ricin' immunotoxin in human B Cell malignancies

CD19 is a B cell glycoprotein (95 kD) expressed on normal and neoplastic human B cells. This antigen is expressed on the cell surface when the Ig heavy chain gene rearranges and is likely to be expressed on the neoplastic clonal cell. An immunotoxin has been constructed with an anti-CD19 monoclonal antibody B4 which reacts with greater than 99% of B cell malignancies.[39] This has been conjugated to ricin in which the carbohydrate binding sites of the ricin B chain have been blocked using chemical agents which form a stable covalent linkage so eliminating its carbohydrate binding activity.[17] The objective of this treatment is to eliminate cell interactions other than those involving antibody. Thus 'blocked' ricin was some 1000 times less cytotoxic for Burkitt's lymphoma cells than natural ricin. Following conjugation to the antibody B4, the immunoconjugate was highly cytotoxic for CD19 antigen positive cells and this cytotoxicity was antigen specific. For example, treatment of Burkitt's lymphoma cells (Namalwa) with 10^{-9} M blocked ricin-antibody conjugate produced 4 to 5 log reduction in cell survival. This cytotoxic effect could be inhibited by treating target cells with unconjugated B4 antibody to block antigen-binding sites. Treatment of tumour cells with galactose to block cell sites binding ricin B chain was ineffective.

Studies in mice and monkeys identified hepatocellular damage as the major toxicity of the immunotoxin, the LD_{50} being 500–1000 µg/kg when administered as a single bolus injection. The maximum tolerated dose administered over 5 days was 200 µg/kg. Following these preclinical studies, a phase I clinical trial has been carried out in 25 patients with CD19 antigen positive B cell malignancies (23 patients with non-Hodgkin's lymphoma, one with acute lymphoblastic leukaemia and one with chronic lymphocytic leukaemia). Most of the patients had disease resistant to salvage treatment and about one-third had failed bone marrow transplantation. Almost all patients had very bulky tumour masses with infiltration of lymphoid organs and bone marrow. Many patients had extranodal disease.

Immunotoxin was administered daily for 5 days as a 1-hour infusion with doses up to 60 µg/kg/day. Pharmacokinetic studies indicated peak serum levels were achieved at the completion of the 1-hour infusion and thereafter rapidly decreased. Although increasing serum levels of immunotoxin were noted in a dose-dependent fashion, the period of detectable conjugate was short, eg 9 to 10 hours at a dose of 50 µg/kg. This probably reflects hepatic clearance of immunotoxin since liver uptake has been reported in experimental animal systems with immunotoxin constructed with ricin A chain. Significantly, hepatotoxicity manifested as elevations in SGOT/SGPT in the range 10 times normal was a major side effect defining maximum tolerated dose (50 µg/kg/day for 5 days). At this dose, reduced serum albumin levels (25%) were noted in most patients.

Tumour responses were determined by bone marrow biopsies, X-ray, CT and gallium scans. One complete response involving disappearance of cervical and mediastinal adenopathy has been noted in 1 patient (greater than 10 months). Partial remissions in 2 patients with extensive bone marrow replacement have been noted and 7 patients had transient or mixed responses.

Immunotoxin treatment produced a 40 to 70% decrease in circulating CD19+ cells which will include B cells and tumour cells. B cell function recovered 2 to 10 days following treatment.

A second phase I trial has been initiated the aim being to maintain significant levels of circulating immunotoxin. Immunotoxin was administered as a bolus infusion of 20 µg/kg over 1 hour, followed by a constant daily infusion (10 to 50 µg/kg daily for 7 days). These are ongoing trials and, at the time of reporting,[17] 8 patients had been treated (4 non-Hodgkin's lymphoma, one CLL and two non-T ALL). Two patients have been reported as partial remissions and one as complete remission.

One of the important side effects noted with many immunotoxins is the production of antibody responses to both the mouse monoclonal antibody (HAMA), and ricin.[37,40] This was also the case with the patients treated with the anti-CD19 antibody-'blocked ricin' immunoconjugate. In the first trial involving daily infusions for 5 days, HAMA and anti-ricin antibodies were detected in 8 patients. A more detailed analysis of this side effect is awaited since the extent of the anti-immunotoxin responses will limit the ability to re-treat patients.

Anti-CD22 monoclonal antibody – ricin A chain immunotoxins in B Cell lymphoma

CD22 is a B cell restricted 2-chain glycoprotein (130 and 140 kD) which, during B cell ontogeny, is first expressed in the cytoplasm at the pre-B cell stage. The marker then is expressed on the cell surface of B cells and it is also expressed on some B cell tumours. Immunotoxins have been constructed for the treatment of B cell lymphoma by conjugation of chemically deglycosylated ricin A chain (dgA) to a murine antibody (RFB4) reacting with CD22 antigen.[25] Two variants of the immunotoxin have been constructed for clinical study. One contains CD22 antibody conjugated to dgA through a hindered disulphide bond; this product being 10- to 20-fold more toxic than whole ricin for cells of a B lymphoblastoid cell line. The other immunotoxin was prepared by linking Fab fragments of the anti-CD22 antibody through a cystine bridge to deglycosylated RTA. This immunotoxin is 2-fold more potent than ricin (Thorpe & Vitetta, unpublished observations). The immunotoxins are in clinical trial with patients with B cell leukaemia/lymphomas. Side effects include a vascular leak syndrome with decreases in serum albumin levels similar to those observed in immunotoxin trials in patients with solid cancers. The generation of low titre antibody responses to the dgA chain has been observed in 2/18 patients, this probably being partly due to the patients being immunosuppressed and also since the immunotoxin is directed against a B lymphocyte antigen. The trials are still ongoing but transient partial or mixed responses (above 50% reduction in tumour mass) have been reported in 60% of patients treated with either anti-CD22-dgA or Fab anti-CD22-dgA (Vitetta & Thorpe, personal communication).

Conclusions

Clinical trials with immunotoxins constructed by conjugation of ricin or ricin A chain to monoclonal antibodies binding to T and B cell associated antigens are only at an early stage of development but these immunotoxins have proved to be effective in the elimination of circulating target cells. This is well illustrated by the efficacy of the anti-CD5 immunotoxin H65-RTA in the elimination of CD5+ peripheral blood lymphocytes[33] and the anti-CD19-ricin immunotoxin for decreasing circulating CD19+ B cells.[17] Further modifications in immunoconjugate design are being considered so as to improve efficacy. These include construction of immunotoxins with a wide range of monoclonal antibodies[24] and the use of antibody fragments.[25,26] Improved blood survival of immunotoxins is also necessary and this has led to the use of ricin A chain components, as well as deglycosylated ricin A chain so as to limit hepatic uptake. Finally, procedures are being designed so as to reduce the impact of patient antibody responses to the monoclonal antibody and toxin components of immunotoxins. This is important if re-treatment schedules are to be designed, although the impact of these responses is still not fully appreciated. For example, antibody production has not been a consistent response in B cells lymphoma patients (Thorpe & Vitetta, unpublished observations) and patients with cutaneous T cell lymphomas have been retreated with H65-RTA without any problem even though anti-immunotoxin antibodies are present.[38] Nevertheless, patients do elicit antibody responses to immunotoxins and these are not desirable. Accordingly, procedures are evolving to reduce the impact of anti-immunotoxin antibodies. These include the construction of human mouse chimeric antibodies which do not provoke significant antibody responses in patients[44] and the design of procedures for down-regulating antibody responses to toxins such as ricin A chain.[45] One anticipates that these refinements will improve the pharmacokinetic properties of immunotoxins and should thus result in better responses.

References

(1) Baldwin RW, Byers, VS. Monoclonal antibodies and immunoconjugates for cancer treatment. In Pinedo HM, Longo DL, Chabner BA eds. *Cancer chemotherapy and biological response modifiers annual*. 9, Amsterdam: Elsevier 1987: 409–31.

(2) Hale G, Clark MR, Marcus R. Remission induction in non-Hodgkin lymphoma with reshaped human monoclonal antibody Campath-1H. *Lancet* 1988; ii: 1394–9.

(3) Bertram JH, Gill PS, Levine AM et al. Monoclonal antibody T101 in T cell malignancy: a clinical, pharmacokinetic and immunological correlation. *Blood* 1986; 68: 752–61.

(4) Vitetta ES, Fulton RJ, May RD, Till M, Urh JW. Redesigning nature's poisons to create anti-tumour reagents. *Science* 1987; 238: 1098–104.

(5) Olsnes S, Sandvig K, Petersen OW, van Deurs B. Immunotoxins – entry into cells and mechanisms of action. *Immunol Today* 1989; 10: 291–5.

(6) Stirpe F, Barbieri L. Ribosome inactivating proteins up to date. *FEBS* Lett 1986; 195: 1–8.

(7) Fitzgerald D, Pastan I. Targeted toxin therapy for the treatment of cancer. *J Natl Cancer Inst* 1989; 81: 1455–63.

(8) Klausner RD. Sorting and traffic in the central vacuolar system. *Cell* 1989; 67: 703–6.

(9) Blakey DC, Wawrzynczak EJ, Wallace PM, Thorpe PE. Antibody toxin conjugates: a perspective. In: Waldmann H ed. *Prog Allergy* Basel:Karger, 1988; 45: 50–90.

(10) Frankel AE, ed. *Immunotoxins*, Norwell, MA. Kluwer Academic, 1988.

(11) Olsnes S, Sandvig K. How protein toxins enter and kill cells. In: Frankel AE, ed. *Immunotoxins*, Norwell, MA. Kluwer, 1988: 39–72.

(12) Endo Y, Mitsui K, Motizuki M, Tsurugi K. The mechanism of action of ricin and related toxic lectins on eukaryotic ribosomes. The site and the characteristics of the modification in 28S ribosomal RNA caused by the toxins. *J Biol Chem* 1987; 262: 5908–12.

(13) Endo Y, Tsurugi K. RNA *N*-glycosidase activity of ricin A chain. *J Biol Chem* 1987; 262: 8128–30.

(14) Marsh JW, Neville Jr, DM. A flexible peptide spacer increases the efficacy of holoricin anti-T cell immunotoxins. *J Immunol* 1988; 140: 3674–8.

(15) Thorpe PE, Ross WJC, Brown ANF et al. Blockade of the galactose-binding sites of ricin by its linkage to antibody. *Europ J Biochem* 1984; 140: 63–71.

(16) Brusa P, Pietribiasi F, Bussolati G et al. Blocked and not blocked whole ricin antibody immunotoxins: intraperitoneal therapy of human tumour xenografted in nude mice. *Cancer Immunol Immunother* 1989; 29: 185–92.

(17) Nadler LM, Breitmeyer J, Coral F, Schlossman SF. Anti-B4 (CD19) blocked ricin immunotoxin therapy after human B cell malignancies. In: Schild G, Haseltine WA, Mann R, eds. *Biotechnology in therapeutics*, Parthenon, 1990: in press.

(18) Wawrzynczak EJ, Watson GJ, Cumber AJ et al. Blocked and non-blocked ricin immunotoxins against CD4 antigen exhibit higher cytotoxic potency than a ricin A chain immunotoxin potentiated with ricin B chain or with a ricin B chain immunotoxin. *Cancer Immunol Immunother* 1990: in press.

(19) Schüt C, Pfüffer U, Siegl E, Walzel H, Franz H. Selective killing of human monocytes by an immunotoxin containing partially denatured mistletoe lectin I. *Int J Immunopharmacol* 1989; 11: 977–80.

(20) Thorpe PE, Wallace PM, Knowles PP et al. New coupling agents for the synthesis of immunotoxins containing a hindered disulfide bond with improved stability in vivo. *Cancer Res* 1987; 47: 5924–31.

(21) Jansen FK, Laurent G, Liance MC et al. Efficiency and tolerance of the treat-

ment with immuno-A-chain toxins in human bone marrow transplantation. In: Baldwin RW, Byers VS, eds. *Monoclonal antibodies for cancer detection and therapy*. Academic Press: London, 1985: 223–48.

(22) Myers DE, Uckun FM, Swain SE, Vallera DA. The effects of aromatic and alkophatic maleimide crosslinkers on anti-CD5 ricin immunotoxins. *J Immunol Methods* 1989; 49: 123–6.

(23) Kernan NA, Byers VS, Scannon PJ et al. Treatment of steroid-resistant acute graft-vs-host disease by in vivo administration of an anti-T cell ricin A chain immunotoxin. *JAMA* 1988; 259: 3154–7.

(24) Carroll SF, Trown PW, Bernhard SL, Staskawicz MO, Kung AHC. Characterization of anti-CD7-RTA30 immunotoxin 4M RTA. *Antibody Immunoconj Radiopharm* 1990; 3: 73.

(25) Ghetie MA, May RD, Till M et al. Evaluation of ricin A chain containing immunotoxins directed against CD19 and CD22 antigens on normal and malignant B cells as potential agents for in vivo therapy. *Cancer Res* 19; 48: 2610–17.

(26) Shen GL, La J-L, Ghetie MA et al. Evaluation of four CD22 antibodies as ricin A chain-containing immunotoxins for the in vivo therapy of human B-cell leukaemias and lymphomas. *Int J Cancer* 1988; 42: 792–7.

(27) Thorpe PE, Wallace PM, Knowles PP et al. Improved antitumour effects of immunotoxins prepared with deglycosylated ricin A chain and hindered disulfide linkage. *Cancer Res* 1988; 48: 6396–403.

(28) Hara H, Luo Y, Seon BK. Efficient transplantation of human non-T-leukaemia cells into nude mice and induction of complete regression of the transplanted distinct tumours by ricin A chain conjugates of monoclonal antibodies SN5 and SN6. *Cancer Res* 1988; 48: 4673–80.

(29) Yokota S, Hara H, Luo Y, Seon BK. Synergistic potentiation of in vivo antitumor activity of anti-human T-leukemia immunotoxins by recombinant α-interferon and daunomycin. *Cancer Res* 1990; 50: 32–7.

(30) Gale RP, Bortin MM, Bekkum DW et al. Risk factors for actue graft-versus-host disease. *Br J Haematol* 1987; 67: 397–406.

(31) Vogelsang GB, Hess AD, Sandos GW. Acute graft-versus-host disease: clinical characteristics in the cyclosporine era. *Medicine* 1988; 67: 163–74.

(32) Martin PJ, Hansem JA, Anasetti C et al. Treatment of acute graft-versus-host disease with anti-CD3-monoclonal antibodies. *Am J Kidney Dis* 1988; 3: 149–52.

(33) Byers VS, Henslee PJ, Kernan NA et al. Use of an anti-pan T-lymphocyte ricin A chain immunotoxin in steroid resistant acute graft versus host disease. *Blood* 1990: in press.

(34) Byers VS. Anti-pan T lymphocyte immunotoxin for therapy of autoimmune diseases: preclinical and clinical development. In: Baldwin RW, Byers VS eds. *Monoclonal antibodies and immunoconjugates in cancer treatment*. Parthenon, Cornforth, UK 1990: in press.

(35) Baldwin RW, Byers VS, Berry N, Pawluczyk I, Garnett MC, Robins RA, Scannon PJ. Endocytosis of ricin A chain immunotoxins recognising human tumor cell surface antigens. *Proc Amer Assn Cancer Res* 1988; 29: 423.

(36) Spitler LE, del Rio M, Khentigan A et al. Therapy of patients with malignant

melanoma using a monoclonal antimelanoma antibody-ricin A chain immunotoxin. *Cancer Res* 1987; 47: 1717–23.

(37) Byers VS, Rodvien R, Grant K et al. Phase I study of monoclonal antibody-ricin A chain immunotoxin Xomazyme 791 in patients with metastatic colon cancer. *Cancer Res* 1989; 49: 6153–60.

(38) Le Maistre CF, Frankel A, Kornfeld S, Rosen S, Scannon P, Byers VS. Phase I/II study of a pan T cell immunotoxin in cutaneous T-cell lymphoma (CTLL). *Blood* 1989; 74: 161.

(39) Nadler LM, Anderson KC, Marti G et al. B4, a human B lymphocyte-associated antigen expressed on normal mitogen activated and malignant B lymphocytes. *J Immunol* 1983; 131: 244–50.

(40) Durrant LG, Robins RA, Ballantyne KC, Austin EB, Baldwin RW. Production of a human monoclonal antibody recognising a determinant on mouse IgG2b from a patient receiving mouse monoclonal antibody for diagnostic imaging. *Clin Exp Immunol* 1989; 75: 258–64.

(41) Press OW, Vitetta ES, Farr AG, Hansen JA, Martin PJ. Evaluation of ricin A chain immunotoxins directed against human T cells. *Cell Immunol* 1986; 102: 10–20.

(42) Preijers FWMB, Tax WJ, DeWitte T et al. Relationship between internalization and cytotoxicity of ricin A chain immunotoxins. *Br J Haematol* 1988; 70: 289–94.

(43) Hertler AA, Schlossman DM, Borowitz MJ, Blythman HE, Casellas, P, Frankel A E. An anti-CD5 immunotoxin for chronic lymphocytic leukemia: enhancement of cytotoxicity with human serum albumin-monensin. *Int J Cancer* 1989; 43: 215–19.

(44) Lo Buglio AF, Wheeler RH, Trang J et al. Mouse/human chimeric monoclonal antibody in man: kinetics and immune response. *Proc Natl Acad Sci USA* 1989; 86: 4220–4.

(45) Byers VS, Clegg JA, Pimm MV et al. Regulation of antibody responses to ricin A chain (RTA) arising following treatment with RTA-immunotoxins. *Antibody Immunoconj Radiopharm* 1990; 3: 72.

(46) Montfort W, Villafranca JE, Monzingo AF et al. The three-dimensional structure of ricin at 2.8 A. *J Biol Chem* 1987; 262: 5398–403.

Alpha interferon: uses and possible mechanisms of action

D W GALVANI and J C CAWLEY

Introduction

It is now almost 20 years since the first clinical trials of interferon α (IFNα) were commenced. In general, the agent has proved to have little part to play in the treatment of common disorders.[1] However, a few unusual neoplasms and chronic viral disorders have proved sufficiently responsive to allow IFNα to be employed as licensed therapy (Table 1). Thus, hairy-cell leukaemia (HCL) and chronic granulocytic leukaemia (CGL) are the most consistently responsive neoplastic disorders, and IFNα may prove to be a therapeutic advance.[2,3] IFNα is not as well established in the treatment of condylomata acuminata and Kaposi sarcoma where there are other therapeutic alternatives.[4] Recently, the courses of chronic hepatitis B and C have been shown to be modified by IFNα therapy, and this may expand the use of IFNα considerably.[5,6]

This chapter describes the biology of the interferons, then deals with the clinical role of IFNα in HCL and CGL. The possible mechanisms underlying the particular sensitivity of these disorders to the cytokine are then considered. Finally, the place of IFNα in other haematological malignancies is also briefly discussed.

The interferons

Definition of an interferon

An interferon (IFN) is a protein which exerts virus non-specific, anti-viral activity, at least in homologous cells, through cellular metabolic processes involving synthesis of RNA and protein.[7]

Types of interferon

The anti-viral activity that was originally described by Lindeman[8] has now been subdivided into three major types of IFN (α, β and γ). Although unified

All correspondence to: DW Galvani, University Department of Haematology, Duncan Building, Royal Liverpool Hospital, Prescot Street, Liverpool L69 3BX, UK.

Cambridge Medical Reviews: Haematological Oncology Volume 1

Table 1. *Therapeutically available IFNα in UK*[a]

Trade name	Type of IFN	Licensed indications
Intron	rh IFNα 2b	HCL, CGL, KS, condylomata acuminata
Roferon	rh IFNα 2a	HCL, KS (AIDS-related), renal cell cancer
Wellferon	lymphoblastoid IFNα N1	HCL

rh IFNα   recombinant human interferon α.
KS   Kaposi sarcoma.
[a]Several companies are developing IFNα which is not yet commercially available.

Table 2. *Molecular biology of the interferons*

Characteristics	IFNα	IFNβ	IFNγ
Synonym	Leucocyte	Fibroblast	Immune
Subtypes	Over 24	None	None
Source	Leucocytes	Fibroblasts	T lymphocytes
Gene	Chromosome 9	Chromosome 9	Chromosome 12
Homology	30% with β	30% with α	10% with α and β
Molecular weight	16–27 kD	20 kD	15–25 kD
Amino acids	165	166	143–146
Glycosylation	+	++	+++
Disulphide bonds	2	1	0
Acid stability	+	+	−
Cell surface receptor	Type I	Type I	Type II
Gene for receptor	Chromosome 21	Chromosome 21	Chromosome 6
Main inducing stimuli	Virus	Virus	Antigen/Mitogen

by anti-viral activity, each type is distinct in its cellular and immunological properties, in particular, anti-viral activity does not necessarily correlate with immunological effect.

The molecular aspects of the three types of interferon are dealt with in Table 2. Both IFNα and β share similar properties and the same cell surface receptor; this led to the term type 1 interferon. IFNγ is quite distinct (cf type 2 interferon), has less potent anti-viral activity but is a strong immunomodulatory cytokine. Table 3 contrasts these cellular biological properties.

It is becoming clearer that interferons are only part of a network of cytokines which is activated in response to different stimuli. Thus, the IFNs cause the release of other cytokines and vice versa. Consequently, the in vivo effect(s) of an IFN represent a combination of direct and indirect responses respectively, mediated by IFN itself, or by secondarily released cytokines.

Table 3. *Cellular biological properties of interferons*

Actions	IFNα	IFNβ	IFNγ
Antiviral	++	++	+
Direct growth inhibition of tumour cells	+	+	+
Increased MHC I expression	+	+	++
Increased MHC II expression	±	±	++
CTL cytotoxicity	+	+	+
NK cytotoxicity	++	++	+
Monocyte cytotoxicity	+	+	++
B Lymphocyte activation	±	±	±
Neutrophil cytotoxicity	−	−	+

CTL, cytotoxic T lymphocyte.
NK,　natural killer cells.

A corollary of these observations is that the in vitro effect of IFNs are, at best, an imperfect guide to what happens in vivo.

Interferon at a molecular level
Interferon receptors Like most cytokines and hormones, an interferon must bind to a specific cell surface receptor to produce an intracellular signal. IFNα receptors are widely distributed on many cell types.[9] The number of receptors per cell may be of relevance to cellular responsiveness,[10] and the degree of receptor occupancy may determine the type of cellular effect.[11] To date, the IFNα/β receptor has not been cloned, but is known to be a glycoprotein of approximately 130 kD.[12] The IFNγ receptor has been cloned and is a glycoprotein containing 489 amino acids.[13]

Signal transduction Conflicting reports connecting the IFNα/β receptor with the phosphoinositol pathway have been published.[14,15] Other evidence suggests that neither cyclic AMP, GMP nor prostaglandin products are involved.[16] There is more substantial evidence linking the IFNγ receptor with protein kinase C activation.[17]

Gene regulation Most IFN-induced genes are activated by all 3 types of IFN. Transcription can be inhibited or stimulated by IFNs. Thus, IFNα/β can stimulate transcription of the 2′5′ oligoadenylate synthetase gene,[18] but inhibits c-*myc* gene transcription.[19,20] Other workers have suggested that IFNs operate at a post-transcriptional control.[21]

Gene products The best studied cell product of IFN stimulation is 2'5' oligoadenylate synthetase. This catalyses the production of 2'5' linked oligonucleotides of adenosine from ATP, this, in turn, activates an endonuclease which degrades mRNA and rRNA halting protein synthesis.[22] This 'interferes' with viral replication but may also be involved in normal cell regulation.

A dsRNA-dependent protein kinase can also be induced which can phosphorylate proteins important in cell division;[23] again, viral and cell replication are inhibited. Numerous other proteins can be up-regulated by the IFNs, and the increased expression of human leucocyte antigens (HLA) by cells exposed to IFNγ is a notable example.

Effects of interferons on cell function
Anti-viral activity IFN-treated cells resist DNA and RNA virus attack in several ways. In addition to endonuclease degradation of RNA, viral attachment and budding may be inhibited, and viral transcription can be reduced by IFN.[22,24]

Cell proliferation and differentiation The anti-proliferative effects of IFNα/β have been extensively studied in human haemic cell lines.[25] For example, in Daudi cells a decrease in c-*myc* expression was associated with growth arrest in G0/G1.[19] This may be relevant to the inhibition of haemopoiesis in vivo, since c-*myc* expression is known to be involved in haemopoietic growth.[20] Both IFNα and γ can stimulate haemic cell lines to differentiate,[26] but the biochemical basis of this differentiating effect is not well understood.

The immune system In vitro NK cytotoxicity is markedly increased, especially by IFNα/β.[27] Initial reports suggested that IFNα therapy may enhance natural killer (NK) activity in vivo,[28] but this is not consistently so. Furthermore, many tumour cells (eg hairy cells) are not susceptible to NK lysis, and it seems unlikely that the beneficial effects of IFNα are mediated by enhanced NK activity.

T lymphocyte cytotoxicity increases following exposure to IFNα or γ in vitro, but proliferation is reduced.[4] Effects on B cell function are complex and are probably dependent on the differentiation/activation state of the given B cell type under investigation.[4] IFNγ was originally termed macrophage activating factor,[29] and is a potent stimulus for macrophage killing. IFNγ increases MHC class II expression on macrophages which may influence T lymphocyte activation.

Measurement of interferon activity
Interferon activity can be expressed in terms of biological effect or mass of protein. Thus, the inhibition of plaque formation in virus-infected cell monolayers can be used to express anti-viral activity of a sample. When

compared to a known standard, units of anti-viral activity can be ascribed to this sample. Alternatively, monoclonal antibodies can be used to quantitate given types of interferon in terms of protein concentration. Both methodologies are valid but give different information.

Pharmacology of IFNα

Although IFNα has been widely studied in the clinic, IFNβ and γ have been employed in far fewer clinical trials. IFNβ and γ are broadly similar to IFNα in terms of pharmacology.

Three main preparations of IFNα are generally available for clinical use in the UK, Table 1 summarizes their titles and indications. All three formulations seem to have similar clinical efficacy, although Wellferon, being a natural cell product, is a mixture of subtypes of IFNα, and may be less immunogenic than the recombinant formulations.[30]

If IFNα is going to be therapeutically effective, it will usually be so at low (1–3 megaU/day) or medium (3–6 megaU/day) doses. Fifty percent of patients cannot tolerate more than 20 megaU daily.[31] Intravenous therapy is not superior to the established subcutaneous route. Thus, in practice, 3–6 megaU daily by the subcutaneous route can achieve anti-tumour effects without severe toxicity. The half-life of IFNα is 12–18 hours and side effects are maximal within 6 hours of subcutaneous administration. However, injecting IFNα in the early evening will result in side effects coinciding with sleep and improved compliance. On 3 megaU daily, serum levels are about 100 U/ml.

Side effects of IFNα therapy are more troublesome with advancing age. Fatigue is the commonest complaint at all ages (90%) and may be a direct effect on the central nervous system. Psychomotor retardation, which is a very rare consequence of IFNα therapy in the elderly, may be the extreme expression of this fatigue syndrome. Fever and 'flu-like symptoms are also common but usually respond to Paracetamol. Nausea and anorexia are seen in two-thirds of patients but tend to be transient. Weight, however, should be regularly monitored. Serum transaminases often rise on commencement of IFNα but jaundice is exceptional. Most of these side effects improve following a few weeks' IFNα therapy. If troublesome, a reduction or temporary cessation of therapy will improve symptoms. Convulsions and coma are indications to stop IFNα therapy altogether.

In patients receiving IFNα therapy for non-haematological disorders, neutropenia and thrombocytopenia may occur. This is a consequence of marrow suppression rather than of redistribution of circulating cells. Reducing the dose schedule usually improves marrow toxicity.

IFNα in hairy cell leukaemia (HCL)

Clinical effects of IFNα

After prolonged administration of IFNα, the peripheral cytopenias of the disease are improved in >80% of patients, whether or not the patient has had a splenectomy.[2] In particular, the neutropenia of HCL is consistently improved and the incidence of serious infection, formally a major cause of death in the disease, is reduced. Hairy-cell variants are generally unresponsive.

The effects of IFNα on the marrow are less striking and HCs are reduced <5% in a minority of cases (probably <10%); even when the HC infiltrate is reduced, considerable fibrosis persists.

These beneficial results are achieved with minimal side effects. Occasionally, neutropenia may significantly worsen early in therapy, but this can now be overcome with G-CSF.[32]

Disease activity slowly returns after cessation of therapy, but will normally respond to reintroduction of IFNα therapy. The optimal duration of therapy is not clear but, since significant improvement in marrow function can occur after between 6–12 months, treatment should probably be continued for at least 1 year.

The different forms of IFNα are probably equally efficacious. Interferon antibodies seem to be more common after IFNα-2a (Roferon) treatment but, although resistance to IFNα-2a in association with neutralizing antibodies has recently been reported in HCL,[33] the clinical significance of such antibodies remains controversial.

IFNα versus other treatment modalities

Deoxycoformycin (dCF) is highly active in HCL (whether or not the patient has had a splenectomy or received IFNα) and produces response rates at least as high as IFNα.[34] Furthermore, when dCF is effective, hairy cells (HCs) are frequently eradicated from the marrow and, on stopping treatment, the disease does not relapse over substantial periods of follow-up. Also, these impressive results are achieved with a relatively small amount of drug (approximately 12 injections of 4 mg/m² over 6 months) and with minimal toxicity.

dCF, therefore, seems to offer a number of advantages over IFNα and probably should be the treatment of choice in the disease. However, dCF is not directly available in the UK, and the drug can only be obtained from the National Cancer Institute (NCI) in the USA for patients resistant to IFNα or as part of an approved clinical trial.

Very recently, impressive clinical responses have been obtained with chloroxyadenosine,[35] an agent related to dCF. However, experience with the drug is still limited, and the supply is restricted to the Scripps Clinic in La Jolla.

Before the recognition that IFNα and dCF are so effective in HCL, splenectomy was the treatment of first choice. If the spleen is substantially enlarged and, if marrow impairment as manifested by marked anaemia is not great, improvement in peripheral cytopenias can be expected following splenectomy. What then is the current place of splenectomy and what is the best overall approach to treatment?

Given that dCF is only available in the UK for patients resistant to IFNα and, given that the latter treatment should be prolonged, it seems reasonable to recommend splenectomy provided that the spleen is substantially enlarged. When the disease eventually recurs, or if there is no response to splenectomy, IFNα therapy should be given. If the spleen is not enlarged, then IFNα should be given from the start. If the disease becomes resistant to IFNα or if the patient becomes intolerant of the agent, dCF (obtained from the NCI) should be given.

Finally, of course, it should be remembered that a small proportion of patients (up to 15%) are asymptomatic and have no peripheral cytopenias – these patients should not be treated.

Mechanism of action of IFNα in HCL

HCs are resistant to the cytolytic effects of NK and lymphokine-activated killer cells (LAK) cells and there is no evidence of generation of cytotoxic T lymphocytes (CTLs) in patients on IFNα.[36,37] It therefore seems unlikely that the beneficial effects of the agent are mediated via its immunomodulatory effects on cytotoxic cells.

Although HCs are not killed by exposure to IFNα, they have substantial numbers of IFNα receptors[10] and the cytokine inhibits HC proliferation in response to a number of growth stimuli such as B cell growth factor (BCGF).[38] It therefore seems likely that IFNα acts via its antiproliferative effect on HCs. However, the proliferative stimuli to HCs in vivo are largely unknown and it remains unclear why HCs, among all neoplastic B cells, are so sensitive to the antiproliferative effects of IFNα.

Recent work in this laboratory has shown that direct contact with macrophages and endothelial cells stimulates HC proliferation and that this proliferation is inhibited by IFNα but not IFNγ (Griffiths & Cawley, unpublished observations). It is tempting to speculate that the long-recognized histological association between marrow macrophages and HCs is relevant to the in vivo proliferation of HCs and that this growth stimulus is specifically inhibited by IFNα.

It is difficult to assess the clinical significance of the demonstration that TNF is an autocrine growth factor for HCs and that its production is inhibited by IFNα,[39] since exactly similar effects are observed in chronic lymphocytic leukaemia (CLL) – a disease which is far less responsive to IFNα than HCL.

IFNα in chronic granulocytic leukaemia (CGL)
Clinical trials of IFNα

IFNα may be effective for initial cytoreduction in CGL, but it is not consistently so. It is probably therefore better to achieve initial control of the disease with hydroxyurea or busulphan as recommended in the current Medical Research Council (MRC) trial. IFNα can then maintain the white cell count in the normal range in 80% of patients, usually at doses of 3 megaU three to seven times per week. Patients with less aggressive disease are more responsive to IFNα and achieve longer survival. Conversely, resistance to IFNα therapy may indicate a poor prognostic group.

The major difference between IFNα and conventional chemotherapy is that the cytokine reduces the Philadelphia positive (Ph+) clone in a significant proportion of patients.[40] Thus, Talpaz showed that half the patients who had responded to IFNα had a reduction in Ph+ marrow metaphases, 10–20% achieving complete karyotypic remission.[3] Other groups are in broad agreement with this, but complete disappearance of the Ph+ clone has been less common.[41,42] This may reflect patient selection or IFNα scheduling. It appears that the best karyotypic results are obtained by administering IFNα at the highest dose that the patient will reasonably tolerate and by maintaining white cell count (WCC) between 2×10^9 and 5×10^9. Easing the schedule may suboptimize karyotypic response, but may be necessary for patient compliance.

The prospect of a karyotypic normal marrow in CGL raises the possibility of autologous bone marrow transplantation (BMT) following IFNα therapy. However, because marrow progenitor growth is so poor following IFNα therapy, reconstitution may be a problem. Harvesting following a period off IFNα therapy may overcome this. These possibilities are being explored by the Houston group. It must be added, however, that the same group have used polymerase chain reaction (PCR) to demonstrate that in those patients with apparent ablation of the Ph+ clone by standard karyotypic means, 90% were positive for the breakpoint cluster region (BCR) rearrangement by PCR (Goldman, personal communication). Whether this will influence prospects for autologous transplantation remains to be seen.

Initial response rates are similar for each of the formulations of IFNα. Recombinant IFNα may stimulate neutralizing antibodies,[42] whether this correlates with loss of clinical efficacy remains to be seen. Such antibodies do not develop with non-recombinant IFNα.[30]

It is clear that even patients who sustain a fall in their Ph+ clone can still develop acute transformation; there is some evidence that this is more likely to be lymphoid.[3] However, some patients with a complete karyotypic response can maintain this status off IFNα therapy. It is too early to say if IFNα therapy will improve survival in CGL and the cytokine needs to be carefully compared with standard therapies. Responses to IFNα will be optimal if the agent is started early in the disease and the highest tolerated maintenance dose is used.

CGL is less responsive to IFNγ than IFNα.[43] Occasional patients will respond to IFNγ and not IFNα. Thus, combination and cross-over trials are under way to optimize response.

Mechanism of action

Immune mechanisms such as NK cytotoxicity are defective in CGL.[44] IFNα therapy does not improve this defect; neither does response correlate with effects on NK activity.[45] Further evidence suggested that NK cells do not lyse normal or CGL myeloid cells. This is in contrast to LAK cells which do influence CGL clonal growth,[46] but evidence suggests that IFNα does not influence LAK generation.[37]

IFNα produces a direct inhibition of normal and CGL colony formation (CFU-GM) which is independent of accessory cells.[47,48] It appears that normal and Ph$^+$ clonal growth, both in terms of colony growth and thymidine incorporation, are equally sensitive to the effects of IFNα. It is possible that presently available assays cannot pick up the differential sensitivity to IFNα that allows Ph$^+$ growth to occur at the expense of Ph$^-$ growth. It has been observed in this laboratory that the mature myeloid progenitors are more sensitive to IFNα than the less mature progenitors.[48] The more mature progenitors are generally more responsive to growth factors. This may be relevant to the mechanism of action of IFNα as it is the mature progenitors that are greatly expanded in CGL.

IFNα receptor expression does not correlate with IFNα clinical responsiveness in CGL.[49] Similarly, resultant induction of 2'5' A synthetase activity does not correlate with disease response.[50] IFNα therapy is associated with a reduction of mRNA for the 210 kD tyrosine kinase of CGL, but whether this reduction is a result of a reduction in the Ph$^+$ clone or of true pathogenic significance is not clear. Secondary cytokine release may also be important, as IFNα stimulates TNF release from macrophages.[51] TNF has been described as a regulator of myelopoiesis, and loss of this control may result in blastic transformation in CGL.[52] Therapeutic IFNα may enhance this TNF effect, potentially delaying acceleration and favouring Ph$^-$ growth.

Recent work has shown that IFNα can have a marked effect on stromal cells in long-term bone marrow culture.[53] It has been suggested that IFNα exposure may alter adhesive properties within the stroma and improve adherence of relatively non-adherent CGL progenitors, thus bringing them back under the influence of normal regulatory mechanisms.[54]

Less responsive disorders

Myeloma

Initial evidence suggesting that IFNα may be beneficial as primary therapy has not gained widespread acceptance, and other workers have suggested that IFNα is not superior to standard therapy.[55-57] In relapsed or resistant disease, an inconsistent response, often requiring increasing doses of IFNα, is seen in up to one-third of individuals.[58,59] Some patients achieve symptomatic and biochemical improvement but the majority show no benefit.

In vitro evidence suggests that IFNα may sensitize myeloma cells to chemotherapeutic agents.[60] Recent clinical work has confirmed that IFNα may be a useful adjunct to chemotherapy but cardiotoxicity has been noted.[61,62]

Most interest now relates to the observation of Mandellis group that IFNα therapy (3 megaU three times a week) may prolong plateau phase and possibly survival.[63] However, the value of IFNα in plateau phase is not yet established and is the subject of a current MRC trial.

Lymphoma

Approximately half of patients with low grade NHL have a reduction in lymphadenopathy in response to IFNα therapy, and there is a degree of dose responsiveness.[64,65] Response is slightly better in previously untreated individuals.[66,67] However, it is not clear that IFNα confers any survival advantage over conventional therapy. Studies are already examining the adjunctive effects of IFNα on conventional therapy.[68] Ozer et al demonstrated that clinical responsiveness did not correlate with immunomodulatory effects of IFNα, which were predominantly suppressive.[69] High grade NHL, whether previously treated or not, is much less responsive to IFNα even at very high doses.[66]

Mycosis fungoides was found to be responsive to high doses of IFNα (ie 50 megaU three times a week) in a trial by Bunn et al.[70] About half of these patients achieved a partial response, but no complete responses were seen. All patients required dose reduction due to IFN toxicity. A more recent study has combined etretinate with doses of IFNα between 18 and 36 megaU daily; two complete responses were obtained, although IFN toxicity again resulted in dose reduction.[71] Thus, IFNα may be useful when other modalities fail in this disease.

Hodgkin's disease has been found to be responsive to IFNα occasionally, although the cytokine has found no real place in the management of this disorder.[66]

Chronic lymphatic leukaemia (CLL)

Early reports suggesting that CLL is generally unresponsive to IFNα have been borne out.[72,73] However, it now appears that early stage CLL can respond to IFNα 3 megaU three times a week, with a fall in circulating lymphocyte count[74] during IFNα therapy, but counts generally return to pretreatment levels once IFNα is stopped. Our experience is that the lymphocyte count can begin to rise during IFNα therapy, and this may be associated with the development of IFNα antibodies.[75] Other groups have observed an improvement in serum IgG, but no progression on therapy.[76] Whether IFNα can significantly alter the course of CLL will require prolonged and careful trials.

Results from this laboratory show that IFNα receptors are maximally expressed on CLL cells during the early phase of the disease.[77] This may account in part for greater responsiveness in early stage disease, but the situation is likely to be more complicated than this because some workers have reported that IFNα can actually promote CLL proliferation in vitro.

Essential thrombocythaemia

Giles et al[78] clearly showed that 3 megaU of IFNα daily can reduce the platelet count to below $600 \times 10^9/l$, with an attendant reduction in ET-related symptoms. This regime was sufficient to induce response in most cases, and 3 megaU three times a week maintained platelet counts below 600. Other studies have now demonstrated a highly significant reduction in thromboembolic and circulatory phenomenon during IFNα therapy.[79] Gugliotta[80] demonstrated that IFNα therapy reduces both the marrow megakaryocyte count and also megakaryocytopoiesis (CFU-Meg 73 ± 18 before IFNα, 29 ± 15 during IFNα). This reduction in platelet production was accompanied by an improvement in platelet function although platelet half-life remained unchanged. Once IFNα therapy is stopped, the platelet count rises again but most patients will achieve a second remission with IFNα.

Minimally responsive disorders
Myelodysplasia (MDS)

As with many diseases, an occasional patient with MDS may respond to IFNα,[81] this may result from inhibition of a leukaemic (sub)clone. The majority of MDS patients treated with IFNα demonstrate a worsening of their cytopenias, but infection risk did not deteriorate.[82,83] Prediction of the rare response is not possible at present, consequently IFNα should not be used for MDS in general.

Myelofibrosis

IFNα can reduce fibroblast growth[53] and, potentially, fibrosis. However, IFNα therapy has no overall benefit in this disease for most patients.[84] Occasional reduction in spleen size and transfusion requirements have been reported with IFNα, but this is unusual.[85]

Conclusions

Following major scientific and clinical investigations, it appears that IFNα has a place in the management of some low proliferative haemic malignancies. Although IFNα is presently enjoying popularity in the treatment of HCL and CGL, other treatment modalities may prove equally efficacious. It is unlikely that IFNα will be used as a single mode of therapy in other haemic malignancies, but it may well be useful as an adjunct to standard therapies. The nature of disease responsiveness probably derives from a direct effect of IFNα on cell proliferation, but the exact nature of this effect is complicated by the cytokine network in vivo.

As one of the first cytokines to be intensively investigated, IFNα has given an important stimulus to research and production of other biological response modifiers. Although the dividend of clinical utility has been limited for IFNα, other cytokine therapies may well make a major contribution to disease management.

References

(1) Galvani DW, Griffiths SD, Cawley JC. Interferon for treatment: the dust settles. *Br Med J* 1988; 296: 1554–6.
(2) Worman C, Catovsky D, Bevan PC et al. Interferon is effective in hairy-cell leukaemia. *Br J Haem* 1985; 60: 759–63.
(3) Talpaz M, Kantarjian HM, McCredie KB et al. Clinical investigation of IFNα in chronic myeloid leukaemia. *Blood* 1987; 69: 1280–8.
(4) Griffiths SD, Galvani DW, Cawley JC. The interferons. In: Hamblin T J ed. *Immunotherapy of disease.* London: Kluwer Academic Publishers, 1989: 43–70.
(5) Brook MO, Petrovic L, McDonald JA, Scheuer PJ, Thomas HC. Histological improvement after anti-viral treatment for chronic hepatitis B infection. *J Hepatol* 1989; 8: 218–25.
(6) Davis GL, Balart LA, Schiff ER et al. Treatment of chronic hepatitis C with recombinant interferon alfa. *N Eng J Med* 1989; 321: 1501–6.
(7) Interferon nomenclature. *Nature* 1980; 286: 110.
(8) Lindemann J, Burke D, Isaacs A. Studies of the production, mode of action and properties of interferon. *Br J Exp Path* 1957; 38: 551–62.
(9) Rubinstein M, Orchansky P. The interferon receptors. *CRC Crit Rev Biochem* 1986; 21: 249–75.
(10) Dadmarz R, Evans T, Secher D, Marshall N, Cawley JC. Hairy-cells possess more interferon α receptors than other lymphoid cell types.*Leukaemia* 1987; 1: 357–61.
(11) Mogensen KE, Bandu MT. Kinetic evidence for an activation step following binding of interferon to the membrane receptors of Daudi cells. *Eur J Biochem* 1983; 134: 355–9.
(12) Thompson MR, Zhange ZQ, Fourniers A, Tan YH. Characterisation of human interferon binding sites on human cells. *J Biol Chem* 1985; 260: 563–71.
(13) Aguet M, Dembic Z, Merlin G. Molecular cloning and expression of the interferon γ receptor. *Cell* 1988; 55: 273–80.

(14) Mehmet H, Morris CME, Taylor-Papadimitriou J, Rozengurt E. Interferon inhibition of DNA synthesis in Swiss 3T3 cells: dissociation from protein kinase C activation. *Biochem Biophys Res Comm* 1987; 145: 1026–32.

(15) Yap WH, Teo TS, McCoy E, Tan YH. Rapid and transient rise in diacylglycerol concentration in Daudi cells exposed to interferon. *Pro Natl Acad Sci USA* 1986; 83: 7765–72.

(16) Tamm I, Lin SL, Pfeffer LM, Sehgal PC. Interferons α and β as cellular regulatory molecules. In: Gresser I, Burke D, Cantell et al. eds. *Interferon 9*. London: Academic Press, 1987: 14–74.

(17) Fan XD, Goldberg M, Bloom BR. Interferon γ-induced transcription is mediated by protein kinase C. *Proc Natl Acad Sci USA* 1988; 85: 5122–30.

(18) Fellous A, Ginsberg I, Littauer UZ. Modulation of tubulin mRNA levels by interferon in human lymphoblastoid cells. *EMBO J* 1982; 7: 835–9.

(19) Einat M, Resnitsky D, Kimchi A. Close link between reduction of c-*myc* expression by interferon and G0/G1 arrest. *Nature* 1985; 313: 597–600.

(20) Resnitsky D, Yarden A, Zipori D, Kimchi A. Autocrine-related interferon controls c-*myc* suppression and growth arrest during haemopoietic cell differentiation. *Cell* 1986; 46: 31–40.

(21) Knight E, Anton ED, Fahey D, Friedland BK, Joual GJ. Interferon regulates c-*myc* expression in Daudi cells at the post-transcriptional level. *Proc Natl Acad Sci USA* 1985; 82: 1151–4.

(22) Williams BRG, Fish EN. Interferon and viruses: in vitro studies. In: Taylor-Papadimitriou J, ed. *Interferons: their impact in biology and medicine*. Oxford: OUP, 1985: 40–60.

(23) Samuel C, Duncan R, Knutsen G, Hershey W. Mechanism of interferon action. *J Biol Chem* 1984; 259: 13451–7.

(24) Staeheli P, Haller O. Interferon-induced Mx protein: a mediator of cellular resistance to influenza virus. In: Gresser I, Burke D, Cantell K et al. *Interferon 8*. London: Academic Press, 1987: 2–24.

(25) Taylor-Papadimitriou J, Rozengurt E. Interferons as regulators of cell growth and differentiation. In: Taylor-Papadimitriou J, ed. *Interferons: their impact in biology and medicine*. Oxford: OUP, 1985: 81–98.

(26) Hemmi H, Breightman TR. Combinations of recombinant interferons and retinoic acid synergistically induce differentiation in HL60. *Blood* 1987; 69: 501–6.

(27) Heberman R, Ortaldo J, Bonnard G. Augmentation by interferon of natural and antibody dependent cell-mediated cytotoxicity. *Nature* 1979; 277: 221–3.

(28) Huddlestone JR, Merigan TC, Oldstone MBA. Induction and kinetics of natural killer cells in humans following interferon therapy. *Nature* 282: 417–18.

(29) Pace JL, Russell SW, Schreiber RD, Altman A, Katz DH. Macrophage activation: priming activity from a T-cell hybridoma is attributable to interferon γ. *Proc Natl Acad Sci USA* 1983; 80: 3782–6.

(30) Galton JE, Bedford P, Scott JE, Brand CM, Nethersell ABW. Antibodies to lymphoblastoid interferon. *Lancet* 1989; ii: 572–3.

(31) Quesada JR, Talpaz M, Rius A, Kurzrock R, Gutterman JU. Clinical toxicity of IFNs in cancer patients: a review. *J Clin Oncol* 1986; 4: 234–43.

(32) Glaspy JA, Baldwin GC, Robertson PA et al. Therapy for neutropenia in hairy-cell leukaemia with recombinant G-CSF. *Ann Int Med* 1988; 109: 789–95.

(33) Steis RG, Smith JW, Urba WJ et al. Resistance to recombinant interferon α 2a in hairy-cell leukaemia associated with neutralising antibodies. *N Eng J Med* 1988; 318: 1409–13.

(34) Kraut EH, Bouroncle BA, Grever MR. Low dose deoxycoformycin in the treatment of hairy-cell leukaemia. *Blood* 1986; 68: 1119–22.

(35) Piro LD, Carrera CJ, Carson DA, Beutler E. Lasting remissions in hairy-cell leukaemia induced by a single infusion of 2-chlorodeoxyadenosine. *N Eng J Med* 1990; 1117–21.

(36) Griffiths SD, Cawley JC. The beneficial effects of α-interferon in hairy-cell leukaemia are not attributable to NK cell mediated cytotoxicity. *Leukaemia* 1987; 1: 372–6.

(37) Griffiths SD, Cawley JC. Interferon and LAK cell activity in hairy-cell leukaemia. *Leukaemia* 1988; 2: 377–81.

(38) Griffiths SD, Cawley JC. The effects of cytokines, including IL-2, IL-4 and IL-6, in hairy cell proliferation/differentiation. *Leukaemia*: in press.

(39) Cordingley FT, Bianchi A, Hoffbrand AV et al. Tumour necrosis factor as an autocrine growth factor for B-cell malignancies. *Lancet* 1988; i: 969–71.

(40) Allan NC, Shepherd PCA. Treatment of chronic myeloid leukaemia. In: Goldman JM, ed. *Chronic Myeloid Leukaemia*, London: Balliere Tindall, 1987: 1031–54.

(41) Alimena G, Morra E, Lazzarino M et al. Interferon α 2b as therapy for chronic myeloid leukaemia: a study of 82 patients treated with intermittent or daily administration. *Blood* 1988; 72: 642–7.

(42) Freund M, Wussow PV, Diedrich H. Recombinant IFNα in chronic myelogenous leukaemia: dose dependency of response and frequency of neutralising antibodies. *Br J Haem* 1989; 72: 350–6.

(43) Kurzrock R, Talpaz M, Kantarjian H, Gutterman JU. Therapy of chronic myelogenous leukaemia with recombinant interferon gamma. *Blood* 1987; 70: 943–7.

(44) Fujiyama Y, Pattengale PK. Characterization of NK cells in patients with chronic myeloid leukaemia. In: Hebermann RB, Callewaert DM, eds. *Mechanisms of cytotoxicity in NK cells*. London: Academic Press, 1985: 521–42.

(45) Galvani DW, Owens W, Nethersell ABW, Cawley JC. The beneficial effects of interferon in CGL are probably not mediated by NK cells. *Br J Haem* 1988; 71: 233–7.

(46) McKinnon S, Hows JM, Goldman JM. In vitro induction of graft versus leukaemia activity following BMT for CGL. *Br J Haem* 1990; 74 (suppl 1): 14.

(47) Broxmeyer HE, Lu L, Platzer E et al. Comparative analysis of the influences of human α, β and γ interferons on CFU-GEMM, BFU-E and CFU-GM progenitor cells. *J Immunol* 1983; 131: 1300–5.

(48) Galvani DW, Cawley JC. Mechanism of action of interferon in CGL: evidence for preferential inhibition of late progenitors. *Br J Haem* 1989; 73: 475–9.

(49) Rosenblum MG, Maxwell BL, Talpaz M et al. In vivo sensitivity and resistance of CML cells to IFNα: correlation with receptor binding and induction of 2'5'-oligoadenylate synthetase. *Can Res* 1986; 46: 4848–52.

(50) Schtalrid M, Blick M, Kurzrock R et al. Variable expression of 2'5' A synthetase and HLA-B genes in CML patients treated with interferon. *Exp Haem* 1989; 17: 609.

(51) Pelus LM, Ottmann OG, Nocka KH. Synergistic inhibition of human CFU-GM progenitor cells by prostaglandin E and recombinant interferon α, β and γ and an effect mediated by TNF. *J Immunol* 1988; 140: 479–84.

(52) Duncombe AS, Heslop HE, Turner M, Meager A, Brenner MK. Autocrine production of TNF inhibits CML growth – a mechanism for chronicity. *Br J Haem* 1989; 71: 169.

(53) Galvani DW, Cawley JC. Effects of interferon α in human long-term bone marrow culture. *Leuk Res*: in press.

(54) Dowding C, Siczkowski M, Osterholz J, Goldman MY, Goldman JM. Interferon α increases glycosaminoglycan synthesis by normal marrow stromal cells. *Br J Haem* 1990; 74 (suppl 1): 3.

(55) Ohno R, Kimura K, Imamura Y et al. Treatment of myeloma with recombinant interferon α 2c. *Can Treat Rep* 1985; 69: 1433–5.

(56) Ludwig H, Cortelezzi A, Scheithauer W et al. Recombinant interferon α 2c versus polychemotherapy (VMCP) for the treatment of multiple myeloma: a prospective randomized trial. *Eur J Can Clin Oncol* 1986; 22: 1111–16.

(57) Ahre A, Bjorkholm M, Mellstedt H et al. Human leukocyte interferon and intermittent high-dose melphalan-prednisolone administration in the treatment of multiple myeloma: a randomised clinical trial from the myeloma group of central Sweden. *Can Treat Rep* 1984; 68: 1331–8.

(58) Oken MM, Kyle RA, Kay NE, Greipp PR, O'Connell MJ. Interferon in the treatment of refractory multiple myeloma: an Eastern Cooperative Oncology Group study. *Leuk & Lymph* 1990; 1: 95–100.

(59) Cooper MR. Interferons in the treatment of multiple myeloma. *Semin Oncol* 1986; 13: 13–20.

(60) Constanzi JJ, Cooper MR, Scarffe JH et al. Phase II study of recombinant interferon in resistant multiple myeloma. *J Clin Oncol* 1985; 3: 654–9.

(61) Oken MM, Kyle RA, Griepp PR et al. Alternating cycles of VBMCP with interferon (rIFNα2) in the treatment of multiple myeloma. *Proc Am Soc Clin Onc* 1988; 7: 868a.

(62) Mellstedt H. Treatment of multiple myeloma with natural α-interferon. *Haematol Oncol* 1988; 6: 187–92.

(63) Mandelli F, Tribalto M, Avvisati G et al. Recombinant interferon as post-induction therapy for responding myeloma patients. *Can Treat Rev* 1988; 15: 43–8.

(64) Merz B. Interferons track record: good in hairy-cell leukaemia, fair in other haematological cancers, poor in solid tumours. *JAMA* 1986; 256: 1242–4.

(65) Steis RG, Foon KA, Longo DL. Current and future uses of recombinant interferon α in the treatment of low-grade non-Hodgkin's lymphoma. *Cancer* 1987; 59: 658–63.

(66) Leavitt RD, Ratanatharathorn V, Ozer H et al. Alfa-2b interferon in the treatment of Hodgkin's and non-Hodgkin's disease. *Sem Oncol* 1987; 14: 18–23.

(67) Wagstaff J, Loynds P, Crowther D. A phase II study of human alpha-2

interferon in patients with low grade non-Hodgkin's lymphoma. *Cancer Chemother Pharmacol* 1986; 18: 54–8.

(68) Rohatiner AZS, Richards MA, Barnett MJ et al. Chlorambucil and interferon for low grade non-Hodgkin's lymphoma. *Br J Can* 1987; 55: 225–6.

(69) Ozer H, Gavigan M, O'Malley J et al. Immunomodulation by interferon in a phase I trial in patients with lymphoproliferative malignancies. *J Biol Response Mod* 1983; 2: 499–515.

(70) Bunn PA, Ihde DC, Foon KA. The role of interferon α 2a in the therapy of cutaneous T-cell lymphoma. *Cancer* 1986; 57: 1689–95.

(71) Thestrup-Pedersen K, Hammer R, Kaltoft K, Sogaard H, Zachariae H. Treatment of mycosis fungoides with recombinant interferon alone and in combination with etretinate. *Br J Derm* 1988; 118: 811–18.

(72) Foon KA, Bottino GC, Abrams PG et al. Phase II trial of interferon in advanced chronic lymphocytic leukaemia. *Am J Haem* 1985; 78: 217–20.

(73) Talpaz M, Rosenblum R, Kurzrock R et al. Clinical and laboratory changes induced by interferon in chronic lymphocytic leukaemia. *Am J Haem* 1987; 24: 341–50.

(74) Rozman C, Monserrat E, Vinolas N et al. Recombinant interferon in the treatment of B-CLL in early stages. *Blood* 1988; 71: 1295–8.

(75) Giles FJ, Worman CP, Gaffar RA et al. Early results of Roferon treatment of chronic lymphoid leukaemia. *Br J Haem* 1990; 74 (suppl 1): 31.

(76) Ziegle-Heitbroch HWL, Schlag R, Flige D, Thiel E. Favourable response of early stage B-CLL patients to interferon α. *Blood* 1989; 73: 1426–30.

(77) Dadmarz R, Cawley JC. Heterogeneity of CLL: high CD23 antigen and IFNα receptor expression are features of favourable disease and of cell activation. *Br J Haem* 1988; 68: 279–84.

(78) Giles FJ, Singer CRJ, Gray AG et al. α interferon for essential thrombocythaemia. *Lancet* 1988; ii: 70–2.

(79) Gisslinger H, Ludwig H, Linkesch W et al. Long-term interferon therapy for thrombocytosis in myeloproliferative diseases. *Lancet* 1989; i: 634–7.

(80) Gugliotta A, Macchi S, Catani L. Evaluation of thrombopoiesis in essential thrombocytosis before and after interferon therapy. *Throm & Haem* 1987; 58: 481–4.

(81) Galvani DW, Nethersell ABW, Bottomley J, Cawley JC. Interferon α in myelodysplasia. *Br J Haem* 1987; 66: 145–6.

(82) Galvani DW, Nethersell ABW, Cawley JC. Interferon α in myelodysplasia: clinical observations and effects on NK cells. *Leuk Res* 1988; 12: 257–62.

(83) Elias L, Hoffman R, Boswell S, Tensen L, Bonnem EM. A trial of recombinant interferon α in the myelodysplastic syndromes. *Leukaemia* 1987; 2: 105–10.

(84) Gastle G, Lang A, Huber C et al. Interferon α for idiopathic myelofibrosis. *Lancet* 1988; i: 765–6.

(85) Wickramsinghe SN, Peert S, Gill DS. Interferon α in primary idiopathic myelofibrosis. *Lancet* 1987; i: 1524–5.

The genetics of the Philadelphia chromosome

R KURZROCK and M TALPAZ

Introduction

Cytogenetic aberrations are a hallmark of malignancy[1] and provide a pointer for the molecular localization of activated cancer genes (oncogenes). The first consistent karyotypic abnormality found to be associated with neoplastic disease was the Philadelphia (Ph) chromosome, an anomaly identified in 1960 by Nowell and Hungerford.[2] Furthermore, the best-studied example of translocation-mediated gene activation occurs in leukaemia patients bearing this abnormality. In these individuals, the Ph translocation $(t(9;22)(q34;q11))$[3] results in transposition of the *abl* proto-oncogene from chromosome 9q34 to 22q11, where it is fused with part of the *bcr* gene.[4-10] The translation product is a chimeric bcr–abl protein with markedly enhanced enzymatic properties. Awareness of these molecular events is crucial to understanding the processes promoting initiation and progression of Ph[+] hematological malignancies. Herein, we will review the molecular biology of the Ph translocation.

Murine leukemia and oncogenes

Virally induced murine leukemias presented investigators with the first clues as to the importance of altered cellular oncogenes. Because, in humans, these alterations could be caused by transfer of cytogenetic material, it followed that translocation breakpoints might yield critical information regarding the residence of cancer-related genes.

The *abl* oncogene was initially discovered through analysis of the viral-*abl* gene of Abelson murine leukemia virus (Ab-MuLV).[11] Ab-MuLV is a replication-defective virus which transforms a wide range of lymphoid and myeloid cells in vitro.[12] In vivo, Ab-MuLV primarily induces nonthymic pre-B lymphomas in susceptible mice;[13,14] however, a variety of other murine

All correspondence to: R Kurzrock, MD, Department of Clinical Immunology and Biological Therapy, Box 41, MD Anderson Cancer Center, 1515 Holcombe Boulevard, Houston, Texas 77030, USA.

Cambridge Medical Reviews: Haematological Oncology Volume 1

hematopoietic neoplasms including plasmacytomas, T-cell lymphomas, myelomonocytic leukemias, and mastocytomas can also be induced.[15-19] Ab-MuLV may therefore cause deregulated proliferation in many hematopoietic lineages in addition to its most frequent target – the immature B-cell.

The Ab-MuLV transforming gene is a fusion product of viral *gag* (core) sequences encoded by Moloney murine leukemia virus (M-MuLV), and a component derived from a normal mouse gene – cellular-*abl*.[12] In other words, viral-*abl* originated from cellular-*abl*, and the Ab-MuLV arose from recombination between M-MuLV and the mouse cellular-*abl* gene, an event resulting in the formation of a chimeric *gag–abl* gene.

There are two main prototypic strains of Ab-MuLV, and they produce viral-*abl* proteins of 120 and 160 kD, respectively.[12,20] The two viruses differ in that the strain producing p120 has an internal in-frame deletion. Transformation by Ab-MuLV is mediated by the viral-abl protein. Both p120*gag–abl* and p160*gag–abl* consist of a truncated cellular-*abl* polypeptide attached in its N-terminus to the viral *gag* (core) protein. In infected cells, the *gag–abl* proteins have cytoplasmic and plasma membrane localization.[21] In addition, *gag–abl* proteins are constitutively active as tyrosine protein kinase enzymes.

Protein kinases catalyze the transfer of the terminal phosphate of adenosine triphosphate (ATP) to the amino acid residue of the substrate protein. Auto-phosphorylation can also occur, in which case the target protein is the enzyme itself. Phosphorylation is a basic cellular mechanism of regulating protein function. Protein kinases usually add phosphate to the amino acids serine or threonine that have a hydroxyl (OH) group to which the phosphate can be linked. Another amino acid that has a hydroxyl group and thus can be phosphorylated is tyrosine; however, phosphotyrosine accounts for less than 1% of cellular phosphoamino acids, indicating that tyrosine is phosphorylated infrequently.

The importance of the tyrosine phosphokinase function is assumed because of the association of this enzymatic property with several growth factor receptors[22] and because loss of the phosphokinase activity of the viral-*abl* protein results in abrogation of its transforming capability.[23] The manner in which the enzymatically enhanced viral-*abl* product modulates growth regulatory circuits has not been clearly defined. However, various in vitro models have supported a spectrum of mechanisms including circumvention of a growth factor/growth factor receptor pathway[24-26] and induction of new growth factors.[27]

Despite the critical part played by the *abl* gene in both in vitro cellular transformation and in vivo tumor production by Ab-MuLV, the complexity of these processes mandates that other variables must also be involved. Indeed, the phenotype of Ab-MuLV-induced malignancies varies with several factors: age and strain of mice, site of virus inoculation, and the helper virus used to package the Ab-MuLV genome. Further, cells transformed by viral-*abl* in vitro often exhibit low tumorigenic properties at first, but evolve to highly malignant cells with time.[28] For lymphocytes to exhibit a fully oncogenic growth phenotype, changes must occur in cellular genes subsequent to expression of viral-*abl*.[28,29] In some instances, Ab-MuLV may only initiate these changes, after which it is no longer needed.

These observations on Ab-MuLV-induced murine malignancies may provide a paradigm for understanding the role of the human cellular-*abl* gene – the cellular counterpart of viral-*abl* gene – in the initiation and phenotypic evolution of CML. In *abl*-related diseases of man, viral mechanisms are presumably not operative. However, the Ph chromosomal translocation may cause alterations in the cellular-*abl* gene analogous to those evoked by viral transduction. A process paralleling that in Ab-MuLV-infected mice is then postulated to occur: changes in abl probably initiate the CML process, but secondary changes are needed to drive the progression of the disease.

Philadelphia chromosome-positive leukemias

The Ph chromosome is found in chronic myelogenous leukemia (CML) (90% of patients), acute lymphoblastic leukemia (ALL) (20% of adult patients and 5% of pediatric patients) and acute myelogenous leukemia (AML) (2% of patients) (Table 1). At the cytogenetic level, the Ph chromosome is indistinguishable in these distinct disorders; at the molecular level, subtle differences are present.

Cytogenetic findings

The Ph chromosome refers to a chromosome 22 with a truncated long arm.[2,3,30] This shortened chromosome occurs as the result of a reciprocal exchange of material between the long (or 'q') arms of chromosomes 22 and 9. Chromosome 22 is broken at band q11; chromosome 9, at band q34. The distal part of the long arm of chromosome 22 is attached to the broken end of chromosome 9, and the distal part of the long arm of chromosome 9 is attached to the broken end of chromosome 22. This configuration is designated a t(9;22)(q34;q11) translocation by standard nomenclature.

In Ph+ CML patients, the Ph translocation is generally found in 100% of bone marrow metaphases. Patients with AML or ALL are more likely to show a mosaic cytogenetic pattern, with both normal diploid and Ph+ metaphases.

Variant translocations There are subgroups of patients with CML and acute leukemia who carry translocations which bear similarities to, but are not identical with, the classic t(9;22)(q34;q11). For instance, some CML patients have complex translocations in which 3, 4, or 5 chromosomes are involved (including chromosomes 9 and 22), or variant translocations in which cytogenetic analysis demonstrates involvement of chromosome 22 and a chromosome other than 9, or vice versa.[31,32] Further, a subset of 'Ph+' ALL patients

Table 1. *Frequency of the Philadelphia translocation (t(9;22) (q34;q11) in various leukemias*

Diagnosis	%-positive patients
Chronic myelogenous leukemia	90
Acute lymphoblastic leukemia	
adult	20
childhood	5
Acute myelogenous leukemia	2

exhibit a shortened chromosome 22, with the break in band q11, but without cytogenetic evidence of a 9q34 anomaly.[33] The opposite also occurs; patients with CML and acute leukemia may have an isolated 9q34 abnormality. There are also individuals with AML and T-cell ALL who carry t(6:9)(p23;q34) and t(7;9)(q36;q34) aberrations, respectively. Recent molecular studies have begun to dissect the genetic correlates of these disparate karyotypes. Current evidence indicates that, regardless of cytogenetic findings, patients with the *bcr–abl* molecular abnormality have a clinical outcome indistinguishable from that of their Ph⁺ counterparts, whereas those patients with distinct molecular events follow a different course.

Clinical features
Chronic myelogenous leukemia CML was originally described in 1845 by Craigie,[34] Bennett,[35] and Virchow[36] as a purulence of the blood with splenomegaly. Today, CML is known to account for about 25% of adult leukemias and has an incidence of 1 case per 100 000 persons per year.[37] Although CML can occur at any age, it is rare in childhood and peaks in the middle 40s. There is no marked sex preponderance.

From the classification standpoint, CML is a myeloproliferative disorder and is nosologically related to polycythemia vera, agnogenic myeloid metaplasia, myelofibrosis, and essential thrombocythemia. Despite the myeloid phenotype of the early stages of CML, the clonal CML progenitor actually arises from neoplastic transformation of a hematopoietic stem cell.[38,39]

The clinical course of CML is triphasic.[40,41] This course exemplifies the multistep process of tumor progression, a phenomenon probably characterizing most malignancies, but less well delineated in other cancers. The disease ineluctably evolves from an idolent benign or chronic phase to a more aggressive accelerated phase, and terminates in blast crisis. The chronic phase is marked by a greatly increased number of committed myeloid precursor cells;[42] this situation is postulated to be a consequence of committed unregulated growth or discordant maturation.[43] Because terminal differentiation of cells is maintained, the salient clinical feature of this stage is a significantly increased number of circulating mature neutrophils. It is not known why the myeloid compartment is preferentially affected in the chronic stage if CML is a stem cell disorder. During this phase, the high white blood cell counts can be readily managed by any one of a variety of nontoxic therapies, and the vast majority of patients maintain a near-normal lifestyle.[44,45] Unfortunately, after a median interval of about 4.0 years (range, several weeks to 27^+ years),[46-48] a more aggressive hematological state of myeloproliferative acceleration develops, wherein the myeloid cell loses its ability for terminal differentiation. In about 80% of cases, new cytogenetic abnormalities also appear.[30] An increase in immature myeloid precursors and clonal evolution are grave signs for they are prescient of the treatment-resistant blast transformation phase, a terminal stage closely resembling Ph^+ acute leukemia.

Blast crisis may have a slow onset following an accelerated phase which lasts about 6 months. Alternatively, the aggressive blastic clone may emerge abruptly. The variables dictating the length of time to blast crisis are unknown. Although clearcut criteria separating the chronic, accelerated, and blast crisis stages are difficult to establish, most clinicians consider the detection of $\geq$ 30% blasts in the bone marrow as indicative of blast transformation.

The blastic clone morphology can reflect any of the hematopoietic lineages arising from the Ph chromosome: myeloid (blasts or, rarely, promyelocytes), T- and B-lymphoid, erythroid, and megakaryocytic.[46,49-56] Accurate classification can be accomplished by the combined use of morphological, cytochemical, enzymatic, immunologic, and molecular techniques. Myeloid and lymphoid blast crisis occur most frequently, and constitute about 65% and 25% of cases, respectively. It is important to be aware of these subtypes because they respond differently to treatment.

Patients rarely die during the chronic phase of CML. Conventional therapy of this disorder includes well-tolerated drugs such as busulfan and hydroxyurea.[57,58] With these agents, the proliferative thrust of the disease can be controlled and hematological remission achieved with few side effects. Unfortunately, the malignant clone remains fully predominant, as evidenced by the persistence of 100% Ph^+ metaphases in bone marrow derived from CML patients in hematological remission. There is no cure fraction, and canonical treatment regimens have minimal impact on survival; progression to blast crisis occurs regardless of hematological response. These observations underscore the importance of developing therapeutic approaches which prevent this terminal event. It is now clear that impeding disease evolution requires eradication of the Ph^+ clone or blocking of the processes that lead to blastic conversion.

Eradication of the Ph$^+$ clone can only be accomplished in select individuals. For instance, interferon-alpha therapy can induce a prolonged complete suppression of the Ph chromosome in a portion of newly diagnosed CML patients; even so, a significant number of resistant patients remain.[45,59-60] Supralethal chemoradiotherapy followed by allogeneic bone marrow transplantation obliterates the malignant clone, and 50% to 70% of CML patients transplanted during the chronic phase are long-term, disease-free survivors. However, patient age (usually >50 years) and a shortage of histocompatible sibling donors makes many CML patients ineligible for bone marrow transplantation. The alternative strategy of preventing disease progression, without elimination of the Ph chromosome, is not clinically feasible because the factors causing blast crisis are unknown.

One of the most fascinating enigmas concerning the malignant evolution of CML is the extraordinary range of time intervals to blast crisis.[47,48] Most patients reach this end-stage in about 4 years; however, blast crisis can occur within several weeks of diagnosis, and a case of ongoing benign phase lasting 27$^+$ years has been reported.[47] Although a host of prognostic variables have been calculated by multivariate regression anayses of large numbers of CML patients, the actual determinants of blast crisis remain elusive. Further, an ongoing debate relates to whether progression is caused by stochastic or by preordained genetic events. The reports[47,61] showing that patients with very long chronic phases (10 to 27 years) also have very long first remissions support the school of thought claiming that the length of time to blast crisis is predetermined.

Ph$^+$ acute leukemia The Ph chromosome was initially believed to be manifested exclusively in CML. However, it is now apparent that a t(9;22) anomaly is present in a small percentage of patients with ALL and AML (Table 1),[30,62,63] and is cytogenetically identical to the t(9;22) of CML. In general, its presence in acute leukemia is a poor prognostic factor.[64]

A question which remains is whether Ph$^+$ acute and chronic leukemia are actually manifestations of the same malignancy or, alternatively, are different disease states with molecularly distinct derangements, despite a cytogenetically similar appearance.[33] These are not merely academic points, since understanding the relationship between chronic and acute Ph$^+$ leukemia may help uncover the pathogenetic events responsible for the conversion of CML from a chronic phenotype (the benign phase) to an acute phenotype (blast crisis). In this regard, several lines of evidence support a single underlying process for Ph$^+$ acute and chronic leukemia.[33,65] The most cogent of these are: (i) the well-documented reports of patients presenting with Ph$^+$ ALL or AML in whom therapy-induced transition to CML occurred; and (ii) the clinical and morphological similarity of Ph$^+$ AML and ALL to the myeloid and lymphoid blast crisis of CML, respectively. Even so, the possibility that Ph$^+$

acute and chronic leukemia are distinct diseases is inferred from their different clinical presentation.

Molecular genetics of the Philadelphia translocation
BCR gene

It is now known that the chromosome 22 breakpoints in Ph+ CML are restricted to a 5.8 kb DNA segment – the breakpoint cluster region (bcr)[6,7] (Fig. 1). Rearrangements within the 5.8 kb bcr have been confirmed in hundreds of published cases of Ph+ CML.[66–73] The specificity of this molecular test is underscored by the observation that bcr rearrangement is never seen in normal individuals, nor in victims of other diseases.

The precise point of breakage within bcr is different in each patient. Bcr sequence deletions (especially in the 3' end) occur in 10% to 20% of patients,[72,74] and mandate the use of probes corresponding to 5' (proximal), as well as 3' (distal), bcr regions, to avoid false-negative results for bcr rearrangement.

The 5.8 kb bcr is part of a gene.[7] This gene has been called the *bcr* gene by some authors and the *phl* gene by others, though the *bcr* nomenclature is currently accepted. The *bcr* gene spans 130 kb, contains 21 exons, and is oriented with its 5' end towards the centromere.[75,76–78] The 5.8 kb bcr segment occupies the central portion of the gene and includes five small exons, termed bcr exons 1 to 5(7) (Fig. 1). Three other chromosome 22 DNA segments, which are highly homologous to the seven 3' exons of the original *bcr* gene, have also been cloned.[79] Because transcripts have not yet been found for these additional DNA segments, it may be that they represent pseudogenes.

The function of the *bcr* gene in normal hematopoiesis is not known. However, it is known that the *bcr* gene codes for 4.5 and 6.7 kb mRNAs (Table 2); some 5' probes also recognize a 1.2 kb mRNA.[8,76,80] The 4.5 and 6.7 kb transcripts are expressed ubiquitously, having been detected in fibroblasts, and myeloid, lymphoid, and epithelial cells.[8,76,80]

The bcr translation product is a 160 kD phosphoprotein (p160[bcr]) with an associated kinase activity.[81,82] Phosphorylation of p160[bcr] occurs on serine or threonine. Because the bcr sequence does not bear significant homology to any known protein kinases, it is possible that p160[bcr] is not itself enzymatically active, but rather that another protein with this activity co-precipitates with it.

The subcellular localization of p160[bcr] has not been established. Computerized predictive hydropathy analysis of *bcr* sequences reveals none of the regions of marked hydrophobicity characteristic of a protein with a transmembrane region,[76] but association with plasma membrane via interplay with other membrane-bound molecules cannot be ruled out.

85

CHROMOSOME 22

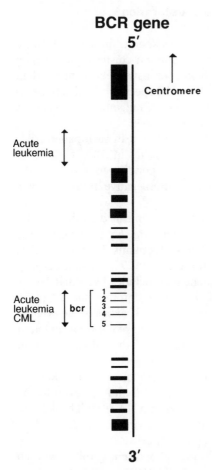

Fig. 1. Schematic representation of the *bcr* gene on chromosome 22. Shaded boxes represent exons. The size of the exons may not be exactly as depicted. Double-headed arrows identify the regions within which breakpoints in Ph+ acute leukemia and CML occur.

ABL gene

The other gene affected by the Ph translocation is the cellular-*abl* gene. In Ph+ CML patients, this gene is transposed from its normal residence on the long arm of chromosome 9 (band q34) to the long arm of chromosome 22 (band q11).[4] Cloning of the normal *abl* gene has revealed that it spans ≥ 230 kb and contains at least 11 exons.[7,8,83,84] It is oriented with its 5' end towards

Table 2. *Molecular consequences of the Philadelphia translocation*

Diagnosis	Chromosome	Messenger RNA	Protein
Normal	9	6.0 and 7.0 kb abl mRNA	$p145^{abl}$
	22	4.5 and 6.7 kb bcr mRNA	$p160^{bcr}$
CML	22q−	8.5 kb bcr–abl mRNA	$p210^{bcr-abl}$
ALL	22q−	8.5 or 7.0 kb bcr–abl mRNA	$p210^{bcr-abl}$ or $p190^{bcr-abl}$
AML	22q−	8.5 or 7.0 kb bcr–abl mRNA	$p210^{bcr-abl}$ or $p190^{bcr-abl}$

Abbreviations: ALL = acute lymphoblastic leukemia; AML = acute myelogenous leukemia; CML = chronic myelogenous leukemia; kb = kilobase.

the centromere. Two alternative first exons (exons 1a and 1b) exist and are governed by independent promoters. Exon 1a is 19 kb proximal to exon 2; exon 1b is a formidable ⩾ 200 kb proximal to exon 2.[8,83] As a result of this genomic configuration, two major *abl* transcripts are produced: 6.0 and 7.0 kb messenger RNAs (mRNA)[85] (Table 2). The 6.0 kb transcript consists of exons 1a through 11; the 7.0 kb transcript begins with exon 1b, skips exon 1a and the immense (in molecular terms) distance to exon 2, and continues with exons 2 through 11. A similar situation occurs in the mouse, where four types of abl message with distinct first exons (designated exons I through IV) exist.[86] All the abl messages share a common set of 3′ exons. Therefore, the splice acceptor site of exon 2 is unusual in its promiscuous accommodation of multiple donors, and in its propensity to jump nearby donor splice sites in favor of those much further away. The ability of *abl* exon 2 to permit this facile interchange of attaching abl DNA sequences may be a critical factor in its malignant potential, for it also allows abl to be fused with non-abl sequences and thus become activated.

To date, only one normal human abl protein has been identified. This protein has a molecular mass of 145 kD, and is termed p145*abl*.[87] The *abl* polypeptide belongs to a family of tyrosine protein kinases. Hence, it is conceivable that p145*abl* may be involved in normal growth control. Analysis of the predicted amino acid sequence of the human *abl* product reveals neither a transmembrane region nor a signal peptide, indicating that *abl* is not a receptor for extracellular factors.[8] Even so, p145*abl* may associate with the plasma membrane via other mechanisms. In this regard, the *abl* protein encoded by the 7.0 kb abl mRNA has a glycine at its N-terminus. Such a structure in several other proteins (the SRC oncogene product and the catalytic unit of cyclic AMP dependent kinase)[88,89] is linked to myristic acid, which is thought to stabilize the interaction of proteins with the lipid bilayer of cell membranes.

BCR-ABL gene

Chronic myelogenous leukemia (chronic phase) Interpatient variability exists in the breakpoints on both chromosomes 22 and 9 in Ph[+] CML. On chromosome 22, the breakpoints span a region of 5.8 kb within bcr (Fig. 1);[6,7] on chromosome 9, they extend over a region of >200 kb at the 5' (proximal) end of the *abl* gene.[83,84] However, *abl* exon 2 is always included in the segment transposed to chromosome 22, and exons 1a and 1b are often included as well. As a consequence of the reciprocal exchange of cytogenetic material between chromosomes 9 and 22, proximal *bcr* sequences (ending within the central 5.8 kb bcr segment) are juxtaposed to abl sequences in a head-to-tail fashion, and thus form a chimeric *bcr–abl* gene on chromosome 22.[8] This aberrant genomic configuration occurs even in CML patients with variant Ph translocations.[90] Therefore, at the molecular level, chromosome 9 is universally involved in CML, regardless of cytogenetic findings. When fused to bcr, the splice acceptor site associated with *abl* exon 2 skips splice donor sites in *abl* exon 1a, and frequently in *abl* exon 1b, to fuse with the splice donor sites of *bcr* exons. *abl* Exons 1a and 1b do not have a splice acceptor site and, hence, cannot fuse with the donor sites within bcr. The result is that *abl* exons 1a and 1b are not included in the *bcr–abl* mRNA, even though they may be part of the *bcr–abl* gene on chromosome 22q-.[9] The 8.5 kb transcript consists of 5' *bcr* exons ending in bcr exon 2 or 3 fused to *abl* exons 2 through 11[8,91] (Table 2). The point of fusion includes a chimeric codon with one nucleotide from bcr exon 2 or 3 and two nucleotides from *abl* exon 2. It is also possible for bcr exon 1 to be fused with *abl* exon 2 in this manner, but fusion of bcr exons 4 or 5 to *abl* exon 2 is not consonant with formation of a *bcr–abl* message because this configuration would result in a reading frameshift.[7]

The translation product is a chimeric protein of 210 kD–$p210^{bcr-abl}$.[92–94] At least two molecular variants of the *bcr–abl* protein are generated: those with and without bcr exon 3.[95] The electrophoretic mobility of these variants is extremely similar, probably because bcr exon 3 is small, containing only 25 amino acids.

The possible mechanisms governing oncogenic activation of the *abl* gene through usurpation of its N-terminus by the *bcr* gene include a change in enzymatic activity, subcellular localization, or substrate affinity. In this regard, $p210^{bcr-abl}$ (regardless of the presence of bcr exon 3) has a much higher tyrosine kinase activity than its normal counterpart $p145^{abl}$, in vitro;[92–95] $p210^{bcr-abl}$ and $p145^{abl}$ also have dissimilar patterns of autophosphorylation and may interact differently with substrates.[87] However, though several candidate substrate phosphoproteins have been identified for $p210^{bcr-abl}$,[96,97] work in this area remains rather limited in scope. Concerning subcellular localization, little is known about the residence of the normal *bcr* and *abl* proteins versus their abnormal *bcr–abl* counterparts. Yet, studies of the four normal mouse *abl* proteins which, as mentioned earlier, differ in their N-termini, may provide insights. Simple overexpression of these proteins is insufficient for transformation of mouse NIH 3T3 cells. However, deletion of a putative regulatory domain (53 N-terminal amino acids) of the mouse abl IV transcript activates its transforming potential fully, both with respect to fibroblast and B-lymphocyte transformation in vitro, and leukemogenicity in vivo.[21] Apparently, deletion of this sequence is also associated with translocation of the *abl* protein from its normal residence in the nucleus to the cytoplasm. It remains speculative as to whether a similar change in subcellular localization between the normal human *abl* protein and the aberrant *bcr–abl* protein exists and can account for the emergence of the leukemic phenotype.

p210$^{bcr-abl}$ is not detected in hematological malignancies other than Ph$^+$ leukemia.[96] The high specificity of p210$^{bcr-abl}$, its altered tyrosine phosphokinase activity, and recent evidence that it can transform hematopoietic cells in vitro[98,99] constitute powerful support for the belief that this protein is directly involved in the malignant process.

Ph$^+$ AML and ALL The bcr status of over 400 cases of Ph$^+$ CML have been documented in the literature and at least 98% of these individuals (including >70 patients with blast crisis) have rearrangement. In contrast, only about 50% of adult Ph$^+$ ALL or AML patients, and 10% of pediatric Ph$^+$ ALL patients demonstrate bcr rearrangement (Table 3). Therefore, Ph$^+$ ALL and AML include both bcr rearrangement-positive (bcr$^+$) and bcr rearrangement-negative (bcr$^-$) subgroups. In general, bcr rearrangement positivity is associated with expression of p210$^{bcr-abl}$. Patients who do not show a rearrangement within the bcr region of the *bcr* gene, nevertheless have a break within this gene, albeit at a more proximal position – the first *bcr* intron[75,100,101,102] (Fig. 1). It is now known that the first intron of the *bcr* gene, like that of the *abl* gene, is large – 68 kb.[78] The breakpoints in Ph$^+$ acute leukemia appear to cluster in the 3′ or distal 35 kb of this intron[78,103] (Fig. 1). In these patients, *bcr* exon 1 is juxtaposed to the *abl* gene. The resultant chimeric gene encodes an abnormal 7.0 kb bcr–abl mRNA consisting of *bcr* exon 1 fused to *abl* exons 2 through 11 (Table 2). The translation product is an 190 kD bcr–abl protein (p190$^{bcr-abl}$).[73,104–106] There is also a third, small (about 10%) subgroup of Ph$^+$ acute leukemia patients who exhibit a rearrangement localizing immediately proximal to the 5.8 kb bcr segment[107] (Fig. 1); the impact of this breakpoint on protein expression is not known.

Initially, p190$^{bcr-abl}$ was discerned in ALL cells, and, hence, was thought to participate in lymphoid leukemogenesis. More recently, this protein has also been detected in Ph$^+$ AML and in acute leukemia with a mixed myeloid/lymphoid phenotype; these data oppose the concept of lineage specificity for p190$^{bcr-abl}$.[107–109]

P190$^{bcr-abl}$ is enzymatically active as a tyrosine protein kinase,[73,110] an

Table 3. *Frequency of bcr rearrangement in Philadelphia-positive leukemia patients*[a]

Diagnosis	Number of patients studied	% positive for bcr rearrangement
CML	>400	98
ALL		
Adult	>75	50
Pediatric	>20	10
AML	13	46

[a]Data compiled from refs 6, 9, 10, 66–78, 100–14.

observation consonant with direct participation of this aberrant protein in the development of t(9;22) leukemia. Indeed, its enzymatic activity is more potent than that of $p210^{bcr-abl}$;[110] this may explain the association of $p190^{bcr-abl}$ with the more aggressive acute leukemia phenotype. As with $p210^{bcr-abl}$, it is not known if the production of $p190^{bcr-abl}$ results in a change in subcellular localization or substrate specificity, and if such phenomena may also provide a mechanism for initiating oncogenic activity.

Ph^+ bcr^+ $(p210^+)$ acute leukemia is strongly reminiscent of CML blast crisis, and both entities carry the identical molecular aberration; therefore, it seems reasonable to postulate that they are a single disease process, with the acute leukemia representing the blast crisis stage of CML in patients who failed to be diagnosed while in the asyptomatic, early benign phase. The corollary to this notion is that Ph^+ bcr^- $(p190^+)$ ALL and AML represent bona fide acute leukemias. Evidence for such assumptions includes the following findings: (i) transition to a chronic phase CML phenotype has been seen in several cases of $p210^+$, but not $p190^+$, acute leukemia[114] (and Kurzrock, unpublished observations), suggesting that the disease was really blast crisis of a previously undiagnosed CML; (ii) bcr positivity and expression of $p210^{bcr-abl}$ are found in nearly all cases of CML, while $p190^{bcr-abl}$ has been reported almost exclusively in acute leukemia rather than in CML; and (iii) the absence of a pre-existing CML state has been documented in the time interval immediately preceding the onset of Ph^+ bcr^- $(p190^+)$ AML.[108] Therefore, expression of $p190^{bcr-abl}$ versus $p210^{bcr-abl}$ may play a critical role in the manifestation of an acute, rather than a chronic, Ph^+ leukemia phenotype. The above hypothesis is especially appealing in the light of recent data indicating that, in an in vitro system using retroviral constructs,[115] $p190^{bcr-abl}$ is a more potent stimulator of hematopoietic transformation and proliferation than $p210^{bcr-abl}$.

It still remains possible that the significant event in Ph^+ leukemogenesis lies solely in the truncation and resultant activation of *abl*. According to this alternate hypothesis, leukemia phenotype is determined by the target cell affected by the t(9;22) translocation, regardless of whether it is p190$^{bcr-abl}$ or p210$^{bcr-abl}$ that is expressed. CML results because of the acquisition of the Ph translocation by a pluripotent stem cell; ALL, by a lymphoid progenitor cell. Research data supporting this proposition have been generated by Turhan and colleagues[116] who have shown that Ph$^+$ bcr$^+$ ALL can originate in either a pluripotent stem cell or a lineage-restricted lymphoid progenitor. The distinct breakpoints associated with the Ph translocation in acute and chronic leukemia may simply be preferentially created or maintained in different hematopoietic cell lineages.

The discovery of two molecularly distinct subgroups of Ph$^+$ acute leukemia prompted a search for clinical distinguishing features. The data gleaned from the literature as well as our prospective study of 30 patients (Kurzrock, unpublished observations) reveals no striking differences between bcr$^+$ (p210$^+$) and bcr$^-$ (p190$^+$) Ph$^+$ acute leukemia patients.[10,107,108,111–113]

Chronic myelogenous leukemia (blast crisis) Since the Ph chromosome is found in the early chronic phase, it seems likely that bcr rearrangement is necessary, but not sufficient, for disease evolution; superimposed secondary genetic driving forces are required.[30]

Cytogenetic and clinical heterogeneity characterizes the blast crisis stage. For example, blasts can have a myeloid, lymphoid, or, less commonly, an erythroid or megakaryocytic morphology. Secondary cytogenetic abnormalities can include an additional Ph chromosome, trisomy of chromosome 8, isochromosome 17(q), trisomy of chromosome 19, and loss of chromosome 7 or the Y chromosome. This heterogeneity suggests that several different subsets of blast crisis exist and that the genetic events in each of these subsets are distinct. It is therefore highly unlikely that any single molecular abnormality will account for blast crisis in all patients. The known cytogenetic anomalies may provide localization clues in the search for relevant molecular perturbations.

To date, several aberrant molecular events have been implicated in the development of blast crisis (Table 4). In this regard, one of the most common manifestations of clonal evolution is the appearance of an additional Ph chromosome. The presence of this aberration can be used to argue for the association of quantitative changes in *abl*-related expression with disease progression. A role for increased *bcr–abl* expression in driving metamorphosis to the blastic phenotype is also supported by the observation of elevated levels of *bcr–abl* mRNA in some individuals with advanced as compared to early CML,[117–119] though this finding has been disputed by at least one group of investigators.[120]

Alternatively, a role for a qualitative change in *bcr–abl* expression has also

Table 4. *Postulated molecular mechanisms of blast crisis*

Mechanism	Refs
Increased expression of the *bcr–abl* message	117–19
Presence of 3' (distal), rather than 5' (proximal) breakpoints within the bcr	67, 123
Emergence of the acute leukemia-associated $p190^{bcr-abl}$ in addition to $p210^{bcr-abl}$	Dhingra K., Talpaz M., Kurzrock R. unpublished observations
Expression of novel *bcr–abl* messages	163
Rearrangement in the p53 gene	134, 135
Elevated expression or amplification of the *myc* proto-oncogene	136, 137
Increased hematopoietic growth factor (interleukin-1β) expression	Wetzler M., Kurzrock R., Talpaz M. unpublished observations

been advanced. Several observations support this concept. First, in some cases, a new bcr rearrangement (albeit with retention of the original rearrangement) can be detected during the course of disease evolution.[72,121] Further, even in those instances in which only a single rearranged bcr band is discerned, the presence of a second *bcr* gene rearrangement which is outside the region recognized by the probe for the 5.8 kb bcr, cannot be ruled out. It is therefore conceivable that an additional recombination event coincides with the development of a second Ph chromosome. Second, all the sequences needed to code for p190[bcr–abl] are included in the *bcr–abl* gene of CML.[75,100,101] In the event that a switch from the exclusive expression of this gene as p210[bcr–abl], to the expression of p190[bcr–abl] in addition to p210[bcr–abl] was possible, would a change in phenotype occur? Recently, we have studied 37 patients with CML and found that 3 (8%) expressed both p190[bcr–abl] and p210[bcr–abl] in the advanced (blast crisis or accelerated) stage, while only p210[bcr–abl] was expressed in the chronic phase (Dhingra K, Talpaz M, and Kurzrock R, unpublished observations). In addition, a CML-type breakpoint (within the 5.8 kb bcr) co-existing with an ALL-type breakpoint (within the first *bcr* exon) has been described in a child with ALL and two Ph chromosomes.[122]

Another controversial theory is that patients with 5' (proximal) breakpoints within the 5.8 kb bcr have a more prolonged survival than those with 3' (distal) breakpoints.[67,72,123–125] The most cogent evidence against this theory is that two alternative 210 kD *bcr–abl* products (those with and those without exon 3[95]) often co-exist in CML patients,[120,127,128] thus obviating the influence of distinct breakpoints within the 5.8 kb bcr.

Finally, several lines of evidence suggest that the role of $p210^{bcr-abl}$ in advanced CML is supplanted by other factors. Convincing arguments against the participation of bcr–abl expression in disease evolution are as follows: (i) we found equivalent expression of $p210^{bcr-abl}$ enzymatic activity in myeloid, lymphoid, and undifferentiated blast crisis.[96] Yet the distinct phenotypes of these disease manifestations should reflect disparate genetic events; (ii) Bartram and colleagues[129] documented deletion of bcr–abl sequences in cells derived from a CML patient entering blast crisis; (iii) we have observed that the growth rate of CML blast crisis cells in vitro can be maintained even in the presence of severely reduced levels of bcr–abl protein and enzymatic activity;[130] and (iv) Young and Witte have demonstrated that, although $p210^{bcr-abl}$ can transform hematopoietic cells in vitro, these cells do not display an aggressive oncogenic phenotype.[131] The latter result is consistent with a role for bcr–abl in the indolent, chronic phase of CML, but not in the virulent blastic phase.

Other oncogenes have also been analyzed in CML blast transformation. LeMaistre et al[132] studied 22 samples derived from CML blast crisis patients and 29 samples from chronic phase CML patients for mutations of codons 12, 13 or 61 of the N-ras, H-ras, and K-ras genes; two blast crisis patients (9%) exhibited mutations, both in the K-ras gene. Collins et al[133] could not, however, identify mutations in any of the 21 cases of CML blast crisis that they analyzed. These data indicate that ras mutations can occur in advanced disease, albeit rarely. Alteration in p53, a gene whose protein product is associated with tumorigenicity, has also been described.[134,135] Ahuja and coworkers found rearrangement in the p53 gene in 7 of 23 patients (30%) with CML blast crisis, but not in patients with other types of leukemias.[134] The myc proto-oncogene has also been analyzed in advanced CML, with investigators reporting both elevated myc RNA expression[136] and myc amplification.[137]

Finally, we have examined cytokine expression in both hematopoietic cells and cultured stromal cells from CML patients at various stages of their disease. Interestingly, interleukin-1β, a potent inducer of other hematopoietic growth factors, was found to be constitutively expressed in both the blood cells and the stromal layer in most myeloid or undifferentiated blast crisis patients, but not in chronic phase CML patients or normal individuals (Wetzler M, Kurzrock R, Talpaz M, unpublished observations). It is therefore possible that autonomous expression of interleukin-1β by the malignant clone in advanced disease induces the bone marrow stromal cells to secrete other growth factors, a chain of events leading to a progressively more virulent phenotype.

Overall, there is still a dearth of data regarding the etiology of blast crisis, and the data which exists is confusing. The conflicting experimental observations, as well as the diverse spectrum of clinical manifestations and cytogenetic changes associated with blast transformation, suggest that multiple molecular pathways lead to this terminal state. Some of these pathways may include aberrant cytokine expression, appearance of the acute leukemia-associated $p190^{bcr-abl}$, and alterations in other oncogenes.

Philadelphia chromosome-negative CML

The Ph chromosome is not discernible in about 5 to 10% of patients with a presumptive diagnosis of CML.[138] Ph-negative (Ph⁻) CML patients usually have a normal karyotype; however, about one-third of these individuals exhibit cytogenetic aberrations such as trisomy of chromosome 8 or, occasionally, a reciprocal translocation between chromosome 9 band q34 and a chromosome other than 22.[139,140]

In the past, the absence of the Ph chromosome in a patient with CML was considered an omen of a poor outcome.[138] There was also some dispute as to whether Ph⁻ CML actually existed, as many of these patients, on careful review, were found to have a myelodysplastic syndrome.[141,142] It is now apparent that Ph⁻ CML is an entity (Fig. 2), and that its clinical course is closely coupled to the presence of subchromosomal changes resulting in a bcr–abl product.[143,144]

Ph⁻, bcr⁺ CML In 1985, Bartram described a Ph⁻ CML patient who exhibited a typical bcr rearrangement and juxtaposition of the *bcr* and *abl* genes.[145] This observation has now been confirmed by several investigators in a total of 48 reported patients;[10,143,146–151] it has also been demonstrated that Ph⁻ bcr⁺ CML patients produce the 8.5 kb bcr–abl mRNA[143] and the 210 kd bcr–abl protein.[146] In Ph⁻ CML, as in Ph⁺ disease,[72,74] deletions in the 3′ region of bcr can occur and result in false negative results for bcr rearrangement;[143] therefore, accurate assessment of bcr status in these patients requires the use of probes encompassing both the 5′ and 3′ segments of the 5.8 kb bcr region.

Ph⁻ bcr⁺ CML patients usually have either a normal cytogenetic profile or an abnormality involving chromosome 9 band q34. The mechanism by which bcr and abl genes are juxtaposed in these patients has been investigated by in situ hybridization. These studies suggest that, in cytogenetically diploid cells, interstitial insertion of the *abl* gene next to the bcr segment of the *bcr* gene on chromosome 22 occurs without reciprocal translocation of genomic material to chromosome 9;[149] in patients with a translocation between 9q34 and another chromosome, a complex three-way set of recombination events is needed to produce the juxtaposition of the *bcr* and *abl* genes.[145]

Ph⁺ bcr⁺ CML patients have clinical and laboratory features that are indistinguishable from those of Ph⁺ CML patients, and both groups respond to hydroxyurea, busulfan, and interferon-alpha therapy in an identical manner.[143,146] Importantly, during hematological remission, CML patients with a diploid karyotype exhibit a normal morphological and cytogenetic

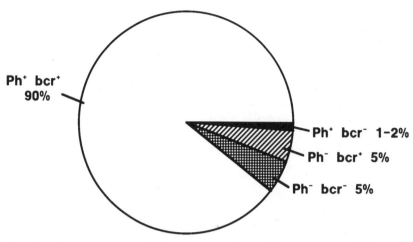

Cytogenetic and molecular changes in chronic myelogenous leukemia

Ph⁺ bcr⁺ 90%

Ph⁺ bcr⁻ 1-2%
Ph⁻ bcr⁺ 5%
Ph⁻ bcr⁻ 5%

Fig. 2. The percentage of CML patients with the Ph chromosome (Ph⁺) and bcr rearrangement (bcr⁺) are shown. The data has been gleaned from the literature and from the patients seen at MD Anderson Cancer Center.

blood and bone marrow profile. Even so, molecular studies will reveal bcr rearrangement, reflecting the persistence of the malignant clone.[143]

Overall, several important concepts have emerged from the molecular investigations of Ph⁻ CML: (i) the ability of molecular techniques to define subchromosomal genomic aberrations in Ph⁻ CML indicates that these methods are a crucial adjunct to clinical and morphological evaluation of disease nosology; (ii) Ph⁺ and Ph⁻ CML with bcr rearrangement have a similar clinical outcome and an identical molecular emblem suggesting that they represent a single disease. Ph⁻ bcr⁺ CML patients should therefore be eligible for therapeutic protocols aimed at Ph⁺ CML patients, including bone marrow transplantation and interferon therapy; and (iii) Ph⁻ bcr⁺ patients should be followed by molecular techniques, since bcr rearrangement may be the only evidence of residual malignancy at the time of hematological remission.

Ph⁻, bcr⁻ CML The question arises as to whether all Ph-negative patients with classic CML will exhibit bcr rearrangement. Intuitively, we have felt that this should be true. Yet, we have now encountered 11 patients with classic chronic phase CML, who have neither a discernible bcr rearrangement nor a *bcr–abl* message[144] (Fig. 2). At the time of diagnosis, these patients presented with splenomegaly, neutrophilia, occasional basophilia and thrombocytosis, a generally low leukocyte alkaline phosphatase score, and a hypercellular bone marrow with an increased myeloid : erythroid ratio, a shift to the left in myeloid maturity, and a pronounced granulocytic hyperplasia. Monocytosis, polycythemia, dysplasia, and disproportionate thrombocytosis were not observed. Cytogenetic analysis revealed that 6 of these patients had a normal diploid karyotype; 5 patients had karyotypic abnormalities (trisomy 21, 2 patients); trisomy 8, 1 patient; trisomy 19, 1 patient; 20q⁻, 1 patient; t(1p⁻;13q⁺), 1 patient; and monosomy 17 with an i(17q), 1 patient) in a fraction of their metaphases. Individuals with Ph⁻, bcr⁻ CML responded to hydroxyurea, busulphan, and interferon-alpha, although the small number of cases precluded a statistically valid comparison of their response rates to those of bcr⁺ patients. Their predicted 50% survival was 37 months by Kaplan and Meir analysis. Distinguishing characteristics appeared to be limited to a higher median age (60 years) at diagnosis than that of bcr⁺ CML patients (46 years), and the occasional presence of B symptoms (fever, weight loss, or night sweats), a finding which is rare in early bcr⁺ CML.

Despite the overall striking resemblance between chronic phase, bcr⁺ and bcr⁻ CML, disease progression manifests differently in these two groups. In bcr⁺ disease, the chronic phase ineluctably yields to a blast transformation phase typified by growing numbers of rapidly proliferating immature cells. In contrast, blast crisis did not occur in the bcr⁻ CML patients; rather, progression was characterized by increasing leukemia burden with profound leukocytosis, organomegaly, extramedullary infiltrates, and eventual bone marrow failure (anemia and thrombocytopenia, with blast counts $<20\%$).

The molecular forces driving Ph⁻, bcr⁻ CML are not known. However, it may be that p210$^{bcr-abl}$ is part of a growth factor, growth factor receptor, signal transduction pathway. Perturbation of any part of this pathway could conceivably result in a disease phenotype similar to bcr⁺ CML. In this regard, p210$^{bcr-abl}$ can transform interleukin-3 dependent hematopoietic cells to factor independence without autocrine secretion of interleukin-3.[99] It is conceivable that interleukin-3, or another growth factor, forms part of the bcr–abl pathway, and that an aberration of this yet to be determined factor or its receptor may result in leukemic proliferation and, hence, Ph⁻ bcr⁻ CML.

Essential thrombocythemia

Essential thrombocythemia is a clonal myeloproliferative disorder characterized by exuberant thrombocytosis with only mild to moderate leukocytosis. Although considered closely related to CML in clinical phenotype, transformation to an acute leukemic process rarely complicates essential throbocythemia. To date, the Ph chromosome has been reported in a small number of patients with this disorder,[152,153] and, further, essential thrombocythemia patients can occasionally exhibit the bcr and abl gene abnormalities typical of CML,[154] even in the absence of the Ph chromosome. In these cases, the disease behaves like CML, in that it has been reported to undergo blast transformation. Because many patients with CML have profoundly elevated platelet counts and therefore could be misdiagnosed as having essential thrombocythemia, it may be advisable that all persons with a tentative diagnosis of essential thrombocythemia be studied at both the cytogenetic and the molecular level.

Distinguishing the Ph translocation from other anomalies at 22q11 and 9q34

Ph⁻ acute leukemias with 9q34 chromosomal abnormalities As mentioned earlier, patients with a CML phenotype may have several types of karyotypic alterations which are variants of the classic t(9;22)(q34;q11) Ph anomalies: (i) complex translocations between ⩾3 chromosomes including 9 and 22; (ii) variant translocations between chromosome 22q11 and a chromosome other than 9; and (iii) variant translocations between chromosome 9q34 and a chromosome other than 22. At the molecular level, these patients exhibit the *bcr–abl* genotype which is pathognomonic for CML, and their clinical outcome mirrors that of their counterparts carrying the standard t(9;22).

Even so, there exist cases of acute leukemias with a 9q34 chromosomal abnormality which does not involve the *abl* gene. For instance, a subgroup of AML patients have a t(6;9)(p23;q34) aberration.[155] Westbrook and coworkers[156] studied these patients and found that, at the molecular level, the break on chromosome 9q34 occurs distal to the *abl* gene and no anomalous *abl* protein is produced. Similarly, in an acute T-cell leukemia line carrying a t(7;9)(q36;q34) abnormality, Westbrook et al[157] demonstrated that the *abl* gene is not involved. The breakpoint in these cells occurs at chromosome 9q34, but is ⩾ 250 kb proximal to the *abl* gene.

ALL with a 22q11 variant chromosomal abnormality There exists a subgroup of 'Ph⁺' ALL patients who display a deletion of the long arm of chromosome 22, with the breakpoint occurring at 22q11, but without cytogenetic evidence of involvement of 9q34. In contrast to the situation in CML, where variant Ph translocations are always associated with production of a *bcr–abl* product,[158] the 22q11 variant of ALL has been shown to encode only the normal p145^{abl} in some patients.[159] It follows that the disruption of chromosome 22 in these patients does not involve the *bcr* gene. It is theoretically possible, but experimentally unproven, that the break occurs in the immunoglobulin lambda light chain, a region on 22q11 known to be rearranged in some lymphoid malignancies. Although systematic correlation of the outcome of *bcr–abl*-positive versus *bcr–abl*-negative, 22q⁻ patients has not been performed, the poor prognosis associated with the t(9;22) in acute leukemias suggests that the 2 subgroups of patients should behave differently. Therefore, even though *bcr–abl* status (p210-positivity versus p190-positivity) in acute leukemia patients carrying a classic Ph chromosome is not currently useful as a predictive test, further molecular assessment of Ph variants in this disease is warranted, and may yield important prognostic information.

Minimal residual disease

Polymerase chain reaction The polymerase chain reaction is a tremendously potent technique which allows amplification of specific DNA or RNA (using cDNA) sequences, and the detection of small numbers (1 malignant cell amongst up to 1×10^6 normal cells) of cells containing these sequences. Currently, this technology can only be applied to the detection of minimal residual disease if a known nucleotide sequence is unique to the malignant cells. Ph+ leukemias are therefore the perfect prototypes on which to use the polymerase chain reaction.

Amplification of cDNA sequences corresponding to the *bcr–abl* mRNA can be easily exploited for determining the presence of residual malignant cells in CML and/or Ph+ acute leukemia. However, extreme caution in preventing false positive results must be implemented by laboratories utilizing the polymerase chain reaction, as the powerful amplification process makes sample contamination a constant hazard.

Employing this technology, several groups have demonstrated *bcr–abl* transcripts in some CML patients in clinical and cytogenetic remission after bone marrow transplantation[128,160] and interferon-alpha therapy (Dhingra K, Kurzrock R, Talpaz M, unpublished observations). It is not yet clear if patients with 'molecular relapse' will eventually develop clinical relapse. However, it may be reasonable to assume that patients with no evidence of disease by polymerase chain reaction are cured of their leukemia. The ease and rapidity with which this technique can be performed also makes it a useful tool for the diagnosis of *bcr–abl*-positivity in acute and chronic leukemias.[161,162]

Conclusions

Over the last few years, a wealth of incisive studies have led to a rapid expansion in our understanding of the molecular basis of Ph+ leukemogenesis. The following concepts have emerged:

1 As a result of the Ph translocation, p160*bcr* and p145*abl* (the normal *bcr* and *abl* gene products) are replaced by p210*bcr–abl*. This aberrant protein constitutes the molecular fingerprint of CML. It is a hybrid product consisting of part of the *bcr* protein and part of the *abl* protein. Because the Ph translocation is present in the early chronic phase, the union of the *bcr* and *abl* genes has been implicated in the initiation of the leukemic process.

2 Approximately 10% of CML patients lack a Ph chromosome. One-half of these individuals have bcr rearrangement and express p210$^{bcr-abl}$ (Fig. 2). Ph$^+$ and Ph$^-$ bcr$^+$ (p210$^+$) CML are identical and should be treated the same. Molecular follow-up of bcr$^+$ CML patients with a diploid karyotype is essential for detection of persistent malignancy after therapy.

3 A phenotypic facsimile of chronic phase CML exists in which bcr rearrangement and a bcr–abl message cannot be discerned.[144] The molecular events in these patients remains to be determined and may provide clues to the biological basis of chronic myeloid leukemogenesis. Ph$^-$ bcr$^-$ CML patients have a distinct clinical course despite their early resemblance to classic CML. They eventually develop bone marrow failure (anemia and thrombocytopenia) accompanied by a markedly increased leukemia burden with elevated white blood cell counts, organomegaly, and extramedullary disease. Blast transformation does not generally occur.[144]

4 Adult Ph$^+$ ALL and AML may be associated with either a 210 kd or 190 kD bcr–abl protein (Table 2). The clinical course of p210$^+$ vs p190$^+$ adult acute leukemia cannot currently be distinguished. In contrast, the vast majority of pediatric Ph$^+$ acute leukemia patients express p190$^{bcr-abl}$, but not p210$^{bcr-abl}$.

5 The CML-associated p210$^{bcr-abl}$ and the acute leukemia-associated p190$^{bcr-abl}$ are probably the first genuine cancer-specific markers. Their enhanced tyrosine phosphokinase enzymatic activity (a property linked to certain growth factor receptors and the transforming capability of some oncogenes) provides a cogent argument for direct involvement of these unique proteins in the process of tumor development.

6 The biological role of p210$^{bcr-abl}$ and p190$^{bcr-abl}$ requires definition. It is not known if these distinct proteins are linked to chronic vs acute Ph$^+$ leukemogenesis or if leukemia phenotype is determined by the transformed target cell regardless of the *bcr–abl* protein generated.

7 The detection of the Ph chromosome in acute leukemia is prescient of a poor prognosis. It will be important to determine if molecular probes can identify a subgroup of Ph$^-$ ALL or AML patients who express p210 or p190 and have a clinical outcome similar to that of Ph$^+$ acute leukemia patients.

8 The secondary molecular forces driving progression of CML to blast crisis are unknown, and may differ from patient to patient. Potential mechanisms include additional changes in the *bcr–abl* product, altered growth factor expression, and abnormalities in other oncogenes (Table 4).

9 The presence of a specific marker – the *bcr–abl* message – permits the analysis of minimal residual disease with the use of the highly sensitive

polymerase chain reaction, a technique capable of detecting up to one leukemia cell amongst one million normal cells.

Finally, studies of the role of the unaltered *bcr* and *abl* genes in hematopoiesis are required if the part played by these genes in normal versus leukemic processes is to be elucidated. The *bcr–abl* gene is cancer-specific and hence its discovery has already spawned a new role for molecular analysis in the diagnostic process. The possibility of exploiting this knowledge for therapeutic purposes merits consideration.

Glossary

3': The end of a gene at which transcription ceases.

5': The end of a gene at which transcription begins.

Exon: A segment of a gene that is represented in the mRNA product.

Intron: A segment of a gene that is not represented in the mRNA product because of its removal as a consequence of the splicing together of sequences (exons) on either side of it.

Kilobase (kb): 1000 base pairs of DNA or 1000 bases of RNA.

N-terminal (amino-terminal): The end of a polypeptide that has an amino acid with a free amino group. Proteins are synthesized starting from the N-terminal amino acid.

Oncogene: A gene that causes cancer. Oncogenes are altered versions of ordinarily benign genes present in normal cells.

Polymerase chain reaction: A method of amplification of nucleotide sequences using a chain reaction technique.

Proto-oncogene: A normal gene with the potential to be activated and hence become a cancer gene (oncogene).

Rearrangement: DNA breakage and subsequent reattachment at a new site.

Splice: The removal of introns and joining of exons in RNA; introns are spliced out whereas exons are spliced together.

Transcription: Synthesis of RNA on a DNA template.

Transformation: The conversion of cells in culture to a state of unrestrained growth reminiscent of that in malignancy.

Translation: Synthesis of protein on the mRNA template.

References

(1) Mitelman F, *Catalog of chromosome aberrations in cancer*. New York: Alan R Liss Inc, 1988.
(2) Nowell PC, Hungerford DA. A minute chromosome in human chronic granulocytic leukemia. *Science* 1960; 132: 1197.

(3) Rowley JD. A new consistent chromosomal abnormality in chronic myelogenous leukemia identified by quinacrine fluorescence and Giemsa staining. *Nature* 1973; 243: 290.

(4) Bartram CR, deKlein A, Hagemeijer A et al. Translocation of the *abl* oncogene correlates with the presence of the Philadelphia chromosome in chronic myelocytic leukaemia. *Nature* 1983; 306: 277.

(5) Heisterkamp N, Stephenson JR, Groffen J et al. Localization of the *abl* oncogene adjacent to a translocation breakpoint in CML. *Nature* 1983; 306: 239.

(6) Groffen J, Stephenson JR, Heisterkamp N et al. Philadelphia chromosomal breakpoints are clustered within a limited region, bcr, on chromosome 22. *Cell* 1984; 36: 93.

(7) Heisterkamp N, Stam K, Groffen J et al. Structural organization of the BCR gene and its role in the Ph translocation. *Nature* 1985; 316: 758.

(8) Shtivelman E, Lifshitz B, Gale RP, Canaani E. Fused transcript of *abl* and *bcr* genes in chronic myelogenous leukemia. *Nature* 1985; 315: 550.

(9) Kurzrock R, Gutterman JU, Talpaz M. The molecular genetics of Philadelphia chromosome-positive leukemias. *N Eng J Med* 1988; 319: 990.

(10) Kurzrock R, Shtalrid M, Gutterman JU, Talpaz M. Molecular diagnostics of chronic myelogenous leukemia and Philadelphia-positive acute leukemia. *Cancer Cells* 1989; 7: 9–13.

(11) Abelson HT, Rabstein LS. Lymphosarcoma: virus-induced thymic independent disease in mice. *Cancer Res* 1970; 30: 2212.

(12) Whitlock CA, Witte ON. The complexity of virus–cell interactions in Abelson virus infection of lymphoid and other hematopoietic cells. *Adv Immunol* 1985; 37: 73.

(13) Siden EJ, Baltimore D, Clard D, Rosenber NE. Immunoglobulin synthesis by lymphoid cells transformed in vitro by Abelson murine leukemia virus. *Cell* 1979; 16: 389.

(14) Boss M, Greaves M, Teich N. Abelson virus-transformed haematopoietic cell lines with pre-B cell characteristics. *Nature* 1979; 278: 551.

(15) Cook W. Rapid thymomas induced by Abelson murine leukemia virus. *Proc Natl Acad Sci USA* 1982; 79: 2917.

(16) Raschke W, Baird S, Ralph P, Nakoinz I. Functional macrophage cell lines transformed by Abelson leukemia virus. *Cell* 1978; 15: 261.

(17) Mendoza GR, Metzger H. Disparity of IgE binding between normal and tumor mouse mast cells. *J Immunol* 1976; 117: 1573.

(18) Risser R, Potter M, Rowe WP. Abelson virus-induced lymphomagenesis in mice. *J Exp Med* 1978; 148: 714.

(19) Potter M, Sklar MD, Rowe WP. Rapid viral induction of plasmacytomas in pristane-primed BALB/c mice. *Science* 1973; 182: 592.

(20) Konopka JB, Witte ON. Activation of the abl oncogene in murine and human leukemias. *Biochem Biophys* 1985; 823: 1.

(21) Van Etten RA, Jackson P, Baltimore D. The mouse type IV c-*abl* gene product is a nuclear protein, and activation of transforming ability is associated with cytoplasmic localization. *Cell* 1989; 58: 669.

(22) Hunter T, Cooper JA. Protein–tyrosine kinases. *Ann Rev Biochem* 1985; 4: 897.

(23) Prywes RP, Foulkes JG, Baltimore D. The minimum transforming region of v-abl is the segment encoding protein-tyrosine kinase. *J Virol* 1985; 54: 114.

(24) Pierce JH, Di Fiore PP, Aaronson SA et al. Neoplastic transformation of mast cells by Abelson-MuLV: Abrogation of IL-3 dependence by a nonautocrine mechanism. *Cell* 1985; 41: 685.

(25) Cook WD, Metcalf D, Micola MA et al. Malignant transformation of a growth factor-dependent myeloid cell line by Abelson virus without evidence of an autocrine mechanism. *Cell* 1985; 41: 677.

(26) Broxmeyer HE, Ralph P, Gilbertson S, Margolis VB. Induction of leukemia associated-inhibitory activity and bone marrow granulocyte-macrophage progenitor cell alterations during infection with Abelson virus. *Cancer Res* 1981; 40: 3928.

(27) Twardzik DR, Todaro GJ, Marquardt H. Transformation induced by Abelson murine leukemia virus involves production of a polypeptide growth factor. *Science* 1982; 216: 894.

(28) Whitlock CA, Witte ON. Abelson virus infected cells can exhibit restricted in vitro growth and low oncogenic potential. *J Virol* 1981; 40: 577.

(29) Lane MA, Neary C, Cooper GM. Activation of a cellular transforming gene in tumors induced by Abelson leukemia virus. *Nature* 1982; 300: 659.

(30) Rowley JD. Chromosome abnormalities in human leukemia. *Ann Rev Genet* 1980; 14: 17.

(31) Sandberg AA. Chromosomes and causation of human cancer and leukemia: XL. The Ph[1] and other translocation in CML. *Cancer* 1980; 46: 2221.

(32) Sonta S, Sandberg AA. Chromosomes and causation of human cancer and leukemia: XXIV. Unusual and complex Ph[1] translocations and their clinical significance. *Blood* 1977; 50: 691.

(33) Catovsky K. Ph[1]-positive acute leukaemia and chronic granulocytic leukemia: one or two diseases? *Br J Haematol* 1979; 42: 493.

(34) Craigie D. Case of disease of the spleen in which death took place in consequence of the presence of purulent matter in the blood. *Edin Med Surg J* 1845; 64: 400–4.

(35) Bennett JH. Case of hypertrophy of the spleen and liver in which death took place from suppuration of the blood. *Edin Med Surg J* 1845; 64: 413–18.

(36) Virchow R. Weisses blut. *Froiep Notizen* 1845; 36: 151–4.

(37) Young JL Jr, Percy CL, Asire AJ et al. Cancer incidence and mortality in the United States. 1973–77. *National Cancer Institute Monograph No. 57.* Bethesda, Maryland. NCI, Surveillance, Epidemiology, and End Results Program, 1978.

(38) Fialkow PJ, Jacobson RJ, Papayannopoulou T. Chronic myelocytic leukemia: clonal origin in a stem cell common to the granulocyte, erythrocyte, platelet and monocyte/macrophage. *Am J Med* 1977; 63: 125.

(39) Barr RD, Fialkow PJ. Clonal origin of chronic myelocytic leukemia. *N Eng J Med* 1973; 289: 307.

(40) Sokal JE. Evaluation of survival data for chronic myelocytic leukemia. *Am J Hematol* 1976; 1: 493.

(41) Cervantes F, Rozman C. A multivariate analysis of prognostic factors in chronic myeloid leukemia. *Blood* 1982; 60: 1298.

(42) Galbraith PR, Abu-Zahra HT. Granulopoiesis in chronic granulocytic leukaemia. *Br J Haematol* 1972; 22: 135.

(43) Strife A, Clarkson B. Biology of chronic myelogenous leukemia: Is discordant maturation the primary defect? *Semin Hematol* 1988; 25: 1.

(44) Koeffler HP, Golde DW. Chronic myelongeous leukemia – new concepts. *N Eng J Med* 1981; 304: 1201, 1269.

(45) Talpaz M, Kurzrock R, Kantarjian HM, Gutterman JU. Recent advances in the therapy of chronic myelogenous leukemia. In: DeVita V, Hellman S, Rosenberg S, eds. *Important advances in oncology*. Philadelphia, Pennsylvania: JB Lippincott Co, 1988: 297–321.

(46) Champlin RE, Golde DW. Chronic myelogenous leukemia: Recent advances. *Blood* 1985; 65: 1039.

(47) Nowell PC, Jackson L, Weiss A, Kurzrock R. Philadelphia-positive chronic myelogenous leukemia followed for 27 years. *Cancer Genet Cytogenet* 1988; 34: 57.

(48) Kantarjian HM, Smith TL, McCredie KB et al. Chronic myelogenous leukemia: A multivariate analysis of the associations of patient characteristics and therapy with survival. *Blood* 1985; 66: 1326.

(49) Griffin JD, Todd RF, Ritz J et al. Differentiation patterns in the blastic phase of chronic myeloid leukemia. *Blood* 1983; 61: 85.

(50) Ekblom M, Borgstrom G, Willebrand E et al. Erythroid blast crisis in chronic myelogenous leukemia. *Blood* 1983; 62: 591.

(51) Bain B, Catovsky D, O'Brien M et al. Megakaryoblastic transformation of chronic granulocytic leukaemia. An electron microscopy and cytochemical study. *J Clin Pathol* 1977; 30: 235.

(52) Bakshi A, Minowada J, Arnold A et al. Lymphoid blast crisis of chronic myelogenous leukemia represent stages in the development of B-cell precursors. *N Eng J Med* 1983; 309: 826.

(53) Hernandez P, Carrot J, Cruz C. Chronic myeloid leukemia blast crisis with T-cell features. *Br J Haematol* 1982; 51: 175.

(54) Sarin PS, Anderson PW, Gallo RC. Terminal deoxymucleotidyl-transferase activities in human blood leukocytes and lymphoblast cell lines. High levels in lymphoblast cell lines and blast cells of some patients with chronic myelogenous leukemia in acute phase. *Blood* 1976; 47: 11.

(55) Rosenthal S, Canellos GP, Gralnick H. Erythroblastic transformation of chronic granulocytic leukemia. *Am J Med* 1977; 63: 116.

(56) Kuriyama K, Gale RP, Tomonaga M et al. CML-T1: A cell line derived from T-lymphocyte acute phase of chronic myelogenous leukemia. *Blood* 1989; 74: 1381.

(57) Rushing D, Goldman A, Gibbs G et al. Hydroxyurea vs busulfan in the treatment of chronic granulocytic leukemia. *Am J Clin Oncol* 1982; 5: 307.

(58) Talpaz M, Kantarjian HM, Kurzrock R, Gutterman JU. Therapy of chronic myelogenous leukemia: Chemotherapy and interferons. *Semin Hematol* 1988; 25: 62.

(59) Talpaz M, Kantarjian HM, McCredie KB et al. Hematologic remission and cytogenetic improvement induced by recombinant human interferon alpha in chronic myelogenous leukemia. *N Eng J Med* 1986; 314: 1065.

(60) Kurzrock R, Gutterman JU, Kantarjian H, Talpaz M. Therapy of chronic myelogenous leukemia with interferon. *Cancer Invest* 1989; 7: 83.

(61) Prischl FC, Haas OA, Lion T, Eyb R, Schwarzmeier JD. Duration of first remission as an indicator of long-term survival in chronic myelogenous leukaemia. *Br J Haematol* 1989; 71: 337–42.

(62) Look TA. The emerging genetics of acute lymphoblastic leukemia: Clinical and biologic implications. *Semin Oncol* 1985; 12: 92.

(63) Poplack DG. Acute lymphoblastic leukemia in childhood. *Pediatr Clin North Am* 1985; 32: 669.

(64) Bloomfield CD, Golman G, Alimena R et al. Chromosomal abnormalities identify high-risk and low-risk patients with acute lymphoblastic leukemia. *Blood* 1986; 67: 415.

(65) Jain K, Arlin A, Mertelsmann R et al. Philadelphia chromosome and terminal transferase positive acute leukemia: similarity of terminal phase of chronic myelogenous leukemia and de novo acute presentation. *J Clin Oncol* 1983; 1: 669, positive chronic myelogenous leukemia: *J Clin Invest* 1986; 78:1392.

(66) Collins SJ. Breakpoints on chromosomes 9 and 22 in Philadelphia chromosome-positive chronic myelogenous leukemia (CML). Amplification of rearranged c-*abl* oncogenes in CML blast crisis. *J Clin Invest* 1986; 78: 1392–6.

(67) Schaefer-Rego K, Dudek H, Popenoe D et al. CML patients in blast crisis have breakpoints localized to a specific region of the bcr. *Blood* 1987; 70: 448.

(68) Boehm TLJ, Drahovsky D. Application of a bcr specific probe in the classification of human leukemia. *J Cancer Res Clin Oncol* 1987; 113: 267.

(69) Benn P, Soper L, Eisenberg A et al. Utility of molecular genetic analysis of bcr rearrangement in the diagnosis of chronic myeloid leukemia. *Cancer Genet Cytogenet* 1987; 29: 1.

(70) Selleri L, Narni F, Emilia G et al. Philadelphia-positive chronic myeloid leukemia with a chromosome 22 breakpoint outside the breakpoint cluster region. *Blood* 1987; 70: 1659.

(71) Hirosawa S, Aoki N, Shibuya M, Onozawa Y. Breakpoints in Philadelphia chromosome (Ph[1]) positive leukemias. *Japan J Cancer Res* 1987; 78: 590.

(72) Shtalrid M, Talpaz M, Kurzrock R et al. Analysis of breakpoints with the BCR gene and their correlation with the clinical course of Philadelphia-positive chronic myelogenous leukemia. *Blood* 1988; 72: 485.

(73) Kurzrock R, Shtalrid M, Romero R et al. A novel c-abl protein in Philadelphia-positive acute lymphoblastic leukemia. *Nature* 1987; 325: 631.

(74) Popenoe D, Shaefer-Rego K, Mears JG et al. Frequent and extensive deletion during the 9,22 translocation in CML. *Blood* 1986; 68: 1123.

(75) Hermans A, Heisterkamp N, von Lindern M et al. Unique fusion of *bcr* and *abl* genes in Philadelphia chromosome positive acute lymphoblastic leukemia. *Cell* 1987; 51: 33.

(76) Hariharan IK, Adams J. cDNA sequences for human *bcr*, the gene that translocates to the *abl* oncogene in chronic myeloid leukemia. *EMBO J* 1987; 6: 115.

(77) Mes-Masson A, McLaughlin J, Daley GQ et al. Overlapping cDNA clones define the complete coding region for the $p210^{c-abl}$ gene product associated with chronic myelogenous leukemia cells containing the Philadelphia chromosome. *Proc Natl Acad Sci USA* 1986; 83: 9768.

(78) Heisterkamp N, Knoppel E, Groffen J. The first *bcr* gene intron contains breakpoints in Philadelphia chromosome positive leukemia. *Nucleic Acids Res* 1988; 16: 10069.

(79) Croce CM, Huebner K, Isobe M et al. Mapping of four distinct bcr-related loci to chromosome region 22q11: order of bcr loci relative to chronic myelogenous leukemia and acute lymphoblastic leukemia breakpoints. *Proc Natl Acad Sci USA* 1987; 84: 7174.

(80) Collins S, Coleman H, Groudine M. Expression of bcr and bcr–abl fusion transcripts in normal and leukemic cells. *Mol Cell Biol* 1987; 7: 2870.

(81) Stam K, Heisterkamp N, Reynold FH, Groffen J. Evidence that the *bcr* gene encodes a 160,000 Dalton phosphoprotein with associated kinase activity. *Mol Cell Biol* 1987; 7: 1955.

(82) Timmons MS, Witte ON. Structural characterization of the *bcr* gene product. *Oncogene* 1989; 4: 559–67.

(83) Bernards A, Rubin CM, Westbrook CA et al. The first intron in the human *abl* gene is at least 200 kilobases long and is a target for translocations in chronic myelogenous leukemia. *Mol Cell Biol* 1987; 7: 3231.

(84) Grosveld G, Berwoerd T, van Agrhoven T et al. The chronic myelocytic cell line K562 contains a breakpoint in bcr and produces a chimeric bcr–abl transcript. *Mol Cell Biol* 1986; 6: 607.

(85) Shtivelman E, Lifshitz B, Gale RP et al. Alternative splicing of RNAs transcribed from the human *abl* gene from the *bcr–abl* fused gene. *Cell* 1986; 47: 277–84.

(86) Ben-Neriah Y, Bernareds A, Paskind M et al. Alternative 5' exons in ABL mRNA. *Cell* 1986; 44: 577.

(87) Konopka JB, Witte ON. Detection of abl tyrosine kinase activity in vitro permits direct comparison of normal and altered *abl* gene products. *Mol Cell Biol* 1985; 5: 3116.

(88) Carr SA, Biemann K, Shoji S et al. N-tetradecanoyl is the NH_2-terminal blocking group of the catalytic subunit of cyclic AMP-dependent protein kinase from bovine cardiac muscle. *Proc Natl Acad Sci USA* 1982; 79: 6128.

(89) Buss JE and Sefton BM. Myristic acid, a rare fatty acid, is the lipid attached to the transforming protein of Rous Sarcoma virus and its cellular homologue. *J Virol* 1985; 53: 7.

(90) Browett PJ, Cooke HMG, Secker-Walker LM, Norton JD. Chromosome 22 breakpoints in variant Philadelphia translocations and Philadelphia-negative chronic myeloid leukemia. *Cancer Genet Cytogenet* 1989; 37: 169.

(91) Gale RP, Canaani E. An 8-kilobase ABL RNA transcript in chronic myelogenous leukemia. *Proc Natl Acad Sci USA* 1984; 81: 5648.

(92) Konopka JB, Watanabe SM, Singer JW et al. Cell lines and clinical isolates derived from Ph¹-positive chronic myelogenous leukemia patients express ABL proteins with a common structural alteration. *Proc Natl Acad Sci USA* 1985; 82: 1810.

(93) Kloetzer W, Kurzrock R, Smith L et al. The human cellular *abl* gene product in the chronic myelogenous leukemia cell line K562 has an associated tyrosine protein kinase activity. *Virology* 1985; 140: 230.

(94) Konopka JB, Watanave SM, Witte ON. An alteration of the human abl protein

in K562 leukemia cells unmasks associated tyrosine kinase activity. *Cell* 1984; 37: 1035.

(95) Kurzrock R, Kloetzer WS, Talpaz M et al. Identification of molecular variants of p210$^{bcr-abl}$ in chronic myelogenous leukemia. *Blood* 1987; 70: 233.

(96) Maxwell SA, Kurzrock R, Parsons SJ et al. Analysis of p210$^{bcr-abl}$ tyrosine protein kinase activity in various subtypes of Philadelphia chromosome positive cells from chronic myelogenous leukemia patients. *Cancer Res* 1987; 47: 1731.

(97) Huhn RD, Posner MR, Rayter SI et al. Cell lines and peripheral blood leukocytes derived from individuals with chronic myelogenous leukemia display virtually identical proteins phosphorylated on tyrosine residues. *Proc Natl Acad Sci USA* 1987; 84: 4408.

(98) McLaughlin J, Chianese E, Witte ON. In vitro transformation of immature hematopoietic cells by the p210 *bcr–abl* oncogene product of the Philadelphia chromosome. *Proc Natl Acad Sci USA* 1987; 84: 6558.

(99) Daley GQ, Baltimore D. Transformation of an interleukin 3-dependent hematopoietic cell line by the chronic myelogenous leukemia-specific p210$^{bcr-abl}$ protein. *Proc Natl Acad Sci USA* 1988; 85: 9312.

(100) ar-Rushdi A, Negrini M, Kurzrock R et al. Fusion of the *bcr* and the c-*abl* genes in Ph-positive acute lymphocytic leukemia with no rearrangement in the breakpoint cluster region. *Oncogene* 1988; 2: 353.

(101) Fainstein E, Marcelle C, Rosner A et al. A new fused transcript in Philadelphia chromosome positive acute lymphocytic leukemia. *Nature* 1987; 330: 386.

(102) van der Feltz MJM, Shivji MKK, Grosveld G, Wiedemann L M. Characterization of the translocation breakpoint in a patient with Philadelphia-positive, bcr-negative acute lymphoblastic leukaemia. *Oncogene* 1988; 3: 215.

(103) Chen SJ, Chen Z, Hillion J et al. Ph^1-positive, bcr-negative acute leukemias: clustering of breakpoints on chromosome 22 in the 3' end of the BCR gene first intron. *Blood* 1989; 73: 1312.

(104) Clark SS, McLaughlin J, Crist WM et al. Unique forms of the abl tyrosine kinase distinguish Ph^1-positive CML form Ph^1-positive ALL. *Science* 1987; 235: 85.

(105) Chan LC, Karhi KK, Rayter SI et al. A novel abl protein expressed in Philadelphia chromosome positive acute lymphoblastic leukemia. *Nature* 1987; 323: 635.

(106) Walker LC, Ganesan TS, Dhut S et al. Novel chimaeric protein expressed in Philadelphia positive acute lymphoblastic leukaemia. *Nature* 1988; 329: 851.

(107) Kurzrock R, Shtalrid M, Gutterman J U et al. Molecular analysis of chromosome 22 breakpoints in Ph-positive acute lymphoblastic leukemia. *Br J Hematol* 1987; 67: 55.

(108) Kurzrock R, Shtalrid M, Talpaz M et al. c-*abl* expression in Philadelphia positive acute myelogenous leukemia. *Blood* 1987; 70: 1584.

(109) Okamura J, Yamada S, Ishi E et al. A novel leukemia cell line, MR-87, with positive Philadelphia chromosome and negative breakpoint cluster region rearrangement coexpressing myeloid and early B-cell markers. *Blood* 1988; 72: 1261.

(110) Lugo TG, Pendergast AM, Muller AJ, Witte ON. Tyrosine kinase activity and

transformation potency of *bcr–abl* oncogene products. *Science* 1990; 247: 1079–82.

(111) Rodenhuis S, Smets LA, Slater RM et al. Distinguishing the Philadelphia chromosome of acute lymphoblastic leukemia from its counterpart in chronic myelogenous leukemia. *N Eng J Med* 1985; 313: 51.

(112) Erikson J, Griffin CA, ar-Rushdi A et al. Heterogeneity of chromosome 22 breakpoints in Philadelphia (Ph$^+$) acute lymphoblastic leukemia. *Proc Natl Acad Sci USA* 1986; 82: 1807.

(113) De Klein A, Hagemeijer A, Bartram CT et al. bcr rearrangement and translocation of the abl oncogene in Philadelphia positive acute lymphoblastic leukemia. *Blood* 1986; 68: 1369.

(114) Morgan GJ, Wiedemann LM, Chan LC, Price CM, Kanfer EJ, Galton DA G. A case of M-bcr-rearranged, Philadelphia-positive AML that relapsed as chronic phase CML. *Blood* 1990; 75: 317–23.

(115) McLaughlin J, Chianese E, Witte ON. Alternative forms of the *bcr–abl* oncogene have quantitatively different potencies for stimulation of immature lymphoid cells. *Mol Cell Biol* 1989; 9: 1866–74.

(116) Turhan AG, Eaves CJ, Kalousek DK et al. Molecular analysis of clonality and bcr rearrangements in Philadelphia chromosome-positive acute lymphoblastic leukemia. *Blood* 1988; 71: 1495.

(117) Romero P, Blick M, Talpaz M et al. c-*sis* and c-*abl* expression in chronic myelogenous leukemia and other hematological malignancies. *Blood* 1986; 67: 839.

(118) Collins SJ, Kubonishi I, Miyoshi I, Groukine M. Altered transcription of the abl oncogene in K562 and other chronic myelogenous leukemia cells. *Science* 1984; 225: 72.

(119) Konopka JB, Clark S, McLaughlin J et al. Variable expression of the translocated *abl* oncogene in Philadelphia-chromosome-positive B-lymphoid cell lines from chronic myelogenous leukemia patients. *Proc Natl Acad Sci USA* 1986; 83: 4049.

(120) Shtivelman E, Gale R, Dreazen O et al. BCR–ABL RNA in patients with chronic myelogenous leukemia. *Blood* 1987; 69: 971.

(121) Bartram CR, de Klein A, Hagemeijer A et al. Additional abl/bcr rearrangements in a CML patient exhibiting two Ph^1 chromosomes during blast crisis. *Leuk Res* 1987; 10: 221.

(122) Heisterkamp N, Jenkins R, Thibodeau S et al. The BCR gene in Philadelphia chromosome positive acute lymphoblastic leukemia. *Blood* 1989; 73: 1307.

(123) Mills KI, MacKenzie ED, Birnie GD. The site of the breakpoint within the bcr is a prognostic factor in Philadelphia-positive CML patients. *Blood* 1988; 72: 1237.

(124) Ogawa H, Sugiyama H, Soma T et al. No correlation between locations of bcr breakpoints and clinical states in Ph^1-positive CML patients. *Leukemia* 1989; 3: 492.

(125) Przepiorka D. Breakpoint zone of bcr in chronic myelogenous leukemia does not correlate with disease phase or prognosis. *Cancer Genet Cytogenet* 1988; 36: 117.

(126) Birnie GD, Mills KI, Benn P. Does the site of the breakpoint on chromosome 22 influence the duration of the chronic phase in chronic myeloid leukemia? *Leukemia* 1989; 3: 545–7.

(127) Lee M-S, LeMaistre A, Kantarjian HM et al. Detection of two alternative bcr-abl mRNA junctions and minimal residual disease in Philadelphia chromosome positive chronic myelogenous leukemia by polymerase chain reaction. *Blood* 1989; 73: 2165.

(128) Lange W, Synder DS, Castro R et al. Detection by enzymatic amplification of bcr–abl mRNA in peripheral blood and bone marrow cells of patients with chronic myelogenous leukemia. *Blood* 1989; 73: 1735.

(129) Bartram CR, Jannsen JWG, Becher R et al. Persistence of chronic myelocytic leukemia despite deletion of rearranged bcr–abl sequences in blast crisis. *J Exp Med* 1986; 164: 1389.

(130) Eisbruch A, Blick M, Evinger-Hodges MJ et al. Effect of differentiation-inducing agents on oncogene expression in a chronic myelogenous leukemia cell line. *Cancer* 1988; 62: 1171.

(131) Young JC, Witte ON. Selective transformation of primitive lymphoid cells by the *bcr–abl* oncogene expressed in long-term lymphoid or myeloid cultures. *Mol Cell Biol* 1988; 8: 4079–87.

(132) LeMaistre A, Lee M-S, Talpaz M et al. *ras* oncogene mutations are rare late stage events in chronic myelogenous leukemia. *Blood* 1989; 73: 889.

(133) Collins SJ, Howard M, Andrews DF et al. Rare occurrence of n-*ras* point mutations in Philadelphia chromosome positive chronic myeloid leukemia. *Blood* 1989; 73: 1028.

(134) Ahuja H, Bar-Eli M, Clarke P et al. p53 gene alterations in blast crisis of chronic myelogenous leukemia. *Cancer Cells* 1989; 7: 117.

(135) Mashal R, Shtalrid M, Talpaz M et al. Rearrangement and expression of p53 in the chronic phase and blast crisis of chronic myelogenous leukemia. *Blood* 1990; 75: 180–9.

(136) Blick M, Romero P, Talpaz M et al. Molecular characteristics of chronic myelogenous leukemia in blast crisis. *Cancer Genet Cytogenet* 1987; 27: 349.

(137) McCarthy DM, Goldman JM, Rassool FV et al. Genomic alterations involving the MYC proto oncogene locus during the evolution of a case of chronic granulocytic leukemia. *Lancet* 1984; ii: 1362.

(138) Ezdinli EZ, Sokal JE, Crosswhite L, Sandberh AA. Philadelphia chromosome-positive and negative chronic myelocytic leukemia. *Ann Intern Med* 1970; 72: 175.

(139) Mintz U, Varkiman J, Golomb HM, Rowley JD. Evolution of karyotypes in Philadelphia (Ph¹) chromosome-negative chronic myelogenous leukemia. *Cancer* 1979; 43: 411.

(140) Lewis JP, Watson-Williams EJ, Lazerson J, Jenks HM. Chronic myelogenous leukemia and genetic events at 9q34. *Hematol Oncol* 1983; 1: 269.

(141) Travis LB, Pierre RV, DeWald GW. Ph¹-negative chronic granulocytic leukemia: a nonentity. *Am J Clin Pathol* 1986; 85: 186.

(142) Pugh WC, Pearson M, Vardiman JW, Rowley JD. Philadelphia chromosome-negative chronic myelogenous leukemia: a morphological reassessment. *Br J Haematol* 1985; 60: 457.

(143) Shtalrid M, Talpaz M, Blick M, Kurzrock R. Philadelphia-negative chronic myelogenous leukemia with breakpoint cluster region rearrangement: molecular analysis, clinical characteristics, and response to therapy. *J Clin Oncol* 1988; 6: 1569.

(144) Kurzrock R, Kantarjian HM, Shtalrid M, Gutterman JU, Talpaz M. Philadelphia chromosome-negative chronic myelogenous leukemia without breakpoint cluster region rearrangement: A chronic myeloid leukemia with a distinct clinical course. *Blood* 1990; 75: 445–52.

(145) Bartram CR, Kleihauer E, de Klein A et al. *abl* and *bcr* are rearranged in a Ph-negative CML patient. *EMBO J* 1985; 4: 683.

(146) Kurzrock R, Blick MB, Talpaz M et al. Rearrangement in the breakpoint cluster region and the clinical course in Philadelphia-negative chronic myelogenous leukemia. *Ann Int Med* 1986; 105: 673.

(147) Morris CM, Reeve AE, Fitzgerald PH et al. Genomic diversity correlates with clinical variation in Ph[1]-negative chronic myeloid leukaemia. *Nature* 1986; 320: 281.

(148) Bartram CR. bcr rearrangement without juxtaposition of abl in chronic myelocytic leukemia. *J Exp Med* 1985; 162: 2175.

(149) Dreazen O, Rassol F, Sparkes R et al. Do oncogenes determine clinical features in chronic myeloid leukemia? *Lancet* 1987; i: 1402.

(150) Wiedemann LM, Karhi KK, Shivji MKK et al. The correlation of breakpoint cluster region rearrangement and p210[phl/abl] expression with morphological analysis of Ph-negative chronic myeloid leukemia and other myeloproliferative disorders. *Blood* 1988; 71: 349.

(151) Melani C, Canepa L, Sessarego M et al. Molecular analysis of the bcr rearrangement in a case of Ph-negative blastic crisis of Ph-positive chronic myelogenous leukemia. *Eur J Haematol* 1989; 42: 32.

(152) Stoll DB, Peterson P, Exten R et al. Clinical presentation and natural history of patients with essential thrombocythemia and the Philadelphia chromosome. *Am J Hematol* 1988; 27: 77.

(153) Palumbo AP, Boccadoro M, Battaglio S et al. Philadelphia-positive thrombocythemia with a complex translocation involving chromosomes 9, 15, and 22. *Cancer Genet Cytogenet* 1989; 39: 77.

(154) Morris CM, Fitzgerald PH, Hollings PE et al. Essential thrombocythaemia and the Philadelphia chromosome. *Br J Haematol* 1988; 70: 13.

(155) Pearson MG, Vardiman JW, LeBeau MM et al. Increased numbers of marrow basophils may be associated with a t(6;9) in ANLL. *Am J Hematol* 1985; 18: 393.

(156) Westbrook CA, LeBeau MM, Diaz MO et al. Chromosomal localization and characterization of c-abl in the t(6;9) of acute nonlymphocytic leukemia. *Proc Natl Acad Sci USA* 1985; 82: 8742.

(157) Westbrook CA, Rubin CM, LeBeau MM et al. Molecular analysis of tcr-β and abl in a t(7;9)-containing cell line (sup-T3) from a human T-cell leukemia. *Proc Natl Acad Sci USA* 1987; 84: 251.

(158) Morris CM, Rosman I, Archer SA et al. A cytogenetic and molecular analysis of five variant Philadelphia translocations in chronic myeloid leukemia. *Cancer Genet Cytogenet* 1988; 35: 179.

(159) Dow LW, Tachibana N, Raimondi SC et al. Comparative biochemical and cytogenetic studies of childhood acute lymphoblastic leukemia with the Philadelphia chromosome and other 22q11 variants. *Blood* 1989; 73: 1291.

(160) Gabert J, Lafage M, Maraninchi D et al. Detection of residual bcr–abl translocation by polymerase chain reaction in chronic myeloid leukemia patients after bone-marrow transplantation. *Lancet* 1989; ii: 1125–8.

(161) Kawasaki ES, Clark SS, Coyne MY et al. Diagnosis of chronic myeloid and acute lymphocytic leukemias by detection of leukemia-specific mRNA sequences amplified in vitro. *Proc Natl Acad Sci USA* 1988; 85: 5698.

(162) Dobrovic A, Trainor KJ, Morley AA. Detection of the molecular abnormality in chronic myeloid leukemia by use of the polymerase chain reaction. *Blood* 1988; 72: 2063–5.

(163) Romero P, Beran M, Shtalrid M, Andersson B, Talpaz M, Blick M. Alternative 5′ end of the *bcr–abl* transcript in chronic myelogenous leukemia. *Oncogene* 1989; 4: 93–8.

Treatment options for remission in acute myeloid leukaemia

A K BURNETT and B LÖWENBERG

Introduction

There has been steady progress over the last two decades in the treatment of acute myeloid leukaemia (AML). Few would not subscribe to the view nowadays that all patients, with the possible exception of the very elderly, should be offered treatment.[1] The combination of an anthracycline with cytosine arabinoside in differing schedules, has steadily increased the rate of remission in young patients to 65 – 80%.[2-6] Such figures are not merely achieved in single leukaemia centres but are now reported from large multi-centre trial experience.[6,7] An important component in this progress has been the improvement in supportive care. Blood product support, improved anti-biotics, nursing expertise, means of reliable venous access and a better under-standing of the problems of neutropenia, have brought patients more consistently through the required period of pancytopenia. Approximately 15% of patients fail to enter remission because of resistant disease.[5,7] In the older patient, the rate of remission is still inadequate (40–50%), and the reasons for failure are primarily those of the reduced tolerance of older patients to the toxicity of intensive chemotherapy.[8]

For the patients who enter complete remission, the challenge in the last few years has been to develop strategies of maintenance of the remission into the long term, to what could operationally be called 'cure'. It is the purpose of the review to examine the options available to such patients. It should be stated first, that the focus is primarily on the younger patient (<55 years). While this represents the largest group of patients entering remission, more than half the patients presenting with the disease are over this age.

Quality of complete remission

Extrapolation from experimental data suggests that clinically apparent relapse occurs with a body load of 10^{12} leukaemic cells, ie approximately 1 kg of

All correspondence to: A K Burnett, Department of Haematology, Glasgow Royal Infirmary, Castle Street, Glasgow G4 0SF, UK.

Cambridge Medical Reviews: Haematological Oncology Volume 1

leukaemia. As cytoreductive therapy takes effect this burden becomes undetectable by conventional microscopy, with the consequence that bone marrow function returns. This may still, however, happen with a body load of 10^{10} leukaemic cells. This highlights the first problem – how best to define remission. Agreed criteria, including less than 5% marrow blasts and normal peripheral blood counts, are conventionally accepted,[9] but, given the insensitivity of morphological diagnosis, cytological remission may reflect states of greatly differing residual leukaemia masses. Thus new techniques are obviously required to provide more precision to classify remissions below the threshold of 10^{10} residual cells.

Assessment of post-remission therapy is bound to be influenced by the efficacy of remission induction therapy and the quality of the resulting remission. If two regimens achieve the same remission percentage, as judged by conventional criteria, the cytoreduction could be consideraly greater in one, than in the other, this could alter the pattern of relapse. Evidence that this may be the case can be found in the United Kingdom MRC AML 8 Trial where two induction schedules (DAT 3+10 VS DAT 5+2) resulted in very similar remission rates, albeit the DAT 5+2 cohort more often required a second pulse, with a longer hospital stay. There later appears, however, to be an increased duration of remission in the more intensively treated group (DAT 3+10).[10] The remission rate may also influence the outcome of post remission therapy in another way. If the rate of remission is relatively low, then it is conceivable that this includes the cases with the most responsive disease, whereas the more 'resistant' cases are excluded. Conversely where higher remission rates are achieved, the larger the proportion of 'more difficult' cases are in remission to be coped with by the post-remission modality. In the light of these arguments, it is obviously difficult to make comparisons between one post-remission treatment and another. Techniques for more accurate quantitative assessment of remission status are a current priority.

The options for post-remission treatment in AML
In giving advice to a patient who has entered remission, a number of questions arise. Should the patient have further chemotherapy only? Should the patient have a bone marrow transplant? If a transplant is considered, is an allogeneic donor preferable to the use of autologous marrow? Does the donor need to be a fully matched sibling? Should the transplant be used in first remission or should it be held in reserve to be applied in second remission, or as the only treatment of relapse? Does post-remission chemotherapy improve the outcome of a transplant? Are there variables in the patient which might suggest that they are more or less suitable to one option rather than to another?

Chemotherapy

Post-remission chemotherapy means either consolidation which could be defined as therapy of sufficient intensity to cause cytopenia – therefore requiring in-patient management, or maintenance, ie treatment given at a frequency or dosage not likely to produce cytopenia, and therefore compatible with out patient therapy, or both.[11]

The possibility exists that, for some patients, modern intensive induction therapy is sufficient treatment in itself, in that the disease is sufficiently sensitive, that the cytoreduction is already fully effective.

One report supports such an idea,[12] but these ultra-responsive patients are not able to be identified by any known prognostic marker. Such randomized trial data as is available clearly points to the desirability of further therapy post-remission. Maintenance chemotherapy is of no, or limited, additional value if at least two post-remission courses of sufficient intensity are applied.[8,13–16] Thus, in this setting, there is no evidence to support the use of further maintenance treatment. When prior therapy has been more gentle, it is possible to demonstrate benefit in maintenance.[17]

The current attitude to post-remission therapy is to favour aggressive, but limited, courses of therapy. The value of aggressive post-remission treatment was demonstrated in the VAPA protocols in adults and children.[18–20] Other studies also suggest benefit in post-induction intensification,[21,22] but, while the median duration of remission tends to improve, it remains to be convincingly shown that this benefit is durable in the 5–10 year term.

There is no clear evidence as to which drugs are most effective at this stage. The use of cytosine–arabinoside in high dose effectively makes it a different drug, and encouraging results have been shown with its use, resulting in five-year remission durations of around 40%.[23] It should be pointed out that these results are not from controlled studies and may be influenced by the accrual of comparatively better risk individuals who have remained in remission sufficiently long to receive high dose treatment, with a favourable influence on outcome. It would be logical to include different drugs in post-remission schedules, of known value in relapsed or refractory AML, for example, amsacrine, etoposide and possibly mitoxantrone.[24,25] Although it is possible that the use of such agents will contribute to survival, these regimens require to be evaluated in comparative studies.

In general, modern chemotherapy offers patients approximately a 25% chance of remaining in remission at five years, by this time, unfortunately, the risk of relapse is not excluded, but is very small. Patients continue to relapse for a further 2 to 3 years, after which relapses are rare.[26] Around this average there may be cohorts of patients who do less badly, for whom it might be reasonable to be a little more optimistic. It should be recognized that such prognostic factors are derived retrospectively from individual protocols of treatment, and may not apply to the same extent to more modern intensive schedules.

Prognostic factors in AML The French–American–British (FAB) morphological classification of AML has been useful in creating a common vocabulary within the subtypes of disease,[27] but the value prognostically has been less convincing. The M2 and M3 subtypes tend to have longer durations of remission while M4, M5 and M6 do less well.[28,29] As will be mentioned later, this pattern of response tends to carry through to autologous or allogeneic transplantation as well.

In recent years, cytogenetic abnormalities have also fallen into patterns which have a general prognostic association, sometimes linked to the FAB subtype.[30,31] For instance, t(15;17), t(8;21) and inversion(16) abnormalities are especially seen in M3, M2 and M4 (with abnormal eosinophils) leukaemias. The t(9;11) or 11q- karyotype is usually associated with M4 or M5 subtypes of AML. Cytogenetic parameters probably have the strongest prognostic significance for treatment outcome in patients with AML, ie both as regards the ability to attain complete remission and the duration of remission and survival. For instance, patients with t(8;21) or inv(16) AML have a greater likelihood of achieving remission.[32–34] Chromosome 16 (del16q 22; inv (16)) abnormalities, and t (15;17) AMLs have a favourable prognosis for survival, 45, XY-Y an intermediate prognosis, and abnormal chromosomes 5 or 7 and Philadelphia positive AMLs the worst prognosis.[33–35] Since these conclusions have been reproduced in different studies irrespective of differences in therapy, they probably represent differences in the biology of AML which are reflected in treatment outcome.

In examining a large number of cases within the UK, MRC and the EORTC Leukaemia Group Trials, age and condition at diagnosis were found to be the major predictors of induction outcome.[7,28] In general, the leukaemias which showed more evidence of myeloid differentiation had higher remission rates, but morphological features did not correlate with the duration of remission.[5,8] While older patients are less likely to achieve remission, in most studies, age does not predict for remission duration.[2,5,16] However patients achieving remission within 1 month generally have significantly longer remissions.[5,8]

Immunophenotyping has become a valuable diagnostic tool in recent years, adding objectivity and precision to the initial classification. In general, it can be expected to identify morphologically unclassifiable cases of AML and bilineage acute leukaemia. The abnormalities of maturation of AML may be evident, not only as an arrest of maturation, but also as maturation asynchrony. The latter condition is apparent as the expression of unusual combinations of surface markers on the AML blasts. The prognostic significance of maturation asynchrony for treatment outcome is not yet known.

Immunophenotyping of AML may also be directed towards AML progenitor cells. It appears that AML clonogenic cells represent a comparatively immature subset among the leukaemic mass. These cells may exhibit maturation antigens in abnormal densities on their surface, or in abnormal configuration as compared to their normal counterparts. This finding indicates that maturation asynchrony also involves the progenitor cell compartment of human AML.[36-38]

As will be discussed later, careful analysis of the immunophenotype of AML has revealed that some cases have inappropriate co-expression of surface proteins identifiable by monoclonal antibodies, recognizing either lymphoid or myeloid antigens, or antigens usually only expressed early or late in normal myeloid lineage development. The prognostic significance of these findings on remission induction or duration is not yet clear.

Nature of remission The most obvious interpretation of remission is that the disease is at a stage beyond current levels of detection. This could still represent a considerable number of cells, eg between 1 cell to 1×10^{10} cells, but, as was discussed before, there is, at present, no way of knowing, due to the lack of sufficiently sensitive detection techniques. However, recently, methods have become available which may bring more precision to current understanding of remission status.

It has recently been realized that AML blasts can abnormally co-express normal antigens which can be detected at single cell level by modern flow cytometry.[39,40] While HLA-DR, CD33, and CD15 all appear in normal myeloid development, co-expression of HLA-DR and CD15 is an abnormal phenotype, similarly CD33 and Tdt, and CD33 with CD7 are useful combinations which can be used to detect cells with a leukaemic phenotype at a low level, eg 1 in 10 000 cells. The potential insight which such techniques offer into the nature of remission has been reported for ALL, where detection of occult blast cells predicted subsequent relapse.

Such phenotypes are potentially available in about 60% of AML patients, but the significance of detecting, or not, such unique cells in what is regarded as a remission marrow, is not yet known.

The nature of remission may be more subtle, and the importance of finding or not finding minimal residual disease present during remission by sophisticated techniques, will take some time to elucidate. It was suggested some time ago[41] that leukaemia in remission might merely be in a phase where it regains the capacity to differentiate apparently normally, until a further genetic event restores its proliferative advantage. This would be analogous to the chronic phase of chronic myeloid leukaemia.

It has similarly been assumed that successful eradication of the bulk of the leukaemic clone would permit re-emergence of normal haemopoiesis. This has been demonstrated to be not always the case. Using markers related to the

X chromosome in females heterozygous for the particular marker, either G6PD (glucose-6-phosphate dehydrogenase) or HPRT (hypoxanthine phosphoribosyl transferase), it has been shown that, in some cases, remission cells are derived from a single clone, assumed to be that of the original leukaemia.[42,43] This may be consistent with the onset of AML in a multi-step process and the reversal of the disease to an earlier evolutionary phase. This suggests that this is not true remission, which should be polyclonal, but an altered, possibly preleukaemic, state of the disease. Again, the implications of such findings for clinical outcome is not yet known, but are under study.

Insight into the nature of AML itself, using such assessments, may provide crucial information relating to the possibility of treatment being effective. In a series of 27 patients presenting with AML who were heterozygotes for G-6-PD, the disease was either of type A or type B enzyme phenotype.[44] On examining the apparently unaffected lineages, it was noted that in 6 cases apparently involved haemopoietic lineages were of that enzyme type, suggesting that, in these cases, the disease originated at stem cell level. In the other cases the remaining haemopoiesis was expressing appropriate heterozygosity – suggesting that the cell of origin of the leukaemia was restricted to within the myeloid lineage. Since G-6-PD heterozygotes with AML are rare, it has not been possible to study this finding in a large number of patients, but newer techniques now permit this. The clinical implications are similarly unclear, but it is of interest to note from these studies that there was a tendency for younger patients to have lineage restricted disease, whereas the multi-lineage patients tended to be elderly. This may be one of the factors which relate to the better outcome in younger people.

Bone marrow transplantation

While there will continue to be argument about what proportion of patients can be cured by chemotherapy, it is sufficiently low to be regarded as unsatisfactory. Allogeneic bone marrow transplantation has been widely used as an alternative for the past decade following the initial reports of its apparent advantage.[45–47]

It is worth remembering that one of the original concepts behind the use of BMT in haematological malignancy was to exploit a possible graft-versus-leukaemia (GVL) effect mediated by the graft.[48] The myeloablation was principally arrived at as that which would reliably permit engraftment[49] not for any known antileukaemic effect. Indeed, very early experience of twin transplantation in relapsed disease suggested that higher doses of total body irradiation alone could not control the disease at this stage.[50] It remains a matter of current controversy what component of the antileukaemic effect is due to the myeloablative protocol, and what is due to a putative GVL effect.

In general, it has been exceptional to find a major difference in the rates of relapse after transplant despite a wide variety of conditioning protocols, which suggests that the high dose treatment could conceivably have a minimal effect beyond ensuring engraftment.[51] Although the evidence is circumstantial, it is probable that a GVL effect does have an important role in curing leukaemia after transplant. The most obvious supportive evidence is the difference in relapse probability between a syngeneic (50–60%) and a T replete allograft (20%).[52] There has been evidence of a direct relationship between the severity of GVHD and the probability of remaining in remission.[53,54] Similarly, where there is no evidence of GVHD, the risk of relapse is the same as that in twins. As will be discussed below, removal to T lymphocytes from the graft to prevent GVHD has also resulted in higher relapse rates in some series.

Allogeneic BMT from an HLA identical MLC non-reactive sibling donor has an 80% chance of eradicating the disease apparently permanently.[55-58] This dramatic potential benefit is substantially curtailed by a number of factors. First, there is only a 1 in 4 chance of any one sibling matching acceptably – in practice the likelihood of finding a suitable donor is 1 in 3. Second, about 30% of patients transplanted die for reasons other than leukaemic relapse, such as pneumonitis and graft-versus-host disease, and these factors tend to increase with age. Most centres, therefore, limit allograft availability to patients under 45 years. These restrictions mean that only about 10% of all patients with AML can be treated this way, of whom half are cured.

Considerable effort has been directed in the last few years, towards trying to eradicate the major causes of transplant related death, namely pneumonitis and graft-versus-host disease.

Pneumonitis Historically at least, as many as 25% of patients undergoing allogeneic BMT developed pneumonitis which was fatal in about half the patients.[59] Approximately half the patients developed cytomegalovirus (CMV) pneumonitis, which was often associated with GVHD as a precipitating factor.[60,61] There is, however, a range of risk – some of which can be acted on – depending on the immunity of the patient and donor with respect to CMV.

CMV status of patient and recipient Cytomegalovirus (CMV) infection particularly pneumonitis has been a major cause of death after allograft. The potential sources of infection are either reactivation of latent virus in those previously exposed (ie seropositive, defined as a titre of > 1 in 4) or transfer in the bone marrow of the donor or in the multiple blood product support. The probability of a seropositive individual developing CMV infection, ie becoming culture positive from throat or urine, is high – probably at least 70%.[62] In this respect there is little difference between an allograft and an autograft, although in the latter there is much less information available. From limited observations we and others have found that, although seropositive autograft recipients excrete virus, they seldom develop CMV disease.[63,64] This difference may result from the considerable immunodeficiency that is especially pronounced after allografting, and is relatively less profound in autograft recipients.

The seropositive patient In a seropositive patient, prevention of CMV disease rests in minimizing the factors that may convert CMV infection to disease. The most important predisposing factor is the presence and severity of acute GVHD.[62] Effective prevention of GVHD may avoid protracted immunosuppression and associated tissue damage, or mechanisms capable of directly reactivating latent CMV.[65] The status of the donor may be influential. Theoretically, immune reconstitution with marrow from a seropositive donor will protect the seropositive host from the dangers of CMV reactivation more effectively than a CMV negative donor marrow, which may be naive to CMV infection. The evidence to support this is conflicting. There appears to be little impact of donor status in the Seattle experience where reactivation (infection) was 70% irrespective of donor status.[62] What may determine whether patients develop pneumonia may be the presence of GVHD. Where the donor marrow has been T-cell depleted, the risk is probably less, but this is not absolutely clear. In addition, the donor status does appear to be important in the context of T-cell depletion,[66] where a seropositive marrow may have a protective influence against pneumonitis (15% disease) compared with a seronegative donor (60% disease) but not on the incidence of reactivation. Other less obvious factors have also been identified as risk factors such as single fraction total body irradiation (TBI), patient age, and prior exposure to chemotherapy agents in addition to cyclophosphamide.

Prevention of CMV pneumonia Apart from the possibility of reliably preventing GVHD, room for manoeuvre in avoiding the defined risk factors in the CMV positive patient, is limited. The mortality of established CMV pneumonitis is in excess of 80%.

Prophylaxis would appear to offer the only immediate hope for the high risk seropositive patient. High titre immunoglobulin therapy has proved to be of little benefit.[67–70] Interferon appears to be effective against some CMV strains.[71] High dose acyclovir has also been reported to be effective, if given in the first month post-transplant, in reducing CMV infection and disease. This benefit appears to favourably influence survival.[72]

More recent experience with the acyclovir derivative ganciclovir appears to offer promise.[73] In the treatment of established disease, marrow suppression can be expected. Another alternative is foscarnet which appears to be less myelosuppressive[74] but is less effective in limited studies.

The seronegative patient There is now convincing data to suggest a clear benefit to the CMV negative patient by providing exclusively CMV negative products post-transplant, particularly if the donor is CMV negative.[63,75] Whether CMV negative products are mandatory in the context of a positive donor is less clear, but this may depend on whether the marrow is fractionated over ficoll-hypague and T-cell depleted (thus perhaps removing antigenic burden) or not.[76] In the Seattle experience, in non-T depleted marrows, negative products did not confer advantage to the negative recipient if the donor marrow was positive.[62]

Graft-versus-host disease

This complication, mediated by a subset of T-cells in the donor's marrow, remains a major risk with a possibility of being directly fatal of about 10%.[77] It is also a major cause of morbidity and immunosuppression and may indirectly contribute to other causes of death such as pneumonitis or infection.

Prevention of graft versus host disease Should T-cells be removed from the donors' marrow? It has become increasingly clear that T-cells in the graft itself make a positive contribution to securing engraftment and preventing leukaemic relapse.

It was a widespread initial experience that removal of T-cells in the absence of any other alteration to standard conditioning protocols resulted in graft failure in up to 20% of cases[78–80] – a rare complication in T replete grafts. Even in patients in whom engraftment was achieved, there has been noted to be a high incidence of mixed chimerism of haemopoiesis of donor and host cells post-transplant.[81] These two observations suggest that some compensatory increase in the conditioning protocol is an essential component of the T-cell depletion technique. We have reported that successful engraftment can be achieved by adding an extra 200 cGy fraction to the radiation regimen, without any increased toxicity.[82] Detailed on-going studies suggest that, even with an increased conditioning protocol that effectively secures engraftment, mixed chimeras are still regularly observed. It is generally accepted that T-cell depletion is highly effective in preventing significant GVHD with the associated advantages of reducing the risk of protracted immunosuppression.[83,84]

There is strong circumstantial evidence to confirm that an 'allogeneic effect', in addition to the cytoreductive effect of the conditioning protocol, is an important component of cure by allograft, it seems likely that this has to be accompanied by clinically significant GVHD. The evidence derives from three aspects. Although the total experience is small, it appears clear that the relapse rate following syngeneic BMT is twice that for recipients of T-cell replete allografts.[52] It was originally pointed out by the Seattle group that, in a heterogeneous risk group of leukaemias, there was a higher statistical probability of remaining in remission the more severe the graft-versus-host disease.[85] For patients with no clinically apparent GVHD, the relapse rate was similar to that seen in twins, confirming the suspicion that graft-versus-host and graft-versus-leukaemia are not separable in man.

There is little doubt that T-cell depletion substantially increases the relapse rate in chronic myeloid leukaemia whether that is defined, haematologically, cytogentically or by very sensitive molecular genetic techniques.[86] The evidence for such an effect in AML in first remission is less clear-cut. In some single centre series, this is apparently not the case but in others relapse is increased.[87-89] Even if there is an increased rate of relapse, this may be compensated for by lower morbidity and reduction in other causes of death. In most individual series, survival is not reduced by T-cell depletion – particularly when graft failure is eliminated by modification of the conditioning protocol.

It is likely that, even when the donor and host pairs are matched at the major loci, and have a negative MLC reaction, they have different levels of risk for GVHD.[90] In the absence of T-cell depletion, GVHD will not develop in 50% of patients. If these patients could somehow be identified in advance, those who would benefit from T-cell depletion could electively receive it. Retrospective analysis of large series can identify factors which positively correlate with increased risk.[91] The most significant predictor of GVHD is if the patient is male and the donor is female, with the risk being more marked if the female had been pregnant or transfused. Risk has usually been assumed to increase with patient age, but, when the female donor factor is removed, increasing age is not a strong predictor.

These factors are not sufficiently reliable to form the basis of policy for each patient. Individually orientated in vitro techniques have been reported which appear promising but require wider confirmation.[92]

It is conceivable that T-cell depletion is only effective in patients with minimal residual disease. In T-replete allografts there is little evidence to suggest that the duration of remission pre-transplant, or the amount of post-remission chemotherapy prior to transplant has any important effect on the outcome of the allograft.

It may be that the heterogeneity of results obtained with T-cell depletion may be related to differences in prior chemotherapy, which, in this context, might be crucial. Chronic phase CML is equivalent to bulk disease and, as clinically now apparent, T-depletion appears to reduce the chances of cure – albeit not as yet of survival. No data are available in AML to clarify this point but this may come to light in the current UK Medical Research Council's trial (which will be referred to later).

It has been suggested that regeneration of cytotoxic T-cells post-transplant may be a component of the antileukaemic effect. These have been demonstrated in recipients of T-depleted grafts and indeed of autografts. In these cells can be shown to kill autologous blast cells.[93]

Because of the problems associated with T-cell depletion, there rem considerable incentive to use alternatives. Cyclosporin with 4 doses of methotrexate (short methotrexate) has proved effective in chronic myeloid leukaemia and is associated with excellent survival but it is of less convincing benefit in AML.[94,95]

Despite the introduction of these modifications to the transplant technique, there is little data to suggest that there has been any substantial improvement in the survival reported a decade ago. T-cell depletion undoubtedly reduces the associated morbidity, but the problems of rejection and relapse may outweigh any benefit. Since rejection can be avoided, it remains to be seen whether it will, in due course, turn out to have been an advance also in terms of survival.

Prognostic factors for allogeneic BMT in AML There are poor prognostic subgroups which can now be identified. In the joint European experience, the FAB subtypes M4 and M5 had an increased relapse rate and survived less well than other types.[58] This reflected the experience of the Minnesota Team.[96]

In the European and International Bone Marrow Transplant Registries in which there is some overlap of patients – age is important. Patients under 20 years have a good prognosis. In children, of course, chemotherapy has a better 5 year outcome than in adults, but this should not deter children – apart from the very young – from allograft for which the results in that group are superior to any alternative. Although most transplant teams restrict the option in first remission to patients under 45, those in the fourth decade do not do less well, and apparently no better, than those remaining on chemotherapy. Precise application of the upper age limit can be difficult and is influenced by other factors such as CMV status, or possibly FAB type. Not undertaking the transplant in first remission or performing an autograft are other choices to which there is no clear answer in this age group. While cytogenetic factors are important predictors of outcome of conventional therapy in AML, data are not yet available to judge how they predict for outcome after transplantation.

Timing of allogeneic transplant It is not infrequent for patients to relapse from first remission while awaiting admission to a transplant unit. This raises the question of how selected the patients actually being transplanted are. It may be that, while the probability of preventing leukaemia is substantially superior following a transplant, the overall survival advantage may not be so dramatic. There are surprisingly few prospective studies of BMT versus chemotherapy that have been conducted from diagnosis, or analysed on an 'intention to treat' basis. Such data as are available are open to criticism, but tend to show an advantage for the transplanted cohorts.[97–100]

For patients who have relapsed, the first decision to be made is whether reinduction should be attempted. As will be illustrated later, achievement of a second remission is far from a foregone conclusion, and largely depends on the duration of the first remission and whether relapse occurred on, or off, chemotherapy. As will also be illustrated later, only a minority (10%) of patients in second remission will be alive after another 3–4 years if treated only by chemotherapy. The European and International Registry data both indicate that an allograft in second remission will salvage about 30% of cases. This, it should be pointed out, is 30% patients undergoing transplant, presumably several patients who relapsed failed to survive until, or were not considered fit for, transplant.

The Seattle Team have shown that the overall outcome of transplanting patients who relapse, without attempting to achieve a further remission, is not different from what they observe in patients in second remission.[101] Since the possibility of achieving a second remission is unpredictable, this would suggest that patients should be electively transplanted in relapse, without attempting chemotherapy. These results of transplantation of relapse have not yet been confirmed in subsequent studies, so to use such data to devise an argument that only relapsed patients should be transplanted for AML is probably premature. The basis of such a proposition is that 30% of patients are cured by first line chemotherapy and transplanted unnecessarily in first remission. If 25–30% of those who relapse can be salvaged by an allograft then around 55–60% of patients can be cured. Another weakness of this argument is that only the occasional chemotherapy series has a 30% 5 year survival, this is not the norm.

Autologous bone marrow transplantation

The majority of patients, under 60 years, who enter remission of disease have no allograft option available to them. For them the only alternative to chemotherapy to be considered is autologous transplantation (ABMT).

The fact that remission bone marrow from leukaemic patients could be used to restore haemopoietic function after myeloablative therapy, was demonstrated by the Houston group in the late 1970s.[102] The approach was to harvest remission marrow for use when relapse occurred. This strategy met with limited long-term success, because, although further remissions were successfully induced, they were not durable. It was not possible to say whether relapse was due to inadequate ablation, or as a result of contamination of the autograft itself. The former explanation would seem highly likely since even an allograft in this situation, with its potential GVL advantages (discussed below), was rarely successful at this advanced stage of the disease.

In analogy with the experience with allogeneic BMT, such an approach with autograft was much more likely to be successful if undertaken at an earlier stage of the disease.

The patient group who would clearly be autograft candidates would include the 2 out of 3 for whom a matched donor could not be found. It was, however, clear from experience of twins receiving myeloablation treatment including TBI, for a variety of haematological malignancies, that the myeloablative protocol was well tolerated in older patients[103] – beyond the age usually accepted for allograft. Initial clinical studies of autograft arbitrarily have set the upper age limit at 60 years.

As well as the potential benefits, there were recognized to be conceptual disadvantages. The ultimate outcome would depend on whether the theoretical disadvantages would cancel out the potential benefits. These currently remain areas of argument in relation to autologous bone marrow transplantation for leukaemia. First, it was thought that the autograft would permit the use of marrow ablative doses of chemotherapy and radiotherapy, thus resulting in a greater therapeutic efficacy than could be achieved with conventional treatment. While this is the main rationale for the development of autologous BMT, it may be too simplistic to attribute the apparent antileukaemic effect to the myeloablative protocol itself. The extreme point of view suggests that the myeloablation in allogeneic bone marrow transplantation makes little contribution, other than securing engraftment, which then facilitates a graft-versus-leukaemia (GVL) effect. There is little convincing evidence that alteration of the preparative protocol reduces subsequent relapse risk, suggesting that, indeed, while there is a certain minimum requirement, dose escalation or addition of other agents is not convincingly beneficial, despite claims made for protocols evaluated in relative small series. This could imply that these intensive schedules of cytotoxic therapy are not very active, or it could indicate that the tested variations of scheduling at this dose level did not add significantly to the power of the original regimens. In a rare randomized study, however, a relationship between TBI dose and relapse has been shown.[104] A similar benefit was demonstrated in a non-randomized retrospective study, where there was variation in the TBI dose.[105]

Somewhat more substantial data derives from the reported association between grade and severity of acute and chronic GVHD and predicted relapse risk in acute leukaemia. This is not conclusively demonstrated for AML in first remission, but there does appear to be an antileukaemia effect in AML associated with chronic GVHD.[106,107] It is of interest to note that, while the overall risk of relapse is around 20%, it is more than double that if the allograft is not associated with either acute or chronic GVHD. In other words, a GVL effect if expressed only occurs in association with GVHD.

Twins transplanted in first remission with syngeneic marrow have experienced relapse in at least 50% of cases.[52] Taken in conjunction with the results of T-cell depletion referred to above, there is therefore strong circumstantial evidence to suggest that the absence of GVHD in the autograft setting will result in a prospect of eradicating residual leukaemia in no more than 50% of cases. Since the overall aim is to produce more survivors from the disease, the outcome will depend on the balance of the negative factors and the potential advantages discussed above.

First, as previously discussed, the intensity of remission induction therapy will influence the level of cytoreduction achieved, even though the proportion of patients achieving remission is not different. Secondly, some further post-remission therapy can be expected to achieve further cytoreduction. Time deliberately spent at this stage will have the benefit not only of reducing the amount of occult disease in the patient, but also in the harvested marrow. The disadvantages of delay and further treatment at this point are that there is a risk of intercurrent relapse anyway, and further treatment may damage the repopulative potential of the marrow. Thirdly, there is clearly no reason to return more marrow than is needed for regeneration. There has been substantial variation in the harvest dose targets set by individual groups and based on preclinical investigations in monkeys, the minimum requirements for an autograft would be 1×10^7 nucleated cells per kilogram of body weight. In man, the minimum cell number required is unknown but extrapolation from the results in subhuman primates, and taking account of the compromised repopulation of haematopoietic stem cells in AML in remission marrow, the usual target is 1×10^8 per kilogram. Ironically, it is usual to aim for 2–4 times this amount if in vitro purging is being carried out.

The concept of maximal in vivo cytoreduction has been taken to its logical conclusion using double autografting, developed principally by the University College Hospital Group, London,[108] whereby the first course of high dose therapy with marrow support is intended to cytoreduce the patient such that the patient at the time of the second auto BMT has a minimal tumour load, as well as the second marrow harvested having minimum contamination.

Purging

Since the majority of patients with AML in remission will eventually relapse, it is assumed that the autograft is necessarily contaminated with residual leukaemia. A successful autograft may therefore depend on effective removal of the leukaemic cells from the reinfused marrow – so-called purging. The question of if, and how, to purge the marrow has received considerable scientific attention but still remains controversial.

For most groups initiating programmes several years ago, no form of purging was available, yet they were not deterred. The positive decision not to purge is still taken by choice, largely based on the belief that mathematically the possibility of reinfusing clonogenic leukaemic cells is small. If, for example, the conventional definition of remission, ie normal peripheral blood counts and less than 5% blast cells in the marrow, represented maximum residual leukaemia cell burden of 10^9 cells, further post-remission treatment (or, indeed, intensive induction treatment) may reduce this to 1×10^7 cells at the time of harvest. A satisfactory harvest dose of 1×10^8 cells/kg probably represents about 1% of total marrow, which, if it is assumed that the leukaemic burden is homogeneously distributed within the marrow – a proposal with little supportive evidence – will contain 10^5 residual leukaemic cells. Of these, about 1% will be clonogenic, and half may be lost during the freezing and thawing process, leaving a potential inoculum to the patient of 5×10^2 clonogenic cells. Little is known about the potential of these cells to seed in an ablated marrow, but, if it is assumed to be 20% successful, only about 100 clonogenic cells may be reinfused.

These figures are hypothetical but similar calculations have been derived experimentally in a myeloid leukaemia model.[109] There are then clearly a number of points that the final reinjected burden could be influenced by, which may be crucially relevant to the overall approach to autograft.

Some effort was made originally by the Houston Group to minimize the risk of autograft contamination using albumin density gradient separation. The major impetus to purging in AML was provided by the Baltimore Group who were able to demonstrate in the Brown Norway rat model a clear effect by treating the contaminated marrow donation with 4 hydroxy-per-cyclophosphamide[110] – an active metabolite of cyclophosphamide. Cyclophosphamide would not be the obvious drug to choose for AML, but this experimental leukaemia which is equivalent to promyelocytic leukaemia in humans is particularly responsive, and the dose exposure achieved under such circumstances has been calculated to be far in excess of what would be achieved with conventional systemic doses.

A number of reports have compared the in vitro sensitivity of leukaemic cell lines with human marrow precursors with equivocal results. There is, indeed, little data to suggest that clonogenic leukaemic cells are more sensitive than marrow precursors.[111] One of the problems of assessing purging methods is the lack of a good in vitro measure of human marrow repopulative ability. Even patients whose CFU-GM precursor cells have been eradicated by in vitro treatment are capable of repopulating. While the cyclophosphamide metabolites can eradicate committed precursors, cells which repopulate long term in vitro cultures survive.[112] This therefore begs the question of what is the appropriate purging dose. This is complicated by the demonstration that there is individual variation in dose responsiveness.[113] The choice is therefore either to treat marrow at a fixed in vitro dose, acknowledging that some over- and under-treatment will take place, or individually to adjust the dose based on a dose–response result obtained on a patients marrow a short time previously, which will mean a dose reduction for some patients.

Immunologically based methods have been limited by the lack of expression of unique leukaemic antigens in AML. In suitable circumstances, monoclonal antibody-based purging techniques, either with complement lysis or mediated by attached ricin, can achieve a 3–4 log kill in vitro. Not only is there heterogeneity of surface phenotypes within the AML subtypes, but it is usual to have different expression between clonogenic and endstage leukaemic cells as mentioned earlier.[36,37] The question is therefore whether targeting early myeloid expression such as CD33 is sufficient to eradicate leukaemic cells. At this level, haemopoietic regeneration can occur.[114]

Another approach in AML is exploiting the fact that leukaemic cells die out more rapidly in vitro culture systems than do normal haemopoietic precursors. This selective advantage for normal has been demonstrated cytogenetically, when only normal haemopoietic cells are sustained. It appears that a relatively short time span, eg 10–14 days in these circumstances is adequate to select for normal cells. While scaling up the process to cope with sufficient cells to make an adequate bone marrow donation presents significant logistic problems, a promising clinical initiative has established the feasibility of such an approach.[115]

Clinical experience of autograft in AML Single centre series and co-operative studies have reported durable survivals of around 45–55% in patients aged up to their mid-50s.[116,117]

The allograft and syngeneic experience represent a yardstick of what is achievable using an uncontaminated marrow. Without significant graft versus host disease, relapse will occur in about half of allograft recipients, and a similar number of syngeneic recipients. This then is the baseline from which autograft can be assessed, representing the extent to which conventional myeloablative regimens can eradicate leukaemia – there being no influence of leukaemic contamination of the graft.

One of the important features is that the autograft procedure has, indeed, proved to be safe for older patients, but, for those in their sixth decade, it is an arduous procedure. This, therefore, is an option for a large proportion of patients with AML.

A major difficulty in evaluating the autograft experience is that the procedure is not usually undertaken until 4–6 months into remission. A relationship between length of time spent in remission pre-autograft, and the probability of relapse post-autograft, has been demonstrated in the pooled data of the European Bone Marrow Transplant Group,[118] although this is not always seen in the single centre experience. Where the autograft was done within 3 months of achieving remission, 65% relapsed, whereas, if the delay was nine months or more, the relapse probability was 25%. There was an approximate gradation of risk at intervening durations of delay. There are two plausible explanations for this effect. First, although the information was not available within the data studied, it is likely that, during the delay, patients

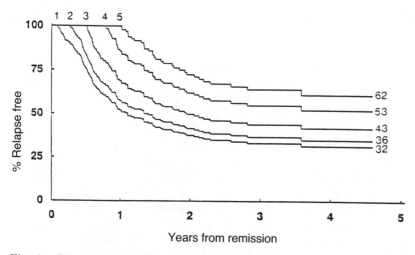

Fig. 1. Time censoring effect on outcome of chemotherapy in first remission of AML. Line 1: disease-free survival (DFS) from CR; line 2: DFS from 4 months; line 3: DFS from 7 months; line 4: DFS from 10 months; line 5: DFS from 2 years. Patients are from UK MRC 8 Trial. (Data provided courtesy of Dr J K H Rees.)

were receiving further chemotherapy. While this is unlikely to be curative, it might have the important cytoreductive effect, which both reduced the bulk of residual disease in the patient, and potential contamination of the autograft. The second, and more probable explanation, is that the transplant done after different delays, selects patients at inherently different risks of relapse.[119,120,121] That such an effect occurs is well illustrated in Figure 1.

In data derived from the UK MRC AML 8 Trial,[7] in which around 25% of remitters continue to be in remission at 5 years, the influence of 'time censoring' cohorts, depending on how long they had been in remission, can be clearly seen. At a delay of 4–6 months, these chemotherapy-treated patients had a prospect of remaining in remission of 36–43%. This is not substantially inferior to the autograft experience. While this illustrates an important point, none of the single autograft series undertakes the graft at an exact time point and will include some earlier (ie higher risk) cases. From a recent prospective study, where auto BMT was applied after 2 post-remission consolidation courses, it became clear that approximately a third of those who remit would get through to autograft and another quarter would have an allograft.[117] This is the first prospective estimation of the numbers of patients who survive in remission long enough, or in good enough condition, to have a transplant as planned at 3–4 months after achieving remission.

One of the impressive features of most series, as they mature to beyond 7 or 8 years, is the apparent absence of late relapses. The overall pattern suggests that relapse beyond 18 months post-autograft is a rare event. This may be one measure to suggest that autograft is an effective treatment.

Factors which influence outcome of autologous BMT Aware that the best results were likely to be obtained in complete remission, most groups initiated studies in patients with AML in first remission up to 60 years of age, usually, but not always, using standard TBI based protocols.[122-125] High dose melphalan has been used as a single agent either as a single or double autograft but the outcome has not been encouraging,[126,127] and, despite in vitro purging, the early experience with the TACC protocol has been similarly poor.[128] Overall, there is little difference between TBI given as a fractionated or single fraction protocol with conventional cyclophosphamide or intermediate dose melphalan. Different groups have used variations of either single or fractionated TBI, with respect to dose rate, fraction size, fraction frequency, and total dose. From all of this, no clear conclusion emerges about which is optimal.[118] Considering the great variability of the physical properties of radiation among different centres and the considerable heterogeneity of other potentially important variables between the series, this is not surprising. Recently, the Rome group developed the BAVC protocol which initially produced impressive results in second remission, but a recent update in first remission does not suggest that it will be a dramatic improvement over what has been achieved with other regimens.[129] There has been surprisingly little experience with the combination of busulphan and cyclophosphamide, either in its original or modified form.[130] The busulphan–cyclophosphamide regimen has been shown to be efficacious in allogeneic BMT in AML in first or second remission. It is also capable of curing a proportion of patients who have relapsed following allogeneic BMT which involved total body irradiation.

Just as at present, there does not appear to be a 'best choice' of ablative protocol so there are relatively few parameters which will predict outcome. The FAB classification produces some stratification of survival if all series are pooled. As consistently appearing from the Registry of the European Bone Marrow Transplant Group, the FAB groups predict for autograft in an approximately similar way as they have done for chemotherapy or allograft.[131] For those with the M3 type, the overall outcome is 60–70%, while M4 and M5 subgroups do less well similarly to allograft experience.

There are virtually no cytogenetic data available on which to base any conclusions, but it is probably over-optimistic to expect that there will be a subgroup for which autograft can particularly be recommended. There appears to be no clear relationship between age and outcome either in terms of survival, ie toxicity, or relapse. As predicted from the twin experience, the procedural related morbidity is acceptable and the mortality around 6–8%.[131] The problems are predominantly those of pancytopenia. Pneumonitis is infrequent and CMV pneumonitis in particular is uncommon, although viral excretion is seen in the seropositive patients.[62,63] There may not be a need to give seronegative blood products to the seronegative, but this is not yet clear.

Persistent thrombocytopenia is typically seen for several weeks or months after autograft for AML, but does not seem to occur in similarly treated ALL autografts – even those in second remission who have, by that time, been exposed to extensive treatment.

In the Glasgow series of TBI treated patients, the overall recovery to $50 \times 10^9/l$ platelets was 103 days, with approximately a third of patients taking longer than 3 months. On analysis of several potentially predictive factors such as previous treatment, marrow dose of cells, or colonable precursors, no factors could be found to explain the delayed recovery in some patients seen in the face of acceptable neutrophil regeneration.[132] Other groups have reported a similar experience.[117] Several patients had platelet specific or HLA reactive antibodies, but this did not directly predict for those who remained thrombocytopenic. Fortunately, the thrombocytopenia has not usually resulted in serious clinical problems, and, in particular, did not correlate in any way with subsequent relapse.

A feature which has shown a strong correlation with outcome has been the growth of a sample of the autograft in the long-term bone marrow culture system.[133] In a relatively small group of patients, it has been noted that, where the marrow continues to generate CFU-GM colonies into the supernatant for more than 4 weeks, the likelihood of relapse was 21%, whereas failure to sustain growth till 4 weeks predicted relapse in 80% of patients. It has more recently been noted that those poor growers who stay in remission can generate growth over a normal irradiated stroma, whereas those who relapsed failed to do so. This observation requires to be confirmed prospectively in a larger number of patients, but one interpretation is that such a technique identifies patients with residual haemopoiesis capable of selectively regenerating following the extreme haemopoietic stress of an autograft, and this regeneration can be established at the expense of the malignant clone.

Purging clinical results The clinical data in relation to purging are difficult to interpret. In the most recent analysis of the pooled data from the European Group, there appears to be a significant reduction in risk of relapse in patients treated with TBI who received marrow purged with a cyclophosphamide derivative.[118] This effect is most obvious in patients transplanted within the first 3 months of remission. Anxiety about the heterogeneity of other variables in this mixed group of patients has been countered by the continuing demonstration of this effect on multivariate analysis. The impact on survival overall is less, because such treatment increases the risk of the procedure by extending the period of cytopenia. It has also been suggested that individually selected dosaging is a more effective approach than simply incubating the collected marrow with a constant dose of the drug, despite the fact that 'adjusted doses' means that about a third of patients received less than they would with a standard dose.

There remain conceptual difficulties with these positive clinical results of purging in first remission. First, although the patient number is small, the relapse rate in syngeneic transplants in first remission is 50–60%.[52] Since this result is virtually superimposable on the autograft experience using unpurged data, this brings into serious doubt what further contribution purging can make. On the other hand, the 20% relapse rate seen with 'adjusted' purging is difficult to understand. Secondly, patients autografted within 3 months of remission have about a 65% relapse risk with unpurged marrow[118] – presumably because they have had limited post-remission cytoreduction or are at an inherently higher risk of relapse – yet, if the autograft is purged, the relapse risk is reduced to 20%, suggesting that virtually all of the relapses originate from the infused marrow, and the purging is 100% effective. It is therefore hard to explain that the clinical results of purging can be explained solely by leukaemia cell eradication.

As already discussed, the options for immunologically based techniques of purging in AML are limited by the lack of a leukaemia specific antibody, but some recent studies have shown encouraging results,[114] although again it remains unclear whether these results are any better than those of non-purged series or auto-BMT based on other purging principles.

The observation that the leukaemic clone selectively dies out in the long-term culture system resulted in the exploitation of this concept as a method of purging. It was developed in Vancouver and Manchester for chronic myeloid leukaemia and AML. While regeneration is delayed, the results in first remission AML patients look encouraging.[115,134] The patients who are considered most suitable for this procedure, ie the ones whose marrow in LTBMC may correspond to those who have a low relapse risk anyway.[133] Differences between the clinical results of these different methodologies of purging have yet to be shown.

It is generally accepted that proving the efficacy of purging in first remission, based on the twin data and the results of unpurged series, will be difficult. The setting in which it might be possible is when the autograft is planned to be done early in remission. Such a study has not yet been initiated.

Autograft in second remission Some investigators have chosen to delay the autograft till after first remission. There is little doubt that the outlook for patients who are successfully reinduced into a second remission is dismal. This is, to some extent, influenced by the duration of the first remission. Only about 10% of patients stay in remission (Fig. 2). The limited experience of autograft in second remission suggests a survival probability of around 30% – not substantially different from that achieved by an allograft.[131]

It is in second remission that the Baltimore group has pioneering experi-

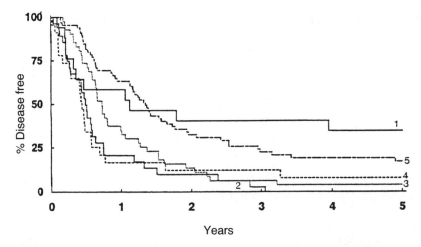

Fig. 2.   The duration of second remission treated with chemotherapy only: stratification by length of first remission. Patient groups are stratified 1–5 on the basis of progressive length of first remission. (Data from UK MRC 8 courtesy of Dr J K H Rees.)

ence of purging using the cyclophosphamide derivative.[135] While this group's initiative has created great interest, it is not clear whether the purging made a major contribution. In a recent report of the combined UK experience, a similar result has been achieved, also using the busulphan/cyclophosphamide protocol with unpurged marrow.[136] What is unclear in the second remission experience is how selected the patients were. Reference to the rate of relapse indicated in Figure 2 indicates that about 20–25% of patients, who had been in second remission for 6 months, survived with chemotherapy alone. So, again, the encouraging data, also reported from the European Group, are open to some criticism on the potential bias introduced by time censoring.

The major influences on second remissions are patient's age and the duration of first remission – which probably reflects whether or not the relapse has occurred on or off treatment. The results of the UK MRC 8th AML Trial on this point are illustrated in Table 1. It will be noted that the second remission rate is only 10% overall in patients relapsing within 6 months, and 14% within 12 months. The age influence is also clear. Since some of these patients then relapse promptly (Fig. 2), the potential pitfalls of such a treatment plan become clearer, and the practicality of such a strategy can only be resolved by a prospective trial.

Clinical trial assessment of autologous BMT There are many questions relating to how, and when, ABMT can be used most effectively, whether with purging or in first or second remission or in relapse. Experience from individual series

131

Table 1. *Second remission rates: relationship to duration of first remission and age*

	Patient age				
Duration of CRI (months)	0–13	14–39	40–59	60+	All ages
1–6	17	8	11	6	10% ($^{17}/_{164}$)
7–12	33	19	17	15	19% ($^{23}/_{123}$)
13–18	17	39	36	6	30% ($^{27}/_{90}$)
19–24	0	70	55	33	53% ($^{42}/_{79}$)
25+	100	61	65	50	61% ($^{45}/_{74}$)

(Data from UK MRC 8 courtesy of Dr JKH Rees.)

certainly justifies its evaluation in major clinical trials which will require to be conducted at a national or international level. Because of the time lapse in remission before patients actually undergo transplant, much has been made of the probability that these patients are selected. If routine chemotherapy trial data are similarly time censored, it can be seen that, for example, from the MRC 8 trial, patients who reach 4 months or 6 months have a 5-year survival of 30% to 40% respectively. Since chemotherapy patients continue to relapse, albeit at a low frequency beyond this point, whereas autograft recipients have not as yet, longer observation times are required. Nevertheless, such analyses point out that the differences between these two strategies may not be as substantial as it initially appeared. Not only does this emphasize the requirement for prospective randomized trial assessment, but it suggests that substantial patient numbers will be required to demonstrate any difference. Trial design will also be constrained by potential patient accrual, for example, substantially more patients will be required to reach a conclusion when the autograft is done at around 6 months into remission than if performed immediately due to the early loss anticipated due to relapse or non-compliance. Two small randomized studies involving an autograft option have been reported, and at least 3 major studies at international level are under way.

The first of the smaller studies has been reported by the French Group.[137] Of 58 patients eligible for allocation to transplantation, or to chemotherapy, 52 were evaluable. Twenty had an identical donor, so 32 were randomized either to autograft ($n = 12$) or intensive chemotherapy ($n = 20$). Every patient who entered remission had a consolidation course. The intensive chemotherapy had 4 courses while the autograft arm comprised a sequence of high dose Melphalan plus ABMT – harvest – a course of chemotherapy – a second high dose Melphalan and ABMT. Anecdotal experience had previously established high dose Melphalan with double autograft as one of the less effective schedules, so it is unfortunate that it was chosen in a randomized trial. The results indicated allograft to be superior to autograft which was superior to intensive chemotherapy. Unfortunately the intensive chemotherapy recipients did poorly. The numbers are far too small to provide useful information.

The Dutch National Study[117] was a comparison of autologous with allogeneic transplantation. The actuarial relapse was 60% versus 34%. A feature of this study was the fact that, for various reasons, including relapse, only 60% of the patients who initially entered remission got a transplant, thus highlighting the logistical difficulties in such a trial. There was no chemotherapy randomization, but those who did not have a transplant did badly with a 10% survival, while the updated projected 4 year survival rates for auto BMT recipient and allo BMT recipients were 35% and 50% respectively.

Of the 3 larger on-going trials, 2 have similar design. In the combined EORTC–GIMEMA study, all patients who enter remission receive 1 further intensive course followed by allogeneic transplant for those with a suitable donor, or a randomization between either 1 further intensification course, or an autologous transplant using either busulphan/cyclophosphamide (for the GIMEMA Group) or cyclophosphamide/TBI. In an interim analysis[138] at the end of 1989, of 495 entrants, 328 (66%) entered complete remission of whom 278 received and survived the intensive consolidation course. Eighty-eight were suitable for allograft but only 55 were allografted for reasons such as toxicity of earlier therapy or relapses while on the waiting list ($n = 18$). For similar reasons, 58 of the available 195 patients were not randomized. Forty-six have so far completed the autograft and 55 the second intensive consolidation. The comparison is therefore allograft vs autograft vs one further consolidation therapy course. The time delay in remission until completion of therapy has been 15.6, 14.3, and 11.4 weeks respectively. The slightly longer delay in the allograft candidates has meant more relapses ($n = 18$) in that arm than in either chemotherapy ($n = 9$) or autograft ($n = 10$). This important trial highlights the difficulties involved in avoiding selection bias by such mechanisms as waiting list delay or treatment-related toxicity. Nevertheless, the size of patient accrual should ensure an answer in due course.

The tenth Medical Research Council Trial in AML opened in 1988. The main aim is that all patients will receive, from diagnosis, 4 intensive courses. After the third, those without an HLA compatible donor will be randomized to receive an autograft (cyclo/TBI) immediately after recovery from the fourth course, or no further therapy after the fourth course until they relapse. If they enter a second remission, they will receive a late autograft. It will, therefore, be possible to compare directly the benefit of an allograft or an autograft or no further treatment on a large population of patients identically treated since diagnosis. In addition, the value and practicality of a late autograft will be assessed. At summer 1990, over 500 patients have joined the trial. Bearing in mind the statistical considerations discussed above, the trial may have to recruit for 5 years.

The new Dutch prospective study intends to assess the value of autograft as additional consolidation in remission. This trial, therefore, comprises an autograft following the completion of on-cross resistant chemotherapy with no further treatment. By mid-summer 1990, 250 patients have been recruited. The preliminary results of the chemotherapy also reveal the practical difficulties of applying autologous BMT to patients who have entered complete remission. The drop-out factors (refusal, complications, relapse, etc) appear quite considerable.

Conclusions

Allogeneic bone marrow transplantation is the first form of treatment, which, when applied in first remission, has shown the potential to cure a substantial number of the eligible patients. The fact that the actual cure falls below the potential cure has consumed much energy of those attempting to minimize the transplant-related risks. There has been little evidence of an overall improvement in the usual survival of 50%. The young patient does well and there can be no argument that it is the present treatment of choice. No matter how safe a procedure it becomes, it is unlikely that it will apply to more than a minority of those with the disease.

For those who lack a donor, the burning issue is whether or not autologous BMT is of value, and, if so, when it should be undertaken. Even for those who are in the latter part of the fourth decade or the fifth decade who have a matched sibling, it is a valid question whether they might be better off with one of the other options. For them, issues such as CMV status or FAB-type might be decisive. The appropriate clinical trials must now be done to resolve some of these issues. Influences such as time-censoring effects have made us realize the potential for bias. None of these studies can be properly done other than on a national, and possibly an international, basis.

Acknowledgement We wish to thank Miss Diane Docherty for her skill and patience in preparing this manuscript.

References

(1) Burge PS, Prankard TAJ, Richards JDM et al. Quality and quantity of survival in acute myeloid leukaemia. *Lancet* 1975; ii: 621–4.

(2) Yates J, Glidewell O, Wiernik P et al. Cytosine arabinoside with danorubicin or adriamycin for therapy of acute myelocytic leukaemia. A CALGB study. *Blood* 1982; 60: 454–62.

(3) Rees JKH, Sandler RM, Challener J, Hayhoe FGJ. Treatment of acute myeloid leukaemia with a triple cytotoxic regimen: DAT. *Br J Cancer* 1977; 36: 770–6.

(4) Gale RP, Foon KA, Cline MJ, Zighelboim J. Intensive chemotherapy for acute myelogenous leukaemia. *Ann Int Med* 1981; 94: 753–7.

(5) Büchner TH, Urbanitz D, Hiddemann, Rühl et al. Intensified induction and consolidation with or without maintenance chemotherapy for acute myeloid leukaemia (AML): Two multicentre studies of the German co-operation group. *J Clin Oncol* 1985; 3: 1583–9.

(6) Löwenberg B, Zittoun R, Kerthofs H, Jehn U et al. In the value of intensive remission-induction chemotherapy in elderly patients of 65+ years with acute myeloid leukaemia: a randomised phase III study of the EORTC leukaemia group. *J Clin Oncol* 1989; 7: 1268–74.

(7) Rees JKH, Swirsky D, Gray RG, Hayhoe FGJ. Principal results of the Medical Research Council's 8th acute myeloid leukaemia trial. *Lancet* 1986; ii: 1236–41.

(8) Zittoun R, Jehn U, Fiere, Haanen L et al. Alternating is repeated post remission treatment in adult myelogenous leukaemia: A randomised Phase III study (AML-6) of the EORTC leukaemia co-operation group. *Blood* 1989; 73: 896–906.

(9) Worsely AM, Galton DAG. Acute myeloid leukaemia: is 'consolidation' therapy necessary? *Br J Haem* 1984; 56: 361–4.

(10) Rees JKH, Gray RG. Post remission therapy in acute myeloid leukaemia (AML): the Medical Research Council experience in the UK. *Bone Marrow Transpl* 1989; 4 (Suppl. 2): 70–1.

(11) Bloomfied CD. Post-remission therapy in acute myeloid leukaemia. *J Clin Oncol* 1985; 3: 1570–2.

(12) Vaughan WP, Karp JE, Burke PJ. Two-cycle time sequential chemotherapy for adult acute nonlymphocytic leukaemia. *Blood* 1984; 64: 975.

(13) Marcus RE, Catovsky D, Goldman JM, Worsely AM, Galton DAG. Maintenance and consolidation therapy in AML. *Lancet* 1984; i: 686–7.

(14) Vogler WR, Winton EF, Gordon DS, Raney MR et al. A randomised comparison of post remission therapy in acute myelogenous leukaemia: a south eastern cancer study group trial. *Blood* 1984; 63: 1039–45.

(15) Sauter C, Berchtold W, Fopp M et al. Acute myelogenous leukaemia: maintenance chemotherapy after early consolidation treatments does not prolong survival. *Lancet* 1984; i: 379–82.

(16) Cassileth PA, Begg CB, Bennett JM et al. A randomised study of the efficacy of consolidation therapy in adult acute non-lymphocytic leukaemia. *Blood* 1984; 63: 843–7.

(17) Cassileth PA, Harrington DP, Hines JD, Oken MM et al. Maintenance chemotherapy prolongs remission duration in adult acute non lymphocytic leukaemia. *J Clin Oncol* 1988; 6: 583–7.

(18) Weinstein HJ, Mayer RJ, Rosenthal DS et al. Treatment of acute myelogenous leukaemia in children and adults. *N Eng J Med* 1980; 313: 473–8.

(19) Weinstein HJ, Mayer RJ, Rosenthal DS, Coral FS, Camitta BM, Gelber RD. Chemotherapy for acute myelogenous leukaemia in children and adults: VAPA update. *Blood* 1983; 62: 315–18.

(20) Weinstein HJ, Mayer RJ, Coral FS et al. Intensive post-remission induction chemotherapy for acute myelogenous leukaemia in children and adults. In:

Löwenberg B, Hagenbeek A, eds. Minimal residual disease in acute leukaemia. Martin Nijhoff 1984: 347–55.

(21) Creutzig U, Ritter J, Riehm H et al. Improved treatment results in childhood acute myelogenous leukaemia: a report of the German co-operative study AML-BFM-78. *Blood* 1985; 65: 298–304.

(22) Büchner T, Urbanitz D, Emmerick B et al. A multicenter study on intensified remission induction therapy for acute myeloid leukaemia. *Leukaemia Res* 1982; 6: 827–31.

(23) Wolff SN, Herzig RH, Fay JW et al. High dose cytarabine and daunorubicin as a consolidation therapy for acute myeloid leukaemia in first remission: long-term follow-up and results. *J Clin Oncol* 1989; 7: 1260–7.

(24) Arlin ZA, Lived TA, Mittelman A, Feldman E et al. A new regimen of amsacrine with high-dose cytarabine is safe and effective therapy for acute leukaemia. *J Clin Oncol* 1987; 5: 371–5.

(25) Hiddemann W, Krentzmann H, Straif K, Ludwig WD et al. High dose cytosine arabinoside and mitoxantrone: a highly effective regimen in refractory acute myeloid leukaemia. *Blood* 1987; 69: 744–9.

(26) Preisler HD, Anderson K, Rai J et al. The frequency of long-term remission in patients with acute myelogenous leukaemia treated with conventional maintenance chemotherapy: a study of 760 patients with a minimal follow-up time of 6 years. *Br J Haem* 1989; 71: 189–94.

(27) Bennett JM, Catovsky D, Danied M-T et al. Proposals for the classification of the acute leukaemias: French–American–British (FAB) co-operative group. *Br J Haematol* 1976; 33: 451–8.

(28) Swirsky DM, de Bastos M, Parish SE, Rees JKH, Hayhoe FGJ. Features affecting outcome during remission induction of acute myeloid leukaemia in 619 adult patients. *Br J Haematol* 1986; 64: 435–53.

(29) Mertlesmann R, Thaler HT, To L et al. Morphological classifications, response to therapy, and survival in 263 adult patients with acute non-lymphocytic leukaemia. *Blood* 1980; 56: 773–81.

(30) Yunis JJ, Brunning RD, Howe RB, Lobell M. High resolution chromosomes as an independent prognostic indicator in adult acute non-lymphocytic leukaemia. *N Eng J Med* 1984; 311: 812–18.

(31) Rowley JD. Biological implications of consistent chromosome rearrangements in leukaemia and lymphoma. *Cancer Res* 1984; 44: 3159.

(32) Berger R, Bernleim A, Ochoa-Noguera ME, Daniel MT et al. Prognostic significance of chromosomal abnormalities in acute non lymphocytic leukaemia: a study of 343 patients. *Cancer Genet Cytogenet* 1987; 28: 293.

(33) Keating MJ, Smith TL, Kantarjian H, Cork A et al. Cytogenetic pattern in acute myelogenous leukaemia: a major reproducible determination of outcome. *Leukaemia* 1988; 2: 403.

(34) Schiffer CA, Lee EJ, Tomisyasa T, Wiernit PH, Testa JR. Prognostic compact of cytogenetic abnormalities in patients with de novo AMLL. *Blood* 1989; 73: 263.

(35) Arthur DC, Berger R, Golomb HM, Swansbury GJ et al. The clinical significance of karyotype in acute myelogenous leukaemia. *Cancer Genet Cytogenet* 1989; 40: 203.

(36) Griffin JD, Löwenberg B. Clonogenic cells in acute myeloblastic leukaemia. *Blood* 1986; 68: 1185–94.

(37) Griffin JD, Mayer RJ, Weinstein HJ et al. Surface marker analysis of acute myeloblastic leukaemia; identification of differentiation-associated phenotypes. *Blood* 1983; 62: 557–63.

(38) Delevel HR, Bot FJ, Touw IP, Löwenberg B. Phenotyping of acute myelocytic leukaemia (AML) progenitors: an approach for tracing minimal number of AML cells among normal bone marrow. *Leukaemia* 1989; 2: 814–20.

(39) Lo Cocco F, Lopen M, Pasqualeti D et al. Terminal transferase positive AML: immunophenotypic characterisation and response to induction therapy. *Haematol Oncol* 1989; 7: 167–74.

(40) Terstappen LWMM, Loken MR. Multidimensional flow cytometric characterisation of normal and leukaemic cells. *Blood* 1988; (Suppl 1): 72, 75.

(41) Powles RL, Selby PJ, Paulu G et al. The nature of remission in acute myeloblastic leukaemia. *Lancet* 1972; ii: 674–6.

(42) Fialkow PJ, Singer JW, Rasking WH et al. Clonal development, stem-cell differentiation, and clinical remission in acute non-lymphocytic leukaemia. *N Eng J Med* 1987; 317: 468–73.

(43) Fearon ER, Burke PJ, Schiffer CA et al. Differentiation of leukaemia cells to polymorphonuclear leukocytes in patients with acute non-lymphocytic leukaemia. *N Eng J Med* 1986; 315: 15–24.

(44) Fialkow PJ, Singer JW, Adamson JW et al. Acute non-lymphocytic leukaemia: heterogeneity of stem cell origin. *Blood* 1981; 57: 1068–73.

(45) Thomas ED, Buckner CD, Clift RA et al. Marrow transplantation for acute non-lymphoblastic leukaemia in first remission. *N Eng J Med* 1979; 301: 597–9.

(46) Powles RL, Morgenstern G, Clink HM et al. The place of bone marrow transplantation in acute myelogenous leukaemia. *Lancet* 1980; i: 1047–50.

(47) Blume KG, Beutler E, Bross KJ et al. Bone marrow ablation and allogeneic marrow transplantation in acute leukaemia. *N Eng J Med* 1980; 302: 1041–6.

(48) Barnes DWH, Corp MJ, Loutit JF, Neal FE. Treatment of murine leukaemia with X-rays and homologous bone marrow. *Br Med J* 1956; 2: 626–30.

(49) Thomas ED, Ashley CA, Lochte HL et al. Homografts of bone marrow in dogs after lethal total-body-irradiation. *Blood* 1959; 14: 720–36.

(50) Thomas ED, Lochte HL, Cannon JH et al. Supralethal whole body irradiation and isologous marrow transplantation in man. *J Clin Invest* 1959; 38: 1709–16.

(51) Santos GW. Marrow transplantation in acute non-lymphocytic leukaemia. *Blood* 1989; 74: 901–8.

(52) Gale RP, Champlin RE. How does bone marrow transplantation cure leukaemia? *Lancet* 1984; ii: 28–30.

(53) Weiden PL, Sullivan K, Flournoy N et al. Antileukemic effect of graft-versus-host disease: contribution to improved survival after allogeneic marrow transplantation. *N Eng J Med* 1981; 304: 1529–33.

(54) Butturini A, Bortin MM, Gale RP. Graft-versus leukemia following bone marrow transplantation. *Bone Marrow Transpl* 1987; 2: 233–42.

(55) Clift RA, Buckner CD, Thomas ED et al. The treatment of acute non-lymphoblastic leukemia by allogeneic marrow transplantation. *Bone Marrow Transpl* 1987; 2: 243.

(56) Dinsmore R, Kirkpatrick D, Flomenberg N et al. Allogeneic bone marrow transplantation for patients with acute non-lymphocytic leukemia. *Blood* 1984; 63: 649.

(57) Bortin MM, Horowitz M, Gale RP. Current status of bone marrow transplantation in humans: report from the International Bone Marrow Transplant Registry. *Nat Immun Cell Growth Regul* 1988; 7: 334–50.

(58) Zwaan FE, Hermans J, Barrett AJ et al. Bone marrow transplantation for acute non-lymphoblastic leukemia. A survey of European group for bone marrow transplantation. *Br J Haematol* 1984; 56: 645–53.

(59) Weiner RS, Bortin MM, Gale RP et al. Interstitial pneumonitis after bone marrow transplantation. *Ann Int Med* 1986; 104: 168–75.

(60) Meyers JD, Flournoy N, Wade JC et al. Biology of interstitial pneumonia after marrow transplantation. In: Gale RP, ed. *Recent advances in bone marrow transplantation*. Alan R Liss Inc, New York, 1983: 405–23.

(61) Miller W, Flynn P, Mccullough J et al. Cytomegalovirus infection after bone marrow transplantation: an association with acute graft-v-host disease. *Blood* 1986; 67: 1162–7.

(62) Meyers JD, Flournoy N, Thomas ED. Risk factors for cytomegalovirus infection after human marrow transplantation. *J Infec Dis* 1986; 153: 478–88.

(63) McKinnon S, Burnett AK, Crawford RJ et al. Seronegative blood products prevent primary cytomegalovirus infection after bone marrow transplantation. *J Clin Path* 1988; 41: 948–50.

(64) Reusser P, Fisher LD, Buchner CD, Thomas ED, Meyers JD. Cytomegalovirus infection after autologous bone marrow transplantation: occurrence of cytomegalovirus disease and effect on engraftment. *Blood* 1990; 75: 1888–94.

(65) Olding LB, Jensen FC, Oldstone MBA. Pathogeneis of cytomegalovirus infection 1. Activation of virus from bone marrow-derived lymphocytes by in vitro allogeneic reaction. *J Exp Med* 1986; 314: 1006–10.

(66) Grob JP, Grundy JE, Prentice HG et al. Immune donors can protect marrow transplant recipients from severe cytomegalovirus infection. *Lancet* 1987; i: 774–6.

(67) O'Reilly RJ, Reich L, Gold J et al. A randomised trial of intravenous hyperimmune globulin for the prevention of cytomegalovirus (CMV) infections following marrow transplantation: preliminary results. *Transpl Proc* 1983; 15: 1405–11.

(68) Meyers JD, Leszczynski J, Szia JA et al. Prevention of cytomegalovirus infection by cytomegalovirus immune globulin after marrow transplantation. *Ann Intern Med* 1983; 98: 442–6.

(69) Kubanek B, Ernst P, Ostendorf P, Schafer U, Wolf H. Preliminary data of a controlled trial of intravenous hyperimmune globulin in the prevention of cytomegalovirus infection in bone marrow transplant recipients. *Transpl Proc* 1985; 17: 468–9.

(70) Winston DJ, Ho WG, Lin C-H et al. Intravenous immune globulin for prevention of cytomegalovirus infection and interstitial pneumonia after bone marrow transplantation. *Ann Intern Med* 1987; 106: 12–18.

(71) Cheeseman SH, Rubin RH, Stewart JA et al. Controlled clinical trial of prophy-

lactic human-leukocyte interferon in renal transplantation. Effects on cytomegalovirus and herpes simplex virus infections. *N Eng J Med* 1979; 300: 1345–9.

(72) Meyers JD, Reed EC, Shepp DH et al. Acyclovir for prevention of cytomegalovirus infection and disease after allogeneic marrow transplantation. *N Eng J Med* 1988; 318: 70–5.

(73) Shepp DH, Dandliker PS, De Miranda P et al. Activity of 9-(2-hydroxy-1-hydroxymethyl ethoxymethyl) guanine (BW B759U) in the treatment of cytomegalovirus pneumonia. *Ann Intern Med* 1985; 103: 368–73.

(74) Klintmalm G, Lonnqvist B, Oberg B et al. Intravenous foscarnet for the treatment of severe cytomegalovirus infection in allograft recipients. *Scand J Infec Dis* 1985; 17: 157–63.

(75) Bowden RA, Sayers M, Gleaves CA, Banaji M, Newton B, Meyers JD. Cytomegalovirus seronegative blood products for the prevention of primary cytomegalovirus infection following marrow transplantation; considerations for blood banks. *Transfusion* 1987; 27: 478–81.

(76) Verdonck LF, De Grann-Hentzen YCE, Dekker AW, Mudde GC, De Gast G C. Cytomegalovirus seronegative platelets and leukocyte-poor red blood cells from random donors can prevent primary cytomegalovirus infection after bone marrow transplantation. *Bone Marrow Transpl* 1987; 2: 73–8.

(77) Gale RP. Graft-versus-host disease. *Immunol Rev* 1985; 88: 193–214.

(78) Mitsuyasu RT, Champlin RE, Gale RP et al. Treatment of Donor Bone Marrow with monoclonal anti-T-cell antibody and complement for the prevention of graft-versus-host disease. *Ann Int Med* 1986; 105: 20–6.

(79) Heit W, Bunjes D, Wiesneth M et al. Ex vivo T-cell depletion with the monoclonal antibody Campath-1 plus human complement effectively prevents acute graft-versus-host disease in allogeneic bone marrow transplantation. *Br J Haemat* 1986; 64: 479–86.

(80) Martin PJ, Hansen JA, Buckner CD et al. Effects of in vitro depletion of T cells in HLA-identical allogeneic marrow grafts. *Blood* 1985; 66: 664–72.

(81) Schouten HC, Sizoo W, Veer Van H, Hagenbeek A, Löwenberg B. Incomplete chimerism in erythroid, myeloid and B lineage after T cell-depleted allogeneic bone marrow transplantation. *Bone Marrow Transpl* 1988; 3: 407–12.

(82) Burnett AK, Hann IM, Robertson AG et al. Prevention of graft-versus-host disease by ex vivo T-cell depletion: reduction in graft failure with augmented total body irradiation. *Leukaemia* 1988; 2: 300–3.

(83) Prentice HG, Blacklock HA, Janossy G et al. Depletion of T lymphocytes in donor marrow prevents significant graft-versus-host disease in matched allogeneic leukaemia marrow transplant recipients. *Lancet* 1984; i: 472–6.

(84) Waldman H, Polliak A, Hale G et al. Elimination of graft-versus-host disease by in vitro depletion of alloreactive lymphocytes with a monoclonal rat anti-human lymphocyte antibody (CAMPATH-1). *Lancet* 1984; ii: 483–6.

(85) Weiden PL, Flournoy N, Thomas ED et al. Anti-leukaemia effect of graft-versus-host disease in recipients of allogeneic marrow grafts. *N Eng J Med* 1979; 300: 1068–73.

(86) Apperley JF, Jones L, Hale G et al. Bone marrow transplantation for patients with chronic myeloid leukaemia: T-cell depletion with Campath-1 reduces the

incidence of graft-versus-host disease but may increase the risk of leukaemia relapse. *Bone Marrow Transpl* 1986; 1: 53–66.

(87) Pollard CM, Powles RL, Millar JL et al. Leukaemia relapse following Campath-1 treated bone marrow transplantation for leukaemia. *Lancet* 1986; ii: 1343–4.

(88) O'Reilly RJ, Kernan N, Collins N et al. Abrogation of both acute and chronic GVHD following transplants of lectin agglutinated, E-Rosette depleted (SBA E) marrow for leukaemia. *Blood* 1986; 68 (Suppl 1): 291a.

(89) Waldmann H, Cobbold S, Hale G. Leukaemic relapse after Campath-1-treated bone marrow transplantation for leukaemia. *Lancet* 1987; i: 44.

(90) Gale RP, Reisner Y. Graft rejection and graft-versus-host disease: mirror images. *Lancet* 1986; ii: 862–3.

(91) Gale RP, Bortin MM, Van Bekkum et al. Risk factors for acute graft-versus-host disease. *Br J Haematol* 1987; 67: 397–406.

(92) Voglesang GB, Hess AD, Berman A et al. Skin explant culture as a model for cutaneous graft-versus-host disease. *N Eng J Med* 1985; 313: 645–50.

(93) Price G, Brenner MK, Prentice HG et al. Cytotoxic effects of tumour necrosis and gamma-interferon on acute myeloid leukaemia blast cells. *Br J Cancer* 1987; 55: 287–90.

(94) Storb R, Deeg HJ, Whitehead J et al. Methotrexate and cyclosporine compared with cyclosporine alone for prophylaxis of acute graft versus host disease after marrow transplantation. *N Eng J Med* 1986; 314: 729–35.

(95) Storb R, Deeg HJ, Pepe M et al. Methotrexate and cyclosporine versus cyclosporine alone for prophylaxis of graft-versus-host disease in patients given HLA-identical marrow grafts for leukemia: long-term follow-up of a controlled trial. *Blood* 1989; 73: 1729–34.

(96) McGlave PB, Haake RJ, Bostrom BC et al. Allogeneic bone marrow transplantation for acute non-lymphocytic leukemia in first remission. *Blood* 1988; 72: 1512–17.

(97) Appelbaum FR, Fisher LD, Thomas ED et al. Chemotherapy v marrow transplantation for adults with acute non-lymphocytic leukemia: a five year follow-up. *Blood* 1988; 72: 178–84.

(98) Conde E, Iriondo A, Rayon C et al. Allogeneic bone marrow transplantation versus intensification chemotherapy for acute myelogenous leukaemia in first remission: a prospective controlled trial. *Br J Haematol* 1988; 68: 219–26.

(99) Champlin R, Ho W, Gale RP et al. Treatment of acute myelogenous leukemia: a prospective controlled trial of bone marrow transplantation versus consolidation chemotherapy. *Ann Int Med* 1985; 102: 285–91.

(100) Begg CB, Pilok L, McGlave PB. Bone marrow transplantation versus chemotherapy in acute non-lymphocytic leukaemia: a meta-analystic review. *Eur J Cancer Clin Oncol* 1989; 25: 1519–23.

(101) Appelbaum FR, Clift RA, Buckner CD et al. Allogeneic bone marrow transplantation for acute non-lymphoblastic leukemia after first relapse. *Blood* 1982; 61: 949.

(102) Dicke KA, Spitzer G, Peters L et al. Autologous bone marrow transplantation in relapsed adult acute leukaemia. *Lancet* 1979; i: 195–210.

(103) Appelbaum FR, Fefer A, Cheever MA et al. Treatment of non-Hodgkin's

lymphoma with marrow transplantation in identical twins. *Blood* 1981; 58: 509–23.

(104) Buckner CD, Clift RA, Appelbaum FR et al. A randomised trial of 12.0 or 15.75 Gy of total body irradiation (TBI) in patients with acute non-lymphoblastic (ANL) and chronic myelogenous leukemia (CML) followed by marrow transplantation [Abstract]. *Exp Hematol* 1989; 17: 522.

(105) Frassoni F, Soarpati D, Bacigalupo A et al. The effects of total body irradiation dose and chronic graft-versus-host disease on leukaemic relapse after allogeneic bone marrow transplantation. *Br J Haematol* 1989; 73: 211–16.

(106) Sullivan KM, Weiden PL, Storb R. Influence of acute and chronic graft-versus-host disease on relapse and survival after bone marrow transplantation from HLA-identical siblings as treatment of acute and chronic leukemia. *Blood* 1989; 73: 1720–8.

(107) Bacigalupo A, Van Lint MT, Frassoni F et al. Graft-versus-leukaemia effect following allogeneic bone marrow transplantation. *Br J Haematol* 1985; 61: 749–51.

(108) Goldstone AH, Anderson CC, Linch DE et al. Autologous bone marrow transplantation following high dose chemotherapy for the treatment of adult patients with acute myeloid leukaemia. *Br J Haematol* 1986; 64: 529–37.

(109) Hagenbeek A, Schultz FW, Martens ACM. *In vitro or in vivo treatment of leukemia to prevent a relapse after autologous bone marrow transplantation in autologous bone marrow transplantation*, Dicke K A, Spitzer G, Jagannath S, eds. Univ of Texas Press: Evinger-Hodges, 1989: 107–12.

(110) Sharkis SJ, Santos GW, Colvin M et al. Elimination of acute myelogenous leukemic cells from marrow and tumor suspensions in the rat with 4-hydroperoxycyclophosphamide. *Blood* 1980; 55: 521–3.

(111) Singer CRJ, Linch DC. Comparison of the sensitivity of normal and leukaemia myeloid progenitors to in-vitro incubation with cytotoxic drugs: a study of pharmacological purging. *Leukaemia Res* 1987; 11(11): 953–9.

(112) Siena S, Castro-Malaspina H, Gulati SC et al. Effects of in vitro purging with 4-hydroperoxycyclophosphamide on the hematopoietic and microenvironmental elements of human bone marrow. *Blood* 1985; 65: 655–62.

(113) Gorin NC, Douay L, Laporte JP et al. Autologous bone marrow transplantation using marrow incubated with ASTA Z 7557 in adult acute leukaemia. *Blood* 1986; 67: 1367–76.

(114) Ball ED, Mills LE, Couglin CT et al. Autologous bone marrow transplantation in acute myelogenous leukemia: in vitro treatment with myeloid cell-specific monoclonal antibodies. *Blood* 1986; 68: 1311–15.

(115) Chang J, Morgenstern G, Deakin D et al. Reconstitution of haemopoietic system with autologous marrow taken during relapse of acute myeloblastic leukaemia and grown in long-term culture. *Lancet* 1986; i: 294–5.

(116) Linch DC, Burnett AK. Clinical studies of ABMT in acute myeloid leukaemia. *Clin Haematol* 1986; 15: 167–86.

(117) Löwenberg B, Verdonck LJ, Dekker AW et al. Autologous bone marrow transplantation in acute myeloid leukaemia in first remission: results of a Dutch prospective study. *J Clin Oncol* 1990; 8: 287–94.

(118) Gorin NC, Aegerter A, Auvert B et al. Autologous bone marrow transplantation

for acute myelocytic leukemia in first remission: a European survey of the role of marrow purging. *Blood* 1990; 75: 1606–14.

(119) Gale RP, Butturini A. Autotransplant in leukaemia. *Lancet* 1989; ii: 315–17.

(120) Burnett AK. Autologous bone marrow transplantation in acute leukaemia. *Leukaemia Res* 1988; 12: 531–6.

(121) Preisler HD, Raza A. Autologous bone marrow transplantation for acute leukaemia in remission. *Br J Haematol* 1986; 65(3): 377–9.

(122) Burnett AK, Tansey P, Watkins R et al. Transplantation of unpurged autologous bone-marrow in acute myeloid leukaemia in first remission. *Lancet* 1984; ii: 1068–70.

(123) Stewart R, Buckner C, Bensinger W et al. Autologous marrow transplantation in patients with acute non-lymphocytic leukemia in first remission. *Exp Hematol* 1985; 13: 267–72.

(124) Löwenberg E, Van der Lelie J, Goudsmith R et al. Autologous bone marrow transplantation in patients with acute myeloid leukaemia in first remission. In: Dicke KA, Spitzer G, Jagannath S, eds. *Autologous bone marrow transplantation III*. Texas: University of Houston, 1987: 3–7.

(125) Carella AM, Martingengo M, Santini G et al. Autologous bone marrow transplantation for acute leukaemia in remission. The Genoa experience. *Haematologica* 1988; 73: 119–24.

(126) Maraninchi D, Gastaut JA, Herve P et al. High dose Melphalan and autologous marrow transplantation in acute leukemias in relapse or remission. *Exp Hematol* 1984; 12 (Suppl 15): 130.

(127) Maraninchi D, Blaise D, Michel G et al. Double unpurged autologous bone marrow transplantation in 41 patients with acute leukemias. In: Dicke KA, Spitzer G, Jagannath S, eds. *Autologous bone marrow transplantation III*. University of Houston, Texas: 1987: 105–10.

(128) Cahn JY, Herve P, Flesch M et al. Autologous bone marrow transplantation (AMBT) for acute leukaemia in complete remission: a pilot study of 33 cases. *Br J Haematol* 1986; 63: 457–70.

(129) Meloni G, De Fabritiis P, Pulsoni A et al. BAVC regimen and autologous bone marrow transplantation in patients with acute myelogenous leukaemia in remission. In: Dicke K A, Spitzer G, Jagannath S, eds. *Autologous bone marrow transplantation III*. Texas: University of Houston, 1987: 9–14.

(130) Santos GW, Tutschka PJ, Brookmeyer R et al. Marrow transplantation for acute non-lymphocytic leukemia after treatment with busulfan and cyclophosphamide. *N Eng J Med* 309: 1347–53.

(131) Gorin NC, Aegerter P, Auvert B. Autologous bone marrow transplantation (ABMT) for acute leukaemia in remission: fifth European survey: evidence in favour of marrow purging. Influence of pre-transplant interval. *Bone Marrow Transpl* 1988; 3 (Suppl 1): 39–41.

(132) Pendry K, Burnett AK, Richmond L J, Pearson C. Mechanisms of thrombocytopenia following autograft for AML. *Br J Haematol* 1990; 74 (Suppl 1): 52.

(133) Burnett AK, Alcorn M, Graham S et al. Correlation of growth of marrow in long-term culture with outcome of autologous bone marrow transplantation. *Bone Marrow Transpl* 1988; 3 (Suppl 1): 335.

(134) Chang J, Morgenstem GP, Coutinho LH et al. The use of bone marrow cells

grown in long-term culture for autologous bone marrow transplantation in acute myeloid leukaemia: an update. *Bone Marrow Transpl* 1989: 4,5.

(135) Yeager AM, Kaiser H, Santor GW et al. Autologous bone marrow transplantation in patients with acute myelogenous leukaemia using ex vivo marrow treatment with 4-hydroperoxy-cyclophosphamide. *N Eng J Med* 1986; 315: 141–7.

(136) McMillan A, Goldstone AH, Powles R et al. British autograft group experience of autologous unpurged bone marrow transplantation (ABMT) with busulphan and cyclophosphamide conditioning in acute myeloid leukaemia beyond first complete remission: implications for AML 10. *Br J Haematol* 1990; 74 (Suppl 1): 20.

(137) Reiffers J, Gaspard MH, Maraninchi D et al. Comparison of allogeneic or autologous bone marrow transplantation and chemotherapy in patients with acute myeloid leukaemia in first remission: a prospective controlled trial. *Br J Haematol* 1989; 72: 57–63.

(138) Zittoun R, Mandelli F, De Witte T et al. Relative value of allogeneic BMT, autologous BMT and intensive chemotherapy during first complete remission (CR) of acute myelogenous leukemia (AML). An interim analysis of the AML8 EORTC-GIMEMA protocol. *Bone Marrow Transpl* 1990; 6 (Suppl 1): 56–8.

Gene rearrangements and minimal residual disease in lymphoproliferative disorders

F E COTTER

Introduction

Lymphoid malignancies are characterized by a proliferation of lymphoid-derived cells and their precursors. The majority of malignant lymphomas and lymphocytic leukaemias are monoclonal in origin[1] and may show either B or T-cell lineage alterations.[2] A clonal population of proliferating cells does not necessarily equate with malignancy but its presence may be of considerable benefit in differentiating between a malignant and a reactive process.[3] The ability to determine the lineage of the clonal population of cells may have clinical significance in the management of the malignancy. Clonality, B or T-cell lineage and the stage of differentiation in lymphoid malignancy has been determined at a molecular level by immunoglobulin gene or T-cell receptor gene rearrangement studies[4-21] and may be of benefit when combined with morphological and immunophenotype analysis.[22] Gene rearrangement studies to provide a clonal marker of the disease are conventionally carried out by Southern analysis[23] using DNA probes to T-cell receptor or immunoglobulin genes. The unique marker is determined and may subsequently be used clinically to determine the presence of the same malignancy in peripheral blood, lymph nodes or tissues suspected of containing the same malignancy at minimal levels.[24-29] Non-malignant lymphocytic proliferations characteristically demonstrate polyclonal antigen receptor gene proliferation on molecular analysis.[2] The advent of the polymerase chain reaction[30] has allowed the detection of minimal disease at a considerably greater level of sensitivity compared to Southern analysis[24,27] and again relies on the individual clonal rearrangement characteristic of the lymphoid malignancy to determine the presence of disease.[26,27,31-37] Non-random chromosome abnormalities have been associated with both B-cell and T-cell malignancies often related to a particular histological group,[38-42] involving the chromosome

All correspondence to: ICRF Department of Medical Oncology, St Bartholomew's Hospital, London EC1A 7BE, UK.

Cambridge Medical Reviews: Haematological Oncology Volume 1
© Cambridge University Press 1991

regions containing immunoglobulin or T-cell receptor genes. These gene rearrangements not only provide a DNA-associated marker of disease but also provide a clue to the induction of malignancy.

Normal rearrangement of immunoglobulin and T-cell receptor genes

Immunoglobulin molecules consist of two identical heavy chains (IgH) and two identical light chains (IgL: either $\varkappa$ or λ).[43,44] There are two varieties of heterodimeric T-cell antigen receptor (TCR) one containing an α and a β chain[45–47] and the other consisting of a γ–δ hetrodimer.[48–51] The chromosomal locations of these genes are shown in Figure 1.[52–55] Antigen receptor specificity depends on a unique amino acid sequence in the antigen binding portion known as the variable region.[56] One of the antigen receptor genes (Ig and TCR), unlike most other genes, must undergo a rearrangement of their DNA before a functional protein can be encoded.[56] The unrearranged germline genes for Ig and TCR are discontinuous coding segments of DNA termed the variable (V), diversity (D for IgH, TCR β and δ genes), joining (J) and constant (C) region genes.[43,44,47,50,52–55]

The Ig and TCR genes may be considered to have evolved from the same supergene family.[57] The antigen receptor genes undergo somatic rearrangement in a sequential manner as an essential step in B- and T-cell lineage commitment. This leads to transcription of a functional Ig or TCR messenger RNA. The highly ordered mechanism is similar for both Ig and TCR genes due to their common evolutionary ancestry. A partially rearranged DJ gene segment is formed by a D segment combining with a J segment as an initiating step for both the IgH and TCR. The variable region gene rearrangement is completed by a second step consisting of the DJ segment combining with a V gene segment and this together with a constant region gene makes up the functional final rearranged antigen receptor gene.[43,44,47,50,52–55]

The IgH locus is initially rearranged in the pre-B-cell and results in synthesis of a μ cytoplasmic heavy chain.[58] IgL-$\varkappa$ gene then attempts to rearrange and produces a μ–$\varkappa$ Ig if successful, however, if a non-functional IgL-$\varkappa$ rearrangement occurs, then the pre-B-cell will attempt IgL-λ gene rearrangement.[59] If there is a failure to produce a functional light chain gene, this leads to a lack of light chain synthesis and the cell will not develop beyond the pre-B stage.[3,59]

The TCR γ chain gene rearranges prior to TCR β[60,61] in the pre-T-cell, while the TCR α gene is the last to rearrange.[62] Although the TCR δ gene probably rearranges at a similar time to TCR γ gene, the exact timing remains uncertain.[21] Failure of functional rearrangement leads to the cell remaining at the pre-T-stage.

During the Ig and TCR gene rearrangements, insertion of up to 20 random nucleotides (N insertions) may occur under the influence of terminal

B - Cell	Chromosome region
IgH	14q32
IgL κ	2p11
IgL λ	22q11

T - Cell	
TCR α–δ	14q11
TCR β	7q32
TCR γ	7p15

Fig. 1.   Germline chromosomal locations for human immunoglobulin (Ig) and T-cell receptor (TCR) genes.

deoxynucleotidyl transferase (TdT) between the junction points.[63-65] Antigen receptor specificity is encoded by the entire VJ or VDJ unit. The number of potential gene permutations with this formation exceeds a billion.[56] Additional specificity may be generated by the presence of N insertions.[63-65] In summary, the ordered mechanism of Ig and TCR rearrangement results in a huge variety of antigen receptors.

Detection of Ig and TCR gene rearrangement
Southern Analysis
DNA rearrangement analysis of the Ig and TCR genes is facilitated by Southern analysis.[23] In brief, DNA from the tissue to be studied is extracted and digested with restriction endonucleolases. Size fractionation by agarose gel electropheresis is followed by transfer of the DNA onto a nylon filter by the method of Southern. Hybridization with a radioactive-labelled DNA probe for the Ig or TCR gene to be studied, precedes exposure of the filter to an autoradiograph. In normal tissue, a germline band of the same size is obtained consistently. A clonal population of cells in the tissue studied is indicated by the presence of any further bands of a different size[4,7] (Fig. 2). Polyclonal proliferations of lymphocytes will show no new specific bands but a vertical smear due to the numerous heterogeneous rearrangement patterns. The sensitivity of this technique allows detection in the region of 1% of clonal cell.[24,27]

147

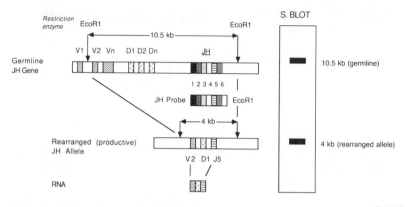

Fig. 2. Schematic representation of the immunoglobulin heavy chain gene (IgH) variable portion rearrangement. This region codes for the immunoglobulin antigen specificity. The germline (unrearranged) and rearranged (productive) portions are shown with EcoR1 restriction enzyme sites indicated by vertical arrows and the size of fragments obtained is shown in kilobases. The representation of germline and clonally rearranged IgH obtained with size selection by Southern analysis (SBlot) and hybridization with a J_H DNA probe is shown on the right.

Polymerase chain reaction (PCR)

Recently, the PCR has been applied to gene rearrangement analysis greatly increasing the level of detection of clonal rearrangements to the region of 1 : 100 000 cells. The ability to amplify exponentially a target sequence of DNA in vitro by enzymatic synthesis (PCR) was first described in 1985.[30] Two synthetically prepared oligonucleotides primers hybridize to opposite strands flanking the region of interest in the target DNA. The intervening sequences are generated by extension from these primers by a DNA polymerase, thus duplicating the target DNA. There is a theoretical doubling of DNA yield for every cycle leading to an amplification of the target DNA by a million-fold (2^{20}) over 20 cycles, a level detectable by gel electrophoresis or Southern analysis.

Detection of immunoglobulin gene rearrangement by PCR This can be applied to a number of B-cell malignancies by the use of synthetic oligonucleotides to a V_H region and the 3' J_H segment consensus sequence. This has been described with a $V_H 251$ oligonucleotide. Detection of Ig gene rearrangement was possible in DNA from 20% of B lineage ALL cases at presentation and in DNA from morphologically normal peripheral blood and bone marrow at follow-up in a number of these patients.[37] Although there is a vast repertoire of V_H genes,[66] by their very nature, it appears that B-cell malignancies are highly restricted in their V_H region selection.[67,68] The $V_H 251$ region, a member of the V_H5 family, is preferentially used in B-cell malignancies[67] facilitating the study of Ig rearrangement by PCR in these cases. The delineation of further preferentially utilized V_H regions in B-cell malignancies, or the use of consensus V_H or D_H[31] flanking region sequence oligonucleotides, will increase the application of PCR for detection of clonal IgH rearrangements to the majority of B-cell neoplasms.

Detection of TCR rearrangements by PCR This is made possible for TCRγ and δ due to the very limited repertoire of V, D, J and C segments in the germline configuration to select from when rearranging. TCRγ contains 15 V_γ segments, of which only 10 undergo rearrangement,[69-74] 5 J_γ and 2 C_γ segments both of which show considerable homology with 2 of the J_γ segments.[75-77] TCRδ has 6 V_δ, 3 D_δ, 3 J_δ segments and 1 C_δ region described.[78-81] The limited selection of segments for rearrangement of TCRγ and δ, while permitting the use of the PCR, with a finite selection of synthetic oligonucleotides[35,36] to detect the limited repertoire of rearrangements, also poses the problem of differentiating clonal from normal rearrangement with this sensitive technique. Direct sequencing of the PCR product will detect the unique clonal 'N insertion' between each rearranged segment which, in turn, acts as the clonal marker for the T-cell malignancy. By this combination of PCR and direct sequencing, it is possible to detect and monitor the clonal population of neoplastic cells in the majority of T-cell malignancies.[35,36]

Gene rearrangements in lymphoproliferative disorders
Southern analysis, with Ig and TCR gene probes, demonstrates, for the majority of lymphoid malignancies, including angioimmunoblastic lympadenopathy (AILD) and some cases of Hodgkin's disease, the presence of a clonal lymphoid population.[3-21,47,54,58,59,82-92] Most of these diseases have consistent patterns of rearrangement.

B-cell malignancies These show clonal IgH and either IgLϰ or IgLλ rearrangements. Only where clonal development has occurred in a very immature B lineage cell will IgH rearrangement alone be observed.[2]

T-cell malignancies These demonstrate clonal rearrangement of TCR γ and β chain genes in nearly all cases and in most additional TCR δ chain genes.[2] TCR γ rearrangement alone may occur in very early T-cell lineage malignancies. The clonal TCR α chain gene rearrangement is considerably more difficult to demonstrate due to the large J_α region in excess of 100 kilobases with over 50 J_α segments.[62]

Hodgkin's disease This appears to demonstrate greater variety of clonal rearrangement patterns.[93-99] A significant number of clonal populations of cells with TCR γ and/or TCR β chain gene rearrangements have been reported. However, cases of Reed–Sternberg cell-rich Hodgkin's disease have shown either TCR γ chain or IgH gene clonal rearrangement.[98,99] In most cases, the intensity of the rearranged band is low suggesting the presence of only a small clonal population of cells. The question arises as to whether this represents a malignant or non-malignant lymphoid clone. At present, the significance of these findings is uncertain.

Mixed lineage These lymphoid malignancies represent those that demonstrate the presence of clonal TCR (usually TCR γ and TCR δ) and IgH gene rearrangements.[12,15,16,18,20,21,100–102] TCR β chain gene rearrangement (predominantly a true marker of T-cell lineage)[60,61] is not usually found as the majority of the mixed lineage lymphoid neoplasms are B-cell malignancies as demonstrated by presence of IgH. TCR γ and TCR δ do not appear to be as lineage restricted.[16,20,21,101] Some cases of AML, particularly the TdT positive variety, show incomplete IgH and/or TCR β gene rearrangement.[87,88] Possibly, where a mixed picture of TCR and IgH rearrangement is observed, it may represent a malignant disorder occurring prior to lineage commitment.

Non-neoplastic gene rearrangements
The detection of a monoclonal proliferation of lymphocytes does not necessarily determine the presence of neoplasia. Non-malignant clonal proliferations occur predominantly in benign lymphoproliferative disorders which predispose to development of non-Hodgkin's lymphoma (NHL). Antigen receptor gene rearrangements have been described in a number of conditions including AILD,[102] *Pityriasis lichenoides et varioliformis acuta*,[103] Castleman's disease[104] and autoimmune diseases such as Sjogren's disease.[105] Immunodeficiency syndromes, both congenital and acquired, also predispose to the development of clonal proliferations, often oligoclonal, as seen in patients heavily immunosuppressed post-cardiac transplantation or with AIDS-related lymphadenopathy,[106,107] when different clonal rearrangements are seen in tissues taken from different sites. If the immunosuppression is removed, the clonal cells regress. Persistence of immunosuppression, however, leads usually to the eventual predominance of a single clonal lymphocytic population and to neoplasia.[108] These findings suggest that, in these patients, a second chromosomal event occurring to one of the clonally rearranged antigen receptor genes leads to malignant transformation. In brief, the presence of a monoclonal population of cells always occurs in lymphoproliferative neoplasias although, alone, it does not determine the presence of neoplasia. It may be, however, a preceding step in its development.

Translocations involving antigen receptor genes
Consistent translocations in lymphoid neoplasia involving antigen receptor genes have been implicated in malignant change. Many of these rearrange-

ments are detectable by Southern analysis, hybridizing with the Ig, TCR or appropriate DNA probes for other genes involved at the point of translocation. The first was described in Burkitt's lymphoma[109] where one of three reciprocal translocations involving the c-*myc* proto-oncogene located on chromosome 8(q24)[110] and the loci for IgH, IgLϰ or IgLλ on chromosomes 14, 2 and 22 respectively occur. In 75% t(8;14) is detected.[111] All three of the translocations lead to elevated expression of c-*myc*.[112,113] The t(11;14)(q13;q21) translocation involving the IgH locus[114] and the *bcl*-1 (B-cell lymphoma/leukaemia-1)[115] locus is seen in CLL,[116] in B-cell lymphomas[117] and in multiple myeloma.[118] The t(14;18)(q32;q21), seen in 85% of follicular lymphomas and in 25% of high grade B-cell lymphomas, involves a J$_H$ segment of the IgH locus and the *bcl*-2 putative proto-oncogene.[56,119–121] Following this translocation, there is greatly enhanced expression of the *bcl*-2 protein analogous to Burkitt's lymphoma.[122] The t(14;19)(q32;q13.1) found in some cases of CLL involves the Cα gene of the IgH locus and the *bcl*-3 putative oncogene on chromosome 19, and again deregulated gene expression occurs.[123] Homology between part of the *bcl*-3 sequence and previously identified yeast genes that regulate the start of cell cycle suggest that this is a true proto-oncogene with a role in leukaemogenesis.[124] Both the t(11;14) and t(14;18) are thought to occur as a mistake during the process of V-D-J joining under the influence of recombinase enzyme responsible for normal V-D-J rearrangement.[125]

Consistent translocations involving the TCR genes predominantly affect the 14q11-12 regions where the TCR α and δ loci are situated. Less frequently, the TCR γ or δ loci on the long arm and short arm respectively of chromosome 7 are involved in T-cell lymphoma associated translocations. The first two recurrent abnormalities defined were the t(8;14)(q24;q11)[126] and inversion 14 [inv(14)(q11q32)],[127] the latter also described in ataxia–telangiectasia.[128] Molecular studies of the t(8;14) show the breakpoint involving a J$_\alpha$ segment on chromosome 14 and result in the C$_\alpha$ gene being translocated to a region immediately 3′ of the c-*myc* gene.[129] This results in deregulation of c-*myc* transcription and is analogous to Burkitt's lymphoma.[130] The inversion 14 is heterogeneous at a molecular level, involving a variable region of the IgH locus and a TCR J$_\alpha$ segment[131] leading to transcription of a hybrid IgH–TCR mRNA.[132,133] The function of the hybrid fusion product in oncogenesis is unknown, although suspicion is high, particularly as the inversion 14 has additionally been described in B-cell lymphoma.[134] Interestingly, there is another recurring translocation in T-cell lymphomas involving the V$_H$ region of the IgH locus and the region containing the TCR β chain gene on chromosome 7, the t(7;14)(q35-q36;q32).[135] It is not clear as yet if the same sequences are involved. Other reciprocal translocations in T-cell malignancies include t(11;14)(p13;q11) involving the TCR δ locus[136,137] with the region on chromosome 11 implicated in the development of Wilm's tumour[137] and the t(10;14)(q24;q11) where a putative proto-onco gene called TCL3 (T-cell leukaemia/lymphoma 3) on chromosome 10 lies proximal to the breakpoint.[138] The t(10;14) is particularly associated with T-ALL and high grade T-cell lymphomas.[138] The significance of translocations involving TCR genes is less clear than for those involving immunoglobulin genes. However, their recurrent involvement leads to speculative implication in the development of malignant transformation. Ultimately, defining the mechanism of oncogenesis at a molecular level may facilitate the use of 'gene therapy'.[139]

Clinical applications of Ig and TCR gene studies

Molecular probes to Ig and TCR genes facilitate rearrangement studies to determine the clonality and lineage of B- or T-cell malignancies. It is possible to distinguish monoclonal from polyclonal proliferations and specify the lymphocytic lineage in B-cell tumours where surface or cytoplasmic immunophenotyping is unhelpful. This is clinically useful in the differentiation between a reactive process, pre-neoplasia, or neoplasia when taken in conjunction with histological appearance and immunophenotyping information.[3] Determination of cell lineage is of importance to ascertain the prognosis, for, in general, T-cell malignancies have a clinically more aggressive outcome than B-cell malignancies.[22,140,141] Assignment of the cell lineage may alter the proposed treatment, as demonstrated by the more intensive treatment for T-cell ALL which, in turn, has led to an improved remission and survival in these patients.

Monoclonal antibodies against $\varkappa$ and λ IgL are capable of detecting a clonal population of B-cells by the presence of restricted IgL surface expression, where there is an abundance of malignant B-cells.[143,144] However, if the malignant B-cells are small in number and reactive B- or T-cells are excessive, detection of a clonal population may not be possible. In addition, monoclonal populations in Null cell ALL and T-cell neoplasms cannot be distinguished by surface immunophenotyping.[141] The problem of determining lineage in lymphoid neoplasms lacking lineage specific surface markers is readily overcome by antigen receptor gene rearrangement studies.[4-21]

The developmental stage of the lymphoid malignancy may also be clarified by gene rearrangement analysis and assist in the classification of the neoplasm. The presence of clonally rearranged TCR γ and TCR δ with surface expression of CD7 indicated the development of clonality early in T-cell commitment or even a pre-T-cell lineage stage, as found in Lennert's lymphoma, large cell anaplastic CD30 positive lymphoma, Null cell ALL and AILD.[20,21] TCR β gene rearranges later in development with concurrent CD2 antigen expression and is found in the majority of T-cell leukaemias and lymphomas.[17,19] Rearrangement of TCR α occurs relatively late in T-cell development representing a later stage of malignant change and is accompanied by CD3, CD4 or CD8 antigens as seen often in T-CLL.[85]

Similarly, clonal rearrangement of IgH alone occurs with early B-cell or even pre-B-cell lineage commitment as found in Null cell ALL[83] and some Hodgkin's disease.[64–70] The additional presence of IgLϰ and finally IgLλ gene rearrangement indicates a B-cell lineage in more mature lymphoid neoplasms such as large cell lymphoma, follicular lymphoma, CLL and hairy cell leukaemia.[2,4,58,83]

In a few cases, clonal rearrangements of both Ig and TCR genes are found in the same population of neoplastic cells, particularly in immature B-cell such as Null cell ALL[12,15,16,18,20,21,100–102] and in occasional cases of non-lymphoid haematological malignancies such as acute myeloid leukaemia.[87,88] This almost certainly reflects a monoclonal cell population arising from early undifferentiated haematopoietic stem cells capable of Ig and TCR gene rearrangement before B- or T-cell lineage commitment. The prognosis is often worse in these patients and may warrant more aggressive therapy.

The gene rearrangements in lymphoid neoplasias follow a precise pattern allowing clonality, cell lineage and maturation stage of malignant change to be defined with a degree of certainty. The information is of use to the clinician in classifying the disease and allows tailoring the treatment according to the probable prognosis. A clonal marker of disease is provided for assessment of treatment outcome by determining the presence or absence of residual disease and to detect recurrence. Peripheral blood, bone marrow, lymph node or suspect tissue may be analysed and reveal the presence of the malignancy related marker even when clinically and morphologically clear of disease.[24–29]

t(14;18) Translocation in lymphomas

The t(14;18)(q32;q21) translocation associated with follicular non-Hodgkin's lymphomas (FCC) and some high grade diffuse NHL[28,32,33,121] was first cloned from a B cell leukaemic cell line.[145] The probe obtained identified the *bcl-2* gene locus on chromosome 18 (band q21) and revealed the involvement of this gene in the t(14;18) translocation of FCC.[146] The translocation involves the *bcl-2* gene at one of two sites on chromosome 18 and the immunoglobulin heavy chain joining region on chromosome 14 (Fig. 3). The first site on chromosome 18 contains 60% of the breakpoints, is approximately 150 bases long at the 3′ untranslated region of the *bcl-2* on exon III and is known as the major breakpoint region (*mbr*).[121,147] The second is known as the minor cluster region (*mcr*) at a distance of approximately 20 kb 3′ of the gene and is a region where a further 25% of breakpoints are found[121,148] (Fig. 4(a)). Occasionally, the breakpoint may occur 5′ to the *bcl-2* gene.[121,149] The coding regions of the *bcl-2* gene are left intact in all t(14;18) translocations so that the *bcl-2*/Ig heavy chain transcript produced continues to encode a normal *bcl-2* protein.[122,150] Molecular analysis of structural abnormalities near, or within, the *bcl-2* gene, particularly the t(14;18) translocation, may be carried out by the use of chromosome 18 DNA probes and Southern analysis. The probes most widely used are shown in Figure 4(a) and were initially described by

Cleary.[147,148] The majority of translocations at the *mbr* may be detected with the use of the PFL1 probe[147] and the PFL3 probe[121] both of which lie within the third exon on the *bcl-2* gene. The PFL2 probe[148] detects the majority of translocations involving the *mcr*. For the majority of lymphomas, the rearranged *bcl-2* fragments co-migrate with rearranged immunoglobulin heavy chain gene fragment as detected by the J_H probe (Fig. 4(b)).[121] With the advent of the PCR using Taq polymerase,[30] the method has been applied to detect the t(14;18) translocation at both the *mbr*[28,31,32] and *mcr*[31,33] with a much higher degree of sensitivity; in the order of 1 : 100 000 cells bearing the alteration. Detection of the translocation is possible on DNA from disease tissue,[151] and the peripheral blood of patients, even on occasions when clinically disease free.[28,32] It is possible to amplify across the breakpoint region for the 14q+ derivative chromosome using synthetic oligonucleotides to the 5′ portion of the *bcl-2* gene flanking the *mbr* or *mcr* region and a consensus sequence from the Ig heavy chain joining region at the 3′ end of the joining exons.[28,32,33] Similarly, it is possible to amplify across the breakpoint of the 18q-derivative chromosome with the use of a heptamer containing oligonucleotide from sequence flanking the unrearranged D_H regions together with a *bcl-2* sequence at the 3′ end of the *mbr* or *mcr* regions.[31] Successful amplification may be determined by gel electrophoresis and ethidium bromide staining showing the presence of an appropriate size-amplified product. This may then be Southern blotted and probed using a *bcl-2* sequence internal to the amplification primer oligonucleotides. A positive signal on the autoradiograph will only be obtained if hybridization of this internal probe occurs due to correct amplification across the breakpoint.[28,33] The precise size of the amplified product may act as a clonal marker for the patient's disease and direct sequencing using the internal oligonucleotide may given an extremely accurate sequence across the translocation, including the 'N' segment, forming a unique marker of clonality.[31,33,152]

The t(14;18) translocation is ideally suited to detection by the PCR technique as the breakpoints at both the *mcr* and *mbr* take place over extremely short segments of the *bcl-2* gene. By this method it should be possible to detect a marker of disease in approximately 85% of patients with FCC. This facilitates an excellent means of detecting minimal disease levels in tissues suspected of containing neoplastic cells, and in the peripheral blood, as well as providing a means of assessing in vitro techniques such as bone marrow purging.[26,28,151]

Minimal residual disease

Leukaemias and lymphomas contrasted sharply with most other malignancies by the fact that, despite widespread dissemination at presentation, many patients may be returned to normality, sometimes permanently, following therapy. Survival correlates closely with the extent to which the disease has

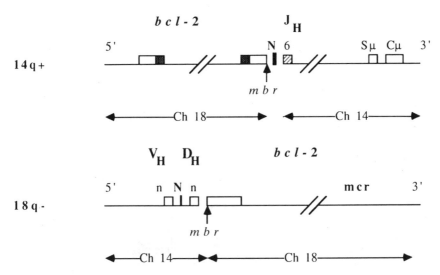

Fig. 3. Schematic diagram of the derivative 14q+ and 18q− chromosomes resultant from the t(14;18) translocation in lymphoma, at the major breakpoint region (*mbr*). V_H, D_H, J_H represent the Ig heavy chain gene variable, diversity and joining regions respectively. N: 'N' segment (insertions of random nucleotides found between the two breakpoints on the derivative chromosome, reminiscent of 'N insertions' between recombining segments in normal IgH rearrangement); Sμ: μ switch region; Cμ: μ constant region; *mcr*: minor cluster region. It is of note that a portion of the J_H segment is deleted on the 18q− derivative chromosome during t(14;18) translocation.

been eliminated, or the completeness of remission. The ability to define the response to therapy as precisely as possible is of considerable practical importance. Techniques permitting the detection of disease at a lower level than conventionally possible might be of benefit to the clinician. It may determine the patient free of disease in whom treatment may stop, from the patient with residual disease at a minimal level but ultimately destined to relapse, for whom alternative strategies of treatment should be considered, allowing an improved probability of eradicating the malignancy. Minimal residual disease (MRD) defines the lowest level of disease detectable by the methods available.[26] The most sensitive techniques are often able to demonstrate molecular and cellular change in the neoplastic cells, in morphologically and cytologically normal tissue.[26,28,32] Tumour-specific markers[153–155] are important in order to devise a strategy for detection of MRD and, in lymphoid malignancies, the presence of a clonal Ig or TCR rearrangement or translocation involving these regions facilitates the use of molecular techniques. There is a need for rapidity, ease and certainty of results, and the PCR offers the best opportunity of attaining these aims.[30] Southern analysis allows similar specificity but is a much lengthier procedure

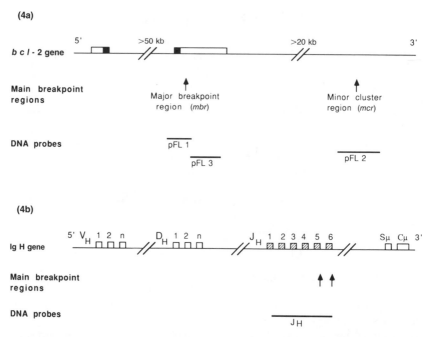

Fig. 4(a) and 4(b). Schematic diagram of the *bcl-2* gene (4(a)) and the Ig heavy chain (IgH) gene (4(b)). The main breakpoint regions are indicated by the arrows. The shaded areas in Figure 4(a) represents the *bcl-2* protein encoding region and lies outside of the breakpoint region. The open boxes represent the untranslated segment of the *bcl-2* transcriptional unit. IgH regions in Figure 4(b) are designated by V_H: variable; D_H: diversity; J_H: joining; $S\mu$: μ switch and $C\mu$: μ constant region.

with a marked loss of sensitivity.[23,24,27] Finally, the means of detecting minimal numbers of neoplastic cells may be helpful in earlier diagnosis or in screening for the early presence of malignancy-related molecular changes in both the predisposed and in the general population.

Methods to detect MRD

Polymerase chain reaction (PCR)

The application of PCR to the detection of minimal residual disease requires the target DNA to be a marker from the tumour cells. This is illustrated well by the t(14;18) in follicular lymphomas and some high-grade diffuse B-cell lymphomas. The PCR is able to detect at least one tumour cell in 10^5 cells.[32,156] The sensitivity may be increased to 1 in 10^6 cells by either enrichment of the sample for tumour cells by the use of flow cytometry followed by PCR or by a 'booster' PCR technique[157] or by utilizing two sets of primers flanking the target DNA. The target DNA should be relatively short.

In contrast, some lymphoid malignancies, predominantly ALL of which 20% have the Philadelphia chromosome, contain alterations involving the bcr gene on chromosome 22 and the c-*abl* gene on chromosome 9, involving longer segments of DNA, sometimes over hundreds of kilobases.[34,156,158] However, the length of DNA sequence may consist mainly of intron sequence that is not expressed in the messenger RNA (mRNA) transcript. This mRNA may be short enough to facilitate the use of the PCR technique to look for alterations over a considerable length within the transcribed exon DNA. Abnormal expression of a chimaeric mRNA (bcr–abl), from the Philadelphia chromosome, is found exclusively in the leukaemic cells.[34,159] The bcr exons involved in the translocation may be separated by over 100 kilobases of intron sequence.[34,156] Utilizing a modified PCR technique, it is possible to detect this abnormal mRNA marker of the disease. Complementary DNA (cDNA) from the chimaeric mRNA is produced by an initial step involving a reverse transcriptase enzyme, followed by the PCR procedure for DNA. Resultant amplification of the cDNA occurs. Amplification from the mRNA is advantageous in that interference from intron sequence does not occur and therefore analysis of changes with longer sections of DNA is possible.[34,156,158] PCR from mRNA will be of most benefit in the detection of MRD for translocations with breakpoint heterogenicity, although further delineation, at a molecular level, of chimeric mRNA transcripts is required before this is of use in lymphoid neoplasia, apart from in those demonstrating the Philadelphia chromosome.

PCR is most suited for detection of target DNA of less than a 1000 nucleotide base pairs.[30] The quantity of DNA required is extremely small,[4] 100 times less than for Southern analysis, while giving at least a 10^3 times greater sensitivity.[24,27,28,32,33,159] In addition, PCR has been applied to small lengths of target DNA allowing the use of this method on degraded DNA, unsuitable for Southern analysis, such as paraffin embedded sections.[151] Retrospective examination of archival material for tumour markers and clonality is thus facilitated for prospective follow-up of patients with MRD. Sequencing reactions, readily carried out directly on the PCR products, allow the tumour specific alterations to be analysed down to the single nucleotide base level. In this way, sequence analysis from tumour material gives a very clear and precise clonal marker for the patient's disease[31,33,35,36] and may be helpful in determining if recurrent disease shows the same clonality as the original tumour. In some cases, it may be possible to use the PCR product as a unique marker for the patient's tumour as shown with amplification of the T-cell receptor in T-cell lymphoid malignancies.[35,36] The use of an immunoglobulin heavy chain variable region consensus sequence in combination with a heavy chain joining sequence has broadened the application of PCR to many B cell lymphoid malignancies.[37] The detection of minimal residual disease by PCR has the advantage of rapidity (approximately 3 hours per reaction), and has greatly increased sensitivity over other techniques and therefore the ability to detect sub-clinical disease at a much earlier stage.[32,34] The main disadvantage lies in the necessity for the neoplastic diseases to have identified flanking sequences of DNA or mRNA that will allow amplification of a tumour-specific marker. PCR is an extremely sensitive method for amplification of a target DNA.[30,32,34] However, it is not directly quantitative. Adaptation of PCR to allow quantitation for detection of proviral DNA has been demonstrated.[160] Application of quantitation techniques to MRD could be of benefit in sequential follow-up, charting progression of disease from an early sub-clinical stage. Further clarification of tumour specific translocations, deletions and alterations will permit greater application of this technique to ascertain the presence or absence of MRD.

Alternative techniques

A number of methods are presently in use for the detection of MRD in addition to PCR. None, however, offers a comparable degree of sensitivity or rapidity. Southern analysis and immunophenotyping are techniques that discern disease at a level of 1 in 100 cells.[24,27,161] The sensitivity of Southern analysis has been improved by initial enrichment for tumour cells by flow cytometry improving the level of detection to 1 in 1000 cells.[159] Immunophenotyping is less specific than molecular analysis requiring therefore a battery of antibodies taking more time while sometimes causing difficulties with the interpretation.[162,163] Monitoring of remission, with other, less sensitive and probably less 'disease-specific' methods have met with only limited success.[24,27,159,161–163] Follow-up of patient in clinical and haematological remission of acute lymphoblastic leukaemia using anti-CALLA antibody to examine the marrow known to have been positive at presentation failed to be of use due to phenotype shift at relapse.[164] However, a study, in which two immunological parameters, tailored to the original phenotype of the blast cells were utilized, produced results highly predictive of relapse[165] with a considerably greater degree of sensitivity. Recently, a technique for rapid RNA transcript sequence analysis of the clonal T cell receptor or immunoglobulin heavy chain rearrangement from malignant B and T lymphocytes was described. This enables the generation of individual tumour probes in lymphomas and leukaemias to facilitate tissue in situ analysis for MRD.[166] However, this technique could be further developed to increase sensitivity of detection of MRD by incorporating the sequence data obtained into the PCR setting. Other techniques, such as digital image microscopy for rare event detection using fluorescence probes, have been developed and are reported to detect 1 in 10000 tumour cells in bone marrow patients with leukaemia but as yet are not generally applicable.[167]

Clinical perspectives in minimal residual disease

Induction therapy in leukaemia and lymphoma is administered in order to obtain a complete remission. However, residual disease cells may still remain and have the ability to regenerate a new tumour mass.[168] The intensity of the induction therapy may influence the length of remission.[169] The detection of a marker for MRD in some cases such as the Philadelphia chromosome following allogeneic transplantation for CML does not necessarily herald relapse[170] but may be a transient marker representing the presence of residual tumour cells with limited capacity for division due to prior treatment. Possibly a failure of an immunological control mechanism,[171] or a second promotional event,[172] may be necessary for further multiplication of the remaining residual tumour cells to occur. Investigation of patients presenting with different stages of lymphoma or leukaemia using flow cytofluorometric analysis for $\varkappa$ or λ light chain expression,[170] or gene rearrangement analysis suggests that clonal evidence of disease may be found in the absence of clinical or morphological findings.[24,27] Studies of the peripheral blood of patients in long-term follow-up of malignant lymphoma using restriction fragment length polymorphisms or PCR for the t(14;18) translocation show persistent abnormalities in a proportion despite continuing clinical remission.[28,32,173] If the abnormalities are present for many years without the evidence of recurrence, their clinical relevance must be queried.[174]

Quantitation of the disease remaining, or determination of increased disease bulk at an early sub-clinical stage, may help delineate those patients requiring further therapy due to early progression while the disease bulk remains small. Those with quiescent disease markers may require no further treatment until evidence of progression is observed.[168,170,174] Southern analysis does allow relative quantitation of the percentage of clonal tumour cells present, although the sensitivity is poor in comparison to PCR and may only precede overt clinical relapse by a short period of time.[24] Adaptation of PCR to quantitation[160] will improve the early detection of clonal proliferation of MRD. However, extreme care is essential with the PCR in the detection of MRD as the sensitivity of the techniques may allow comtamination to contribute to rogue results. Direct sequencing of the PCR products will provide unique clonal markers down to the base sequence level for an individual tumour and help reduce the possibility of a false positive result.

There is little evidence that prolonged periods of maintenance chemotherapy are likely to increase the numbers of cures[174,175] and in some cases might decrease it.[176] Induction of a second remission for relapse following consolidation or maintenance chemotherapy is considerably more difficult.[177] Treatment involving intensification of early post-remission therapy in childhood ALL improves disease for survival[178] and, similarly, allogeneic BMT in childhood ALL in second complete remission shows improved disease-free survival compared to chemotherapy alone.[179] Intensification of therapy with autologous bone marrow support in second remission with or without bone marrow purging has been shown to improve disease-free survival in a number of haematological malignancies including AML,[170,180,181] ALL[178] and FCC[182] although further follow-up is required. The role of autologous or allogeneic BMT in the management of MRD as yet remains unclear.[183] Overall, it appears that early intensification of therapy post-induction of CR where MRD can be detected, or in bad prognostic groups, may improve disease-free survival in both leukaemia and lymphoma.

Recent data suggest that an alternative approach to MRD management utilizing cytokines such as interferon and interleukin-2 may be of benefit.[184-186] Interferon in chronic myeloid leukaemia has been shown to induce a Philadelphia negative status following prolonged treatment.[184] Successful treatment of murine renal carcinomas has been observed using flavone acetic acid and interleukin-2 in combination to augment natural killer cell activity,[187] revealing good synergy in the anti tumour effect. The addition of cytokines to treatment protocol for MRD may have significant therapeutic potential.[188] The role of cytokines particularly in MRD look promising although the scheduling, dosage and combinations requires further consideration. An alternative experimental approach to the elimination of minimal residual leukaemia has involved the use of monoclonal antibody with specific anti-leukaemic cell activity. Leukaemic rats were prepared with non-curative doses of busulfan and cyclophosphamide followed by syngeneic bone marrow transplantation and treatment with monoclonal antibody. A large proportion of the group treated with monoclonal antibody were cured while all the control group that received no monoclonal antibody therapy died of leukaemia relapse.[189]

Ultimately defining the gene defect and mechanism of disease may permit the use of therapy directly targeted at the molecular changes. Lymphoid malignancies particularly demonstrating translocations involving Ig or TCR genes such as the t(8;14) of Burkitt's lymphoma, t(14;18) of follicular lymphoma and t(8;14) of T-cell neoplasms where deregulation of gene transcription has been associated with malignant transformation may be amenable to treatment by 'gene therapy'. In vitro experiments with an antisense oligodeoxynucleotides has successfully demonstrated the ability to decrease c-*myc* protein levels and thus malignant proliferation in cell lines containing the abnormal c-*myc* transcripts while leaving the normal c-*myc* protein expression and cell growth unaltered in control normal cells.[139] If in vivo trials of this form of 'gene therapy' are successful, it will offer great potential for possible curative treatment in an often bad prognostic group of patients, particularly those with MRD destined to relapse. It will become essential if this form of treatment is to be considered to define precisely, at a molecular level, the disease-associated gene rearrangements.

In summary, techniques enabling detection of minimal residual disease in lymphoid malignancies provide pointers towards groups of patients potentially curable with further modalities of treatment. Molecular techniques detecting clonal Ig or TCR rearrangements are generally of most use, with the exception of follicular lymphoma with the clearly defined t(14;18), particularly when detectable by the PCR. Monitoring of peripheral blood lymphocytes, bone marrow or suspect tissue is possible. Early post-remission intensification of therapy appears to improve survival while prolonged maintenance therapy may be of poor proven benefit. The use of monoclonal antibodies, cytokines in combination with other modalities of treatment and possible 'gene therapy' in the future, while still experimental, offer interesting prospects for the future management of MRD.

Conclusions

Gene rearrangement analysis of both antigen receptor genes and non-random chromosomal translocations in lymphoid malignancies, at present, provide excellent clonal markers of disease in the majority of cases. This allows improved classification of disease and provides a prospective marker of disease in order to monitor disease regression or progression even at a subclinical level when incorporated into a PCR strategy. However, even more important is the unravelling of the neoplastic process. Antigen receptor gene rearrangement studies indicate a high incidence of involvement in lymphoid malignancies often splicing a receptor gene into another gene resulting in deregulation of expression of the gene involved. This is demonstrated well for c-*myc* in both B- and T-cell malignancies and for *bcl*-1, -2 and -3 in B-cell malignancies. The implication in oncogenesis is strong particularly in the light of tumour-specific inhibition of lymphoma growth by an antisense oligodeoxynucleotide in a Burkitt's lymphoma cell line. Gene rearrangement studies in lymphoid malignancies are not only useful in providing disease markers but should point the way forward to future tumour-specific and hopefully curative treatments by defining and understanding the disease process at a molecular level.

Acknowledgements I thank Professor J S Malpas and Bryan Young for their helpful comments and Mary Cotter for helping in the manuscript preparation.

References

(1) Fialkow P. Cell lineages in hematopoietic neoplasia studied with glucose-6-phosphate dehydrogenase cell markers. *J Cell Physiol* 1982; Suppl. 1: 37–43.
(2) Griesser H, Tkachuk D, Reis MD, Mak TW. Gene rearrangements and translocations in lymphoproliferative diseases. *Blood* 1989; 73: 1402–15.
(3) Waldmann TA. The arrangement of immunoglobulin and T-cell receptor genes in human lymphoproliferative disorders. In: Dixon FJ, ed. *Adv Immunol* 1987; 40: San Diego: Academic, 247.
(4) Arnold A, Cossman J, Bakhshi A, Jaffe ES, Waldmann TA, Korsmeyer SJ.

Immunoglobulin gene rearrangements as unique clonal markers in human lymphoid neoplasms. *N Eng J Med* 1983; 309: 1593–9.

(5) Korsmeyer ST, Waldmann TA. Immunoglobulin genes: Rearrangement and translocation in human lymphoid malignancy. *J Clin Immunol* 1984; 4: 1–11.

(6) Cleary ML, Chao J, Warnke R, Sklar J. Immunoglobulin gene rearrangement as a diagnostic criterion of B-cell lymphoma. *Proc Natl Acad Sci USA* 1984; 81: 593–7.

(7) Minden M D, Toyonaga B, Ha K et al. Somatic rearrangement of T-cell antigen receptor gene in human T-cell malignancies. *Proc Natl Acad Sci USA* 1985; 82: 1224–7.

(8) Minden MD, Mak TW. The structure of the T-cell antigen receptor genes in normal and malignant T cells. *Blood* 1986; 68: 327–36.

(9) Flug F, Pelicci PG, Bonetti F, Knowles DMII, Dalla Favera T. T-cell receptor gene rearrangements as markers of lineage and clonality in T-cell neoplasms. *Proc Natl Acad Sci USA* 1985; 82: 3460–4.

(10) O'Connor NT, Wainscoat JS, Weatherall DJ et al. Rearrangement of the T-cell receptor β-chain gene in the diagnosis of lymphoproliferative disorders. *Lancet* 1985; i: 1295–7.

(11) Rabbitts TH, Stinson A, Forster A et al. Heterogeneity of T-cell receptor β chain gene rearrangements in human leukemias and lymphomas. *EMBO J* 1985; 4: 2217–24.

(12) Tawa A, Hozumi N, Minden M, Mak TW, Gelfand EW. Rearrangement of the T-cell receptor β-chain gene in non-T, non-B acute lymphoblastic leukemia of childhood. *N Eng J Med* 1986; 313: 1033–7.

(13) Knowles DM, Dalla Favera R, Pelicci PG. T-cell β chain gene rearrangements. *Lancet* 1985; i: 159–60.

(14) Foa R, Pelicci PG, Migone N et al. Analysis of the T-cell receptor beta chain (Tβ) gene rearrangements demonstrates the monoclonal nature of the T-cell chronic lymphoproliferative disorders. *Blood* 1986; 67: 247–50.

(15) Griesser H, Feller A, Lennert K, Minden M, Mak TW. Rearrangement of the β chain of the T-cell antigen receptor and immunoglobulin genes in lymphoproliferative disorders. *J Clin Invest* 1986; 78: 1179–84.

(16) Griesser H, Feller A, Lennert K et al. The structure of the T-cell γ chain gene in lymphoproliferative disorders and lymphoma cell lines. *Blood* 1986; 68: 592–4.

(17) Greenberg JM, Quertermous T, Seidman JG, Kersey JH. Human T cell γ-chain gene rearrangements in acute lymphoid and non-lymphoid leukemia: Comparison with the T-cell receptor β chain gene. *J Immunol* 1986; 137: 2043–9.

(18) Hara J, Benedict SH, Mak TW, Gelfand EW. T cell receptor α-chain gene rearrangements in B-precursor leukemia are in contrast to findings in T-cell acute lymphoblastic leukemia: Comparative study of T-cell receptor gene rearrangement in childhood leukemia. *J Clin Pathol* 1987; 80: 1770–7.

(19) Norton JD, Campana D, Hoffbrand AV et al. Correlation of immunophenotype with rearrangement of T-cell antigen receptor β and γ genes in ALL of adults. *Leukemia* 1988; 2: 27–34.

(20) Tkachuk DC, Griesser H, Feller AC, Lennert K, Mak TW. Rearrangement of the T-cell delta locus in lymphoproliferative disorders. *Blood* 1988; 72: 353–7.

(21) Hara J, Benedict SH, Champagne E et al. T-cell receptor γ gene rearrangements in acute lymphoblastic leukemia. *J Clin Invest* 198; 82: 1974–82.

(22) Krajewski AS, Myskow MW, Cachia PG, Salter DM, Sheehan T, Dewar AE. T-cell lymphoma: morphology, immunophenotype, and clinical features. *Histopathology* 1988; 13: 19–41.

(23) Southern EM. Detection of specific sequences among DNA fragments separated by gel electrophoresis. *J Mol Biol* 1975; 98: 503–17.

(24) Brada M, Mizutani S, Molgaard H et al. Circulating lymphoma cells in patients with B and T non-Hodgkin's lymphoma detected by immunoglobulin and T-cell receptor gene rearrangement. *Br J Cancer* 1987; 56: 147–52.

(25) Cotter FE, Hall PA, Young BD, Lister T A. Simultaneous presentation of T- and B-cell malignant lymphoma with *bcl-2* gene involvement. *Blood* 1989; 73: 1387–8.

(26) Cotter FE, Price C, Young BD, Lister TA. Minimal residual disease in leukaemia and lymphoma. *Ann Oncol* 1990; 1: 167–70.

(27) Katz F, Ball L, Gibbons B, Chessells J. The use of DNA probes to monitor minimal residual disease in childhood acute lymphoblastic leukaemia. *Br J Cancer* 1989; 73: 173–80.

(28) Lee M, Chang KS, Cabanillas F, Freireich EJ, Trujillo JM, Stass SA. Detection of minimal residual cells carrying the t(14;18) by DNA sequence amplification. *Science* 1987; 237: 175–8.

(29) Horning SJ, Galili N, Cleary M, Sklar J. Detection of non-Hodgkin's lymphoma in the peripheral blood by analysis of antigen receptor gene rearrangements: results of a prospective study. *Blood* 1990; 75: 1139–45.

(30) Saiki RK, Gelfand DH, Stoffel S et al. Primer-directed enzymatic amplification of DNA with a thermostable DNA polymerase. *Science* 1988; 239: 487–91.

(31) Cotter F, Price C, Zucca E, Young BD. Direct sequence analysis of the 14q+ and 18q− chromosome junctions in follicular lymphoma. *Blood* 1990; 75: 131–5.

(32) Crescenzi M, Seto M, Herzig GP, Weiss PD, Griffith RC, Korsmeyer SJ. Thermostable DNA polymerase chain amplification of t(14;18) chromosome breakpoints and detection of minimal residual disease. *Proc Natl Acad Sci USA* 1988; 85: 4869–73.

(33) Ngan Bo-Yee, Nourse J, Cleary ML. Detection of chromosomal translocation t(14;18) within the minor cluster region of *bcl-2* by polymerase chain reaction and direct genomic sequencing of the enzymatically amplified DNA in follicular lymphoma. *Blood* 1989; 73: 1759–62.

(34) Lange W, Synder DS, Castro R, Rossi JJ, Blume KG. Detection by enzymatic amplification of bcr–abl mRNA in peripheral blood and bone marrow cells of patients with chronic myelogenous leukemia. *Blood* 1989; 73: 1735–41.

(35) Hansen-Hagge TE, Yokota S, Bartram CR. Detection of minimal residual disease in acute lymphoblastic leukemia by in vitro amplification of rearranged T-cell receptor δ chain sequences. *Blood* 1989; 74: 1762–7.

(36) d'Auriol L, Macintyre E, Galibert F, Sigaux F. In vitro amplification of T cell gamma gene rearrangements: a new tool for the assessment of minimal residual disease in acute lymphoblastic leukemias. *Leukemia* 1989; 3: 155–8.

(37) Deane M, Norton JD. Detection of immunoglobulin gene rearrangement in B lymphoid malignancies by polymerase chain reaction gene amplification. *Br J Haemat* 1990; 74: 251–6.

F E Cotter

(38) Levine EG, Arthur DC, Frizzera G, Peterson BA, Hurd DD, Bloomfield CD. There are differences in cytogenetic abnormalities among histologic subtypes of the non-Hodgkin's lymphomas. *Blood* 1985; 66: 1414–19.

(39) Koduru PR, Filippa DA, Richardson ME et al. Cytogenetic and histologic correlations in malignant lymphoma. *Blood* 1987; 69: 97–102.

(40) Yunis JJ, Frizzera G, Oken MM, McKenna J, Theologides A, Arnesen M. Multiple recurrent genomic defects in follicular lymphoma: a possible model for cancer. *N Eng J Med* 1987; 316: 79–84.

(41) Cabinallas F, Pathak S, Trujillo J et al. Frequent nonrandom chromosome abnormalities in 27 patients with untreated large cell lymphoma and immunoblastic lymphoma. *Cancer Res* 1988; 48: 5557–64.

(42) Le Beau MM. Chromosomal abnormalities in non-Hodgkin's lymphomas. *Seminars in Oncol* 1990; 17: 20–9.

(43) Leder P. The genetics of antibody diversity. *Sci Am* 1982; 246: 102–15.

(44) Alt F, Blackwell K, Yancopoulos GD. Development of the primary antibody repertoire. *Science* 1987; 238: 1079–87.

(45) Yanagi Y, Yoshikai Y, Leggett K, Clark SP, Alexander I, Mak TW. A human T-cell-specific cDNA clone encodes a protein having extensive homology to immunoglobulin chains. *Nature* 1984; 308: 145–9.

(46) Yanagi Y, Chan A, Chin B, Minden M, Mak TW. Analysis of cDNA clones specific for human T cells and α and β chains of the T cell receptor heterodimer from a human T-cell line. *Proc Natl Acad Sci USA* 1985; 82: 3430–4.

(47) Toyonaga B, Mak TW. Genes of the T-cell antigen receptor in normal and malignant T cells. *Ann Rev Immunol* 1987; 5: 585–620.

(48) Lefranc MP, Forster A, Baer T, Stinson MA, Rabbitts TH. Diversity and rearrangement of the human T cell rearranging γ genes: nine germ-line variable genes belonging in two subgroups. *Cell* 1986; 45: 237–46.

(49) Takihara Y, Champagne E, Griesser H et al. Sequence and organization of the human T-cell δ chain gene. *Eur J Immunol* 1987; 18: 283.

(50) Takihara Y, Tkachuk D, Michalopoulous E et al. Sequence and organization of the diversity, joining, and constant region genes of the human T cell δ chain locus. *Proc Natl Acad Sci USA* 1988; 85: 6097–101.

(51) Brenner MB, McLean J, Dialynas DP et al. Identification of a putative second T-cell receptor. *Nature* 1986; 322: 145–9.

(52) Toyonaga B, Yoshikai Y, Vadasz V, Chin B, Mak TW. Organization and sequences of the diversity, joining, and constant region genes of the human T-cell receptor β chain. *Proc Natl Acad Sci USA* 1985; 82: 8624–8.

(53) Yoshikai Y, Clark SP, Taylor S, Sohn U, Minden MD, Mak TW. Organization and sequences of the variable, joining and constant region genes of the human T-cell receptor α chain. *Nature* 1985; 316: 837–40.

(54) Reis MD, Griesser H, Mak TW. Gene rearrangements in leukemias and lymphomas. In: Hoffbrand AV, ed. *Recent advances in haematology*. 1988, vol 5, Edinburgh: Churchill Livingstone, 99.

(55) Siu G, Clark S, Yoshikai Y. The human T-cell antigen receptor is encoded by variable, diversity, and joining gene-segments that rearrange to generate a complex V gene. *Cell* 1984; 37: 393–401.

(56) Tonegawa S. Somatic generation of antibody diversity. *Nature* 1983; 302: 575–81.

(57) Hood L, Kronenberg M, Hunkapiller T. T-cell antigen receptors and the immunoglobulin supergene family. *Cell* 1985; 40: 225–9.

(58) Korsmeyer SJ, Hieter PA, Ravetch JV, Poplack DG, Waldmann TA, Leder P. Developmental hierarchy of immunoglobulin gene rearrangements in human leukemic pre-B cells. *Proc Natl Acad Sci USA* 1981; 78: 7096–100.

(59) Korsmeyer SJ, Hieter P, Sharrow SO, Goldman CK, Leder P, Waldmann TA. Normal human B cells display ordered light-chain gene rearrangements and deletions. *J Exp Med* 1982; 156: 975–85.

(60) Raulet DM, Garman RD, Saito H, Tonegawa S. Developmental regulation of T-cell receptor gene expression. *Nature* 1985; 314: 103–7.

(61) Samelson LE, Lindsten T, Fowlkes BJ, van den Elsen P, Terhorst C, Davis MM. Expression of genes of the T-cell antigen receptor complex in precursor thymocytes. *Nature* 1985; 315: 765–8.

(62) Yoshikai Y, Clark SP, Taylor S et al. Organisation and sequences of the variable, joining and constant region genes of the human T-cell receptor α-chain. *Nature* 1985; 316: 837–40.

(63) Alt F, Baltimore D. Joining of immunoglobulin heavy chain gene segments: implications from a chromosome with evidence of three D-J_H fusions. *Proc Natl Acad Sci USA* 1982; 79: 4118–22.

(64) Desiderio S, Yancopoulos G, Paskind M et al. Insertion of N regions into heavy-chain genes is correlated with expression of terminal deoxynucleotidyl transferase in B cells. *Nature* 1984; 311: 752–5.

(65) Roth DB, Chang Xiu-Bao, Wilson JH. Comparison of filler DNA at immune, nonimmune, and oncogenic rearrangements suggests multiple mechanisms of formation. *Molecular and Cellular Biology* 1989; 9 (7): 3049–57.

(66) Malynn BA, Berman JE, Yancopoulos GD, Bona CA, Alt FW. Expression of the immunoglobulin heavy-chain variable gene repertoire. *Current Topics in Microbiol & Immunol* 1987; 135: 75–94.

(67) Humphries CG, Shen A, Kuziel WA, Capra JD, Blattner FR, Tucker PW. A new human immunoglobulin V_H family preferentially rearranged in immature B cell tumours. *Nature* 1988; 331: 446–9.

(68) Berman JE, Mellis SJ, Pollock R et al. Content and organization of the human Ig V_H locus: definition of three new VH families and linkage to the Ig C_H locus. *EMBO J* 1988; 7: 727–38.

(69) Lefranc MP, Rabbitts TH. Two tandemly organized human genes encoding the T-cell constant region sequences show multiple rearrangement in different T-cell types. *Nature* 1985; 16: 464–6.

(70) Quertermous T, Murre C, Dialynas D et al. Human T-cell γ chain genes: organization, diversity and rearrangement. *Science* 1986; 231: 252–5.

(71) Lefranc MP, Forster A, Rabbitts TH. Rearrangement of two distinct T-cell gamma chain variable region genes in human DNA. *Nature* 1986; 319: 420–2.

(72) Forster A, Huck S, Ganem N, Lefranc MP, Rabbitts TH. New subgroups in the human T rearranging Vγ gene locus. *EMBO J* 1987; 6: 1945–50.

(73) Chen Z, Font MP, Loiseau P et al. The Vγ locus: cloning of new segments and study of Vγ rearrangements in neoplastic B and T cells. *Blood* 1988; 72: 776–83.

(74) Font MP, Chen Z, Bories JC et al. The Vγ locus of the human T-cell receptor γ gene: repertoire polymorphism of the first variable gene segment subgroup. *J Exp Med* 1988; 168: 1383–94.

(75) Lefranc MP, Forster A, Rabbitts TH. Genetic polymorphism and exon changes of the constant regions of the human T-cell rearranging gene γ. *Proc Natl Acad Sci USA* 1986; 83: 9596–600.

(76) Quertermous T, Strauss WM, Van Dongen JJM, Seidman JC. Human T cell γ chain joining regions and T cell development. *J Immunol* 1987; 138: 2687–90.

(77) Huck S, Lefranc MP. Rearrangements to the JP1, JP and JP2 segments in the human T-cell rearranging gamma gene (TRG) locus. *FEBS Lett* 1987; 224: 291–5.

(78) Hata S, Brenner M, Krangel M. Identification of putative human T cell receptor δ complementary DNA clones. *Science* 1987; 238: 678–82.

(79) Rakiyara Y, Champagne E, Griesser H et al. Sequence and organization of the human T cell δ chain gene. *Eur J Immunol* 1988; 18: 283–7.

(80) Hockett RD, de Villartay JP, Pollock K, Pozlack DG, Cohen DJ, Koismeyer S. Human T-cell antigen receptor (TcR) δ chain locus and elements responsible for its deletion are within the TcR α chain laws. *Proc Natl Acad Sci USA* 1988; 85: 9694–8.

(81) Saganarayana K, Hata S, Devlin P et al. Genomic organization of the human T cell receptor α/δ locus. *Proc Natl Acad Sci USA* 1988; 85: 8166–70.

(82) Sehnbauter BA, Pardoll DM, Burke PJ, Graham ML, Vogelstein B. Immunoglobulin gene rearrangements in remission bone marrow specimens from patients with acute lymphoblastic leukemia. *Blood* 1986; 67: 835–8.

(83) Korsmeyer SJ, Arnold A, Bakhshi A et al. Immunoglobulin gene rearrangement and cell surface antigen expression in acute lymphocytic leukemias of T-cell and B-cell precursor origins. *J Clin Invest* 1983; 71: 301–13.

(84) Hu E, Trela M, Thompson J et al. Detection of B-cell lymphoma in peripheral blood by DNA hybridization. *Lancet* 1985; ii: 1092–5.

(85) Davey MP, Bongiovanni KF, Kaulfersch W et al. Immunoglobulin and T-cell receptor gene rearrangement and expression in human lymphoid leukemia cells at different stages of maturation. *Proc Natl Acad Sci USA* 1986; 83: 8759–63.

(86) Tawa A, Benedict SH, Hara J, Hozumi N, Gelfand EW. Rearrangement of the T-cell receptor γ-chain gene in childhood acute lymphoblastic leukemia. *Blood* 1987; 70: 1933–9.

(87) Cheng GY, Minden MD, Toyonaga B, Mak TW, McCulloch E. T-cell receptor and immunoglobulin gene rearrangements in acute myeloblastic leukemia. *J Exp Med* 1986; 163: 414–24.

(88) Seremetis SV, Pelicci PG, Tabilio A et al. High frequency of clonal immunoglobulin or T-cell receptor gene rearrangements in acute myelogenous leukemic expressing terminal deoxyribonucleotidyl transferase. *J Exp Med* 1987; 165: 1703–12.

(89) van Dongen JJM, Wolvers-Tettero ILM, Wassenaar F, Borst J, van den Elsen P. Rearrangement and expression of T-cell receptor delta genes in T-cell acute lymphoblastic leukemias. *Blood* 1989; 74 (1): 334–42.

(90) Yumura-Yagi K, Hara J, Terada N et al. Analysis of molecular events in leukemic cells arrested at an early stage of T-cell differentiation. *Blood* 1989; 74: 2103–11.

(91) Hara J, Yumura-Yagi K, Tawa A et al. Molecular analysis of acute undifferentiated leukemia: two distinct subgroups at the DNA and RNA levels. *Blood* 1989; 75: 1738–46.

(92) Saltman DL, Ross JA, Banks RE, Ross FM, Ford AM, Mackie MJ. Molecular evidence for a single clonal origin in biphenotypic concomitant chronic lymphocytic leukemia and multiple myeloma. *Blood* 1989; 74: 2062–5.

(93) Griesser H, Feller AC, Mak TW, Lennert K. Clonal rearrangements of T-cell receptor and immunoglobulin genes and immunophenotypic antigen expression in different subclasses of Hodgkin's disease. *Int J Cancer* 1987; 40: 157–60.

(94) Sundeen J, Lipford E, Uppenkamp M et al. Rearranged antigen receptor genes in Hodgkin's disease. *Blood* 1987; 70: 96–103.

(95) Falk MH, Tesch H, Stein H et al. Phenotype versus immunoglobulin and T-cell receptor genotype of Hodgkin-derived cell lines. Activation of immature lymphoid cells in Hodgkin's disease. *Int J Cancer* 1987; 40: 262–9.

(96) Knowles DM, Neri A, Pelicci PG et al. Immunoglobulin and T-cell receptor β-chain gene rearrangement analysis of Hodgkin's disease: implications for lineage determination and differential diagnosis. *Proc Natl Acad Sci USA* 1986; 83: 7942–6.

(97) Roth MS, Schnitzer B, Bingham EL, Harnden CE, Hyder DM, Ginsburg D. Rearrangement of immunoglobulin and T-cell receptor genes in Hodgkin's disease. *Am J Pathol* 1988; 131: 331–8.

(98) O'Connor NTJ, Crick JA, Gatter KC, Mason DY, Falini B, Stein H S. Cell lineage in Hodgkin's disease. *Lancet* 1987; ii: 158.

(99) Weiss LM, Strickler JG, Hu E, Warnke RA, Sklar J. Immunoglobulin gene rearrangements in Hodgkin's disease. *Human Pathol* 1987; 17: 1009.

(100) Aisenberg AC, Wilkes BM, Jacobson JO. Rearrangement of the genes for the β and γ chains of the T-cell receptor is rarely observed in adult B-cell lymphoma and chronic lymphocytic leukemia. *J Clin Invest* 1987; 80: 1209–14.

(101) Hara J, Benedict SH, Champagne E, Mak TW, Minden M, Gelfand EW. Comparison of T-cell receptor α, β and γ gene rearrangement and expression in T-cell acute lymphoblastic leukemia. *J Clin Invest* 1988; 81: 989–96.

(102) Lipford EH, Smith HR, Pittaluga S et al. Clonality of angioimmunoblastic lymphadenopathy and implications for its evolution to malignant lymphoma. *J Clin Invest* 1987; 79: 637–42.

(103) Weiss LM, Wood GS, Ellisen LW, Reynolds TC, Sklar J. Clonal T-cell populations in *Pityriasis lichenoids et Varioliformis acuta* (Mucha–Habermann disease). *Am J Pathol* 1987; 126: 417–21.

(104) Hanson CA, Frizzera G, Patton DF et al. Clonal rearrangement for immunoglobulin and T-cell receptor genes in systemic Castleman's disease. *Am J Pathol* 1987; 131: 84.

(105) Fishleder A, Tubbs R, Hesse B, Levine H. Uniform detection of immunoglobulin-gene rearrangement in benign lymphoepithelial lesions. *N Eng J Med* 1987; 316: 1118–21.

(106) Cleary ML, Sklar J. Lymphoproliferative disorders in cardiac transplant recipients are multiclonal lymphomas. *Lancet* 1984; ii: 489–93.

(107) Shearer WT, Ritz J, Finegold MJ et al. Epstein–Barr virus associated B-cell proliferations of diverse clonal origins after bone marrow transplantation in a 12-year old patient with severe combined immunodeficiency. *N Eng J Med* 1985; 312: 1151–9.

(108) Lipford EH, Smith HR, Pittaluga S, Jaffe ES, Steinberg AD, Cossman J.

Clonality of angioimmunoblastic lymphadenopathy and implications for its evolution to malignant lymphoma. *J Clin Invest* 1987; 79: 637–42.

(109) Manolov G, Manolova Y. Marker band in one chromosome 14 from Burkitt's lymphoma. *Nature* 1972; 237: 33–4.

(110) Dalla-Favera R, Bregni M, Erikson J, Patterson D, Gallo RC, Croce CM. Assignment of the human c-*myc* oncogene to the region of chromosome 8 which is translocated in Burkitt's lymphoma cells. *Proc Natl Acad Sci USA* 1982; 79: 7824–7.

(111) Croce CM. Chromosome translocations and human cancer. *Cancer Res* 1986; 46: 6019–23.

(112) Erikson J, Nishikura K, ar-Rushdi A et al. Translocation of a $\varkappa$ immunoglobulin locus to a region 3' of an unrearranged c-*myc* oncogene enhances c-*myc* transcription. *Proc Natl Acad Sci USA* 1983; 80: 7581–5.

(113) Nishikura K, ar-Rushdi A, Erikson J, Watt R, Rovera G, Croce CM. Differential expression of the normal and of the translocated human c-*myc* oncogene in B cells. *Proc Natl Acad Sci USA* 1983; 80: 4822–6.

(114) Erikson J, Finan J, Tsujimoto Y, Nowell P C, Croce C M. The chromosome 14 breakpoint in neoplastic B cells with the t(11;14) translocation involves the immunoglobulin heavy chain locus. *Proc Natl Acad Sci USA* 1984; 81: 4144–8.

(115) Tsujimoto Y, Yunis J, Onorato-Showe L, Erikson J, Nowell PC, Croce CM. Molecular cloning of the chromosomal breakpoint of B-cell lymphomas and leukemias with the t(11;14) chromosome translocation. *Science* 1984; 224: 1403–6.

(116) Nowell PC, Shankey TV, Finan J, Guerry D, Besa E. Proliferation, differentiation, and cytogenetics of chronic leukemic B lymphocytes cultured with mitomycin-treated normal cells. *Blood* 1981; 57: 444–51.

(117) Yunis JJ. The chromosomal basis of human neoplasia. *Science* 1983; 221: 227–36.

(118) van den Berghe H, Vermaelen K, Louwagie A, Criel A, Mecucci C, Vaerman JP. High incidence of chromosome abnormalities in IgG3 myeloma. *Cancer Genet Cytogenet* 1984; 11: 381–7.

(119) Fukuhara S, Rowley JD, Variakojis D, Golomb HM. Chromosome abnormalities in poorly differentiated lymphocytic lymphoma. *Cancer Res* 1979; 39: 3119–28.

(120) Tsujimoto Y, Cossman J, Jaffe E, Croce CM. Involvement of the *bcl*-2 gene in human follicular lymphoma. *Science* 1985; 228: 1440–3.

(121) Weiss LM, Warnke RA, Sklar J, Cleary ML. Molecular analysis of the t(14;18) chromosomal translocation in malignant lymphomas. *N Eng J Med* 1987; 317: 1185–9.

(122) Seto M, Jaeger U, Hockett RD et al. Alternative promoters and exons, somatic mutation and deregulaton of the *bcl*-2-Ig fusion gene in lymphoma. *EMBO J* 1988; 7: 123–31.

(123) Ueshima Y, Bird ML, Vardiman J, Rowley J. A 14;19 translocation in B-cell chronic lymphocytic leukemia: a new recurring chromosome aberration. *Int J Cancer* 1985; 36: 287–90.

(124) Ohno H, Takimoto G, McKeithan TW. The candidate proto-oncogene *bcl*-3 is

related to genes implicated in cell lineage determination and cell cycle control. *Cell* 1990; 60: 991–7.

(125) Tycko B, Sklar J. Chromosomal translocations in lymphoid neoplasia: a reappraisal of the recombinase model. *Cancer Cells* 1990; 1: 1–8.

(126) Ueshima Y, Rowley JD, Variakojis D et al. Cytogenetic studies on patients with chronic T-cell leukemia/lymphoma. *Blood* 1988; 63: 1028–38.

(127) Zech L, Gahrton G, Hammarstrom L et al. Inversion of chromosome 14 marks human T-cell chronic lymphocytic leukemia. *Nature* 1984; 308: 858–60.

(128) Fiorilli M, Carbonari M, Crescenzi M, Russo G, Aiuti F. T-cell receptor genes and ataxia telangiectasia. *Nature* 1985; 313: 186.

(129) Shima E, LeBeau MM, McKeithan TW et al. Gene encoding the α chain of the T-cell receptor is moved immediately downstream of c-*myc* in a chromosome 8;14 translocation in a cell line from a human T-cell leukemia. *Proc Natl Acad Sci USA* 1986; 83: 3439–43.

(130) Erikson J, Finger L, Sun L et al. Deregulation of c-*myc* by translocation of the α-locus of the T-cell receptor in T-cell leukemias. *Science* 1986; 232: 884–6.

(131) Baer R, Forster A, Rabbitts TH. The mechanism of chromosome 14 inversion in a human T cell lymphoma. *Cell* 1987; 50: 97–105.

(132) Baer R, Chen K-C, Smith SD, Rabbitts TH. Fusion of an immunoglobulin variable gene and a T-cell receptor constant gene in the chromosome 14 inversion associated with T-cell tumors. *Cell* 1985; 43: 705–13.

(133) Denny CT, Yoshikai Y, Mak TW, Smith SD, Hollis GF, Kirsch IR. A chromosome 14 inversion in a T-cell lymphoma is caused by site specific recombination between immunoglobulin and T-cell receptor loci. *Nature* 1986; 320: 549–51.

(134) Denny CT, Hollis GF, Hecht F et al. Common mechanism of chromosome inversion of B- and T-cell tumors: relevance to lymphoid development. *Science* 1986; 234: 197–200.

(135) Russo G, Isobe M, Pegoraro L et al. Molecular analysis of a t(7;14)(q35;q32) chromosome translocation in a T cell leukemia of a patient with ataxia telangiectasia. *Cell* 1988; 53: 137–44.

(136) Williams DL, Look AT, Melvin SL et al. New chromosomal translocations correlate with specific immunophenotypes of childhood acute lymphoblastic leukemia. *Cell* 1984; 36: 101–9.

(137) Lewis WH, Michalopoulos EE, Williams DL, Minden MD, Mak TW. Breakpoints in the human T-cell antigen receptor alpha chain locus in two T-cell leukemia patients with chromosomal translocations have breakpoints within the human T-cell antigen receptor α-chain locus. *Nature* 1985; 317: 544–6.

(138) Kagan J, Finan J, Letofsky J, Emmanuel CB, Nowell PC, Croce CM. α-chain locus of the T-cell antigen receptor is involved in the t(10;14) chromosome translocation of T-cell acute lymphoid leukemia. *Proc Natl Acad Sci USA* 1987; 84: 4543–6.

(139) McManaway ME, Neckers LM, Loke SL et al. Tumour-specific inhibition of lymphoma growth by an antisense oligodeoxynucleotide. *Lancet* 1990; i: 808–11.

(140) Hui PK, Feller AC, Pileri S, Gobbi M, Lennert K. New aggressive variant of suppressor/cytotoxic T-CLL. *Am J Clin Pathol* 1987; 87: 55–9.

(141) Suchi T, Lennert K, Tu LY et al. Histopathology and immunocytochemistry of

169

peripheral T cell lymphomas: a proposal for their classification. *J Clin Pathol* 1987; 40: 995–1015.

(142) Hoelzer D, Thiel E, Loffler H et al. Intensified therapy in acute lymphoblastic and acute undifferentiated leukemia in adults. *Blood* 1984; 64: 38–47.

(143) Foon KA, Todd RF III. Immunologic classification of leukemia and lymphoma. *Blood* 1986; 68: 1–31.

(144) Stein H, Lennert K, Feller AC, Mason DY. Immunohistological analysis of human lymphoma: correlation of histological and immunological categories. *Adv Cancer Res* 1984; 42: 67–147.

(145) Tsujimoto Y, Fingler LR, Yunis J, Nowell PC, Croce CM. Cloning of the chromosomal breakpoint of neoplastic B cells with the t(14;18) chromosome translocation. *Science* 1984; 226: 1403–6.

(146) Tsujimoto Y, Cossman J, Jaffe E, Croce CM. Involvement of the *bcl-2* gene in human follicular lymphoma. *Science* 1985; 228: 1097–9.

(147) Cleary ML, Sklar J. Nucleotide sequence of t(14;18) chromosomal breakpoint in follicular lymphoma and demonstration of a breakpoint cluster region near a transcriptionally active locus on chromosome 18. *Proc Natl Acad Sci USA* 1985; 82: 7439–43.

(148) Cleary ML, Galili N, Sklar J. Detection of a second t(14;18) breakpoint cluster region in human follicular lymphomas. *J Exp Med* 1986; 164: 315–20.

(149) Tsujimoto Y, Bashir MM, Givol I, Cossman J, Jaffe E, Croce CM. DNA rearrangements in human follicular lymphoma can involve the 5' or the 3' region of the *bcl-2* gene. *Proc Natl Acad Sci USA* 1987; 84: 1329–31.

(150) Hua C, Zorn S, Jensen JP et al. Consequences of the t(14;18) chromosomal translocation in follicular lymphoma: deregulated expression of a chimeric and mutated *bcl-2* gene. *Oncogene Res* 1988; 2: 263–75.

(151) Price CG, Cotter FE, Curling OM et al. Polymerase chain reaction to confirm extranodal progression of follicular lymphoma. *Lancet* 1989; i: 1132.

(152) Bakhshi A, Wright JJ, Graninger W et al. Mechanism of the t(14;18) chromosomal translocation: structural analysis of both derivative 14 and 18 reciprocal partners. *Proc Natl Acad Sci USA* 1987; 84: 2396–400.

(153) Sampi K. Significance of tumor markers in the treatment of cancer: hematologic malignancy. *Gan-To-Kagaku-Ryoho* 1987; 14 (11): 3041–5.

(154) Collins SJ. Direct sequencing of amplified genomic fragments documents N-*ras* point mutations in myeloid leukemia. *Oncogene Res* 1988; 3: 117–23.

(155) Lyons J, Janssen JW, Bartram C, Layton M, Mufti GJ. Mutation of Ki-ras and N-ras oncogenes in myelodysplastic syndromes. *Blood* 1988; 71: 1707–12.

(156) Evinger-Hodges MJ, Spinolo JA, Spencer V, Nieto P, Dicke KA. Detection of minimal residual disease in acute myelogenous leukemia by RNA-in situ hybridization. *Bone Marrow Transpl* 1989; 4 (1): 13–15.

(157) Ruano G, Fenton W, Kidd KK. Biphasic amplification of very dilute DNA samples via 'booster' PCR. *Nucleic Acid Res* 1989; 17: 5407.

(158) Sarkar G, Sommer SS. Access to a messenger RNA sequence or its protein product is not limited by tissue or species specificity. *Science* 1989; 244 (4902): 331–4.

(159) Bregni M, Siena S, Neri A et al. Minimal residual disease in acute lymphoblastic leukemia detected by immune selection and gene rearrangement analysis. *J Clin Oncol* 1989; 7: 338–43.

(160) Abbott MA, Poiesz BJ, Byrne BC, Kwok S, Sninsky JJ, Ehrlich GD. Enzymatic gene amplification: qualitative and quantitative methods for detecting proviral DNA amplified in vitro. *J Infect Dis* 1988; 158: 1158–69.

(161) Henni T, Vidaud M, Bretagne S, Goosens M. Detection of residual disease in onco-hematology: the contribution of molecular biology. *Pathol Biol Paris* 1988; 36: 91–5.

(162) Bernard A. The limitations in utilizing phenotypic markers to detect minimal residual disease in acute leukaemias (ALL). *Pathol Biol Paris* 1988; 36: 17–20.

(163) Visser JW, Martens AC, Hagenbeek A. Detection of minimal residual disease in acute leukemia by flow cytometry. *Ann NY Acad Sci* 1986; 468: 268–75.

(164) Greaves MF, Paxton AM, Jannossy G, Pain C, Johnson S, Lister TA. Acute lymphoblastic leukaemia associated antigen III alterations in expression during treatment and relapse. *Leukemia Res* 1980; 4: 1.

(165) Campana D, Coustan-Smith E, Jannossy G. Immunological methods of minimal disease detection. *Blood* 1990; 76: 797–800.

(166) Seibel NL, Kirsch IR. Tumour detection through the use of immunoglobulin gene rearrangements combined with tissue in situ hybridization. *Blood* 1989; 74: 1791–5.

(167) Lee BR, Haseman DB, Reynolds CP. A digital image microscopy system for rare-event detection using fluorescent probes. *Cytometry* 1989; 10: 256–62.

(168) Monnat RJ, Loeb LA. Mechanisms of neoplastic transformation. *Cancer Invest* 1989; 1: 175–83.

(169) Misset JL, De Vassal F, Auclair H et al. Improvement of results for poor risk childhood acute lymphoblastic leukemia (ALL): 80% three year acturial plateau of first remissions [Abstract]. *Proc Am Assn Cancer Res* 1982; 23: 124.

(170) Arthur CK, Apperley JF, Gou AP. Cytogenetic events after BMT for CML in chronic phase. *Blood* 1988; 71: 1179–86.

(171) Olsson L, Mathe G, Reizenstein P. The biologic and immunologic response to tumors. In: Berkharda, Karrer, Mathe, eds. *Anti-neoplastic chemotherapy*. New York: Grune & Stratton, 1984: 308–19.

(172) Diamond L, O'Brien TG, Baird WM. Tumor promoters and the mechanism of tumor promotion. *Adv Cancer Res* 1980; 32: 1–74.

(173) Fearon ER, Burke PJ, Schiffer CA, Zehnbauger BA, Vogalstein B. Differentiation of leukemic cells for polymorpholeucocytes in patients with ANLL. *N Eng J Med* 1986; 315: 15–24.

(174) Champlin R, Jacobs A, Gale RP et al. Prolonged survival in acute myelogenous leukaemia without maintenance chemotherapy. *Lancet* 1984; i: 894–5.

(175) Sackmann-Muriel F, Svarch E, Pavlovsky S et al. Alternating pulses of vincristine-prednisone with cytarabine-cyclophosphamide versus vincristine-prednisone in the maintenance therapy of acute lymphoblastic leukemia. *Cancer Treat Rep* 1984; 68: 581–6.

(176) Lister TA, Gregory W, Rohatiner AZS et al. Short term chemotherapy for acute myelogenous leukaemia. In: Lowenberg, Hagenbeek, eds. *Minimal residual disease in acute leukemia*. Boston: Nijhogg, 1984: 141–8.

(177) Rothing HJ, Kramer HP, Sedlacek HH. Development of new drugs for the treatment of leukemia [Abstract]. *XVIIth Int Congr Intern Med Kyoto* 1984: 32.

(178) Champlin R, Gale RP. Acute lymphoblastic leukemia: recent advances in biology and therapy. *Blood* 1989; 73 (8): 2051–66.

(179) Torres A, Martinez F, Gomez P et al. Allogenic bone marrow transplantation versus chemotherapy in the treatment of childhood acute lymphoblastic leukemia in second complete remission. *Bone Marrow Transpl* 1989; 4: 609–12.

(180) Linch DC, Goldstone AH. Autologous bone marrow transplantation in acute leukaemia. *Bone Marrow Transpl* 1987; 2 (3): 219–25.

(181) Yeager AM, Kaizer H, Santos GW. Autologous bone marrow transplantation in patients with acute nonlymphocytic leukemia using ex vivo marrow treatment with 4-hydroperoxycyclophosphamide. *New Eng J Med* 1986; 315: 141–7.

(182) Rohatiner AZS, Barnett MJ, Arnott S et al. Ablative therapy supported by autologous bone marrow transplantation with in vitro treatment of marrow in patients with B-cell malignancy. In: *Modern trends in human leukaemia VII.* Neth, Gallo, Greaves and Kabisch, eds. Berlin, Heidelberg: Springer-Verlag, 1987: 59–62.

(183) Ernst P, Maraninchi D, Jacobsen N et al. Marrow transplantation for non-Hodgkin's lymphoma: a multi-centre study from the European co-operative bone marrow transplant group. *Bone Marrow Transpl* 1986; 1: 81–6.

(184) Alimena G, Morra E, Lazzarino M et al. Interferon alpha-2b as therapy for Ph'-positive chronic myelogenous leukemia: a study of 82 patients with intermittent or daily administration. *Blood* 1988; 72: 642–7.

(185) Quesada JR, Reuben J, Manning JT et al. Alpha interferon for induction of remission in hairy-cell leukemia. *N Eng J Med* 1984; 310: 15–18.

(186) Rosenberg SA, Lotze MT, Muul LM et al. Observations on the systemic administration of autologous lymphokine-activated killer cells and recombinant interleukin-2 to patients with metastatic cancer. *N Eng J Med* 1985; 313: 1485–92.

(187) Hornung RL, Back TC, Zaharko DS, Urba WJ, Longo DL, Wiltrout RH. Augmentation of natural killer activity, induction of IFN and development tumor immunity during the successful treatment of established murine renal cancer using flavone acetic acid and IL-2. *J Immunol* 1988; 141: 3671–9.

(188) Talmadge JE, Black PL. Immunotherapy of metastatic disease. *Semin Thromb Hemost* 1988; 14: 79–87.

(189) Wagner JE, Johnson RJ, Santos GW, Kim BK, Shin HS. Systemic monoclonal antibody therapy for eliminating minimal residual leukemia in a rat bone marrow transplant model. *Blood* 1989; 73: 614–8.

Controversies in therapy for the low grade lymphomas

P McLAUGHLIN, F CABANILLAS and
A C NEWLAND

Introduction

Classification of the lymphomas has been challenging because of the great diversity of clinical and histological features of these diseases. Recent insights into the immunological and chromosomal characteristics of the lymphomas have also had a major impact on our thinking about these diseases. Numerous classifications have been proposed including systems relying mainly on morphology (eg Rappaport[1]) and others which attempt to incorporate immunologic concepts (eg Kiel,[2] Lukes & Collins[3]). Unfortunately, the reproducibility of these classifications is poor, with significant inter- and intra-pathologist variability. An attempt to overcome this difficulty was proposed with the development of the 'Working Formulation',[4] which was devised to act as a link between the various classifications. The Working Formulation does not take into account immunological data, but it has been widely accepted in many recent studies, and thus serves as a useful link among large clinical databases.

The recognition of a follicular pattern in lymph node biopsies, as emphasized in the Rappaport classification, is highly reproducible[5,6] and has been transposed to the Working Formulation classification. It is the follicular lymphomas that comprise the majority of low grade lymphomas. The low grade lymphomas (LGL) represent 30–45% of all cases of malignant lymphomas. They consist of diffuse small lymphocytic lymphoma (20% of LGLs), follicular small cleaved (55%) and follicular mixed lymphoma (25%). A small fraction of follicular lymphomas (follicular large cell type) are considered to be of intermediate grade, and these will be addressed only in passing in this review.

The low grade lymphomas are usually responsive to therapy but are highly prone to relapse. While paradoxically considered 'favorable' diseases by

All correspondence to: Dr P McLaughlin, MD Anderson Cancer Center, 1515 Holcombe, Box 68, Houston, Texas 77030, USA.

Cambridge Haematological Reviews: Haematological Oncology Volume 1 many, they remain among the few categories of lymphoma in which cure is considered unlikely. The variety of management options that can be effective, including periods of deferral of therapy, has made selection of therapy often a matter of philosophy as much as science. The typical indolent pace of these diseases provides the opportunity to make unhurried, thoughtful decisions about the management of these patients. However, we should strive to make those management decisions systematically, based on objective data as much as possible, and in a way that furthers the knowledge needed to make future treatments better. In this chapter, the status of current scientific research, the accomplishments and failures of currently available therapies, and some possible directions for future treatment of these diseases will be reviewed.

Biology

The follicular lymphomas all derive from B lymphocytes, and the vast majority (about 98%) of diffuse small lymphocytic lymphomas (DSL) are also of B cell origin. This homogeneity of the LGL categories contrasts with the phenotypic diversity found in most categories of diffuse lymphoma. In the follicular lymphomas, benign T-cells are consistently found around the malignant follicle.[7,8] This admixture of normal cells highlights the need for excisional biopsy of an intact node to establish the diagnosis: fine needle aspiration can often identify a monomorphic B cell population, but the architecture will always be missed, and occasionally the sampling can miss or underestimate the monoclonal B cell population.

Surface marker studies of the low grade lymphomas are useful to confirm the B cell phenotype, and also to screen for the aberrant expression of markers, such as CD5 in many cases of DSL and the closely related entity, chronic lymphocytic leukemia (CLL).[9] Characterization by markers can occasionally help in the categorization of lymphomas, and is likely to become increasingly important as monoclonal antibody and other targeted therapies are developed.

The low grade lymphomas usually have a low growth fraction.[10,11] Partly because of this slow proliferation, they have been difficult to culture in vitro. Nucleic acid flow cytometry studies reveal a low frequency of aneuploidy, a low S phase, and a low RNA index.[12]

A characteristic and consistent chromosome translocation (t(14;18)) is present in 80–90% of follicular lymphomas.[13] The breakpoint region (18q21) involved in this translocation is considered to be the site of an oncogene, designated bcl-2.[14,15] Cytogenetic studies in DSL are more limited than in the related entity CLL, in which the most common numerical abnormality is trisomy 12 and the most common structural abnormalities include 14q+ or aberrations on 6q and 11q.[16] In DSL, trisomy 12 may not be as frequent as in CLL, but translocations at 14q32 are common.[17] In CLL, a small fraction of patients (less than 10%) have t(11;14); this breakpoint region on chromosome 11 is also considered to be the site of an oncogene, designated bcl-1.[18]

The impact of molecular genetic studies on our understanding of the biology of the LGL has been substantial, and the promise for future advances seems great. Among the 80–90% of follicular lymphomas that have t(14;18) translocations, about 60% of breakpoints occur in the bcl-2 gene at the so-called major breakpoint region, and many others can be characterized by probes for the minor cluster region.[19] Thus, analysis of bcl-2 promises to be a useful marker in the majority of cases of follicular lymphoma, although, as yet, it is unclear if these rearrangements are of prognostic significance. The protein product of the bcl-2 gene has been studied using polyclonal antisera, and preliminary studies have indicated that the protein is membrane-associated, partly in the nuclear membrane and partly in the cell wall.[20] This protein is present in some normal B cells as well. The further characterization of this protein will hopefully lead to new insights that can be exploited therapeutically.

Another molecular genetic technique that is applicable to some of the LGL is the polymerase chain reaction (PCR). For those LGL that have rearrangement of bcl-2 within the major breakpoint region, the PCR technique can be applied to enhance the ability to detect subclinical circulating tumor cells.[21] Currently, it is possible to detect 1 in 10^5 cells with bcl-2 rearrangement with this technique. The current shortcomings of this technique appear to be twofold: (1) it may be too sensitive for practical applications with currently available therapies, since even patients in complete clinical response who have no indication for therapy can have persistent bcl-2 rearrangement detectable by the PCR technique; and (2) there is currently no precise way to monitor the efficiency of the reaction, so that attempts at quantitative measurements based on the number of amplifications (a 'titer') are imperfect. Further improvements of this technique may allow quantification of the number of residual circulating tumor cells, which could guide treatment decisions.

Etiology and incidence

The follicular lymphomas differ from DSL and most other categories of lymphoma in several respects. There is a slight female preponderance for the follicular lymphomas in many studies,[22,23] which contrasts with the male preponderance for most other categories of malignant lymphoma. Also, follicular lymphomas are common only in the western world, being very infrequent in Asia and in the Middle East.

The median age at diagnosis for the LGL is in the range of 50–60 years; patients are rarely younger than 20.

For the majority of patients with LGL, there are no clear etiological factors.

175

Patients with primary immunodeficiency states such as ataxia telangiectasia have a high risk of lymphomas, but it is the intermediate and high grade lymphomas that make up the majority of cases that follow both primary and acquired immunodeficiency states.

Clinical presentation and staging

The presentation of patients with low grade lymphoma is usually with a history of gradually progressive adenopathy. The nodes often wax and wane, and the clinical course is often quite prolonged. Extranodal presentations are uncommon, although there is often focal disease in the bone marrow, and microscopic involvement of the liver is often seen when liver biopsies are done. When adequately staged, about 15–20% will be stage I–II at presentation, and the remainder stage III-IV (Table 1).

Since the great majority of patients have advanced stage disease, the utility of the Ann Arbor staging system for stratifying prognostic groups is somewhat limited. In fact, while some studies show an impact of stage on prognosis,[24,25] others show a similar outcome for patients with stages III and IV as well as stage II disease.[26,27] Thus, other clinical parameters have been explored as potential prognostic factors.[28-31] Features such as bulky abdominal disease, distribution of extranodal involvement, beta-2-microglobulin, and serum lactic dehydrogenase should be assessed. At MD Anderson, a model has been developed for stage IV patients which stratifies groups according to number of extranodal sites, size of nodes, and extent of marrow involvement. This model identifies subsets of stage IV patients with significantly different survivals, ranging from 73% at 10 years for low burden (nodal disease <5 cm, and only 1 extranodal site, exclusive of extensive marrow disease) to 24% at 10 years for high burden (nodes >5 cm and 2 or more extranodal sites), and 40% at 10 years for those with intermediate burden.[28] The frequent finding of subclinical monoclonal excess on studies of peripheral blood lymphocytes by both surface marker and gene rearrangement studies is noteworthy but thus far not well defined as a prognostic factor.[32-34]

Staging laparotomy is rarely an issue, since so few patients have localized disease and since there are often medical contraindications to laparotomy in this age-group. However, the majority of patients with clinical stage I–II disease will be found to have occult abdominal disease if laparotomy is done.[35] This high likelihood of occult dissemination may be an important issue in planning therapy for patients with clinical stage I–II disease.

Results of treatment

Comparisons of treatment trials at different centers for patients with low grade lymphomas can be difficult. Overall survival can be influenced by many factors other than the initial choice of therapy, including intercurrent

Table 1. *Stage by cell type*[4]

	Stage at presentation (%)			
Cell type	I	II	III	IV
Diffuse small lymphocytic	3	8	8	81
Follicular small cleaved	8	10	16	66
Follicular mixed	15	12	28	46

illness in this older patient population, the changing efficacy of patient support measures over time, and the efficacy of secondary therapy. Individualized treatment and stringent patient eligibility for innovative therapy or for observation without therapy can select patient subsets that are impossible to compare with uniformly managed unselected patient populations. While individualization may often be a reasonable strategy in practice, the most reliable data on the efficacy of a particular treatment approach must be derived from studies of large patient populations who receive uniform management and are followed for long periods of time. An important and reliable parameter of the efficacy of primary therapy is the time to treatment failure, which is not affected by secondary therapy. Thus, the frequency and stringency of patient monitoring is another factor that deserves careful attention.

Many studies combine patients with DSL, FSC, and FM when reporting the results of treatment; patients with FLC are also included in some series. Many series describe little or no difference in survival among the 3 categories of low grade lymphoma. Others note a slightly longer median survival for patients with FSC. A study from the National Cancer Institute suggested the potential for cure for patients with FM when treated with COPP (cyclophosphamide, vincristine, procarbazine, and prednisone);[36] others have failed to confirm this result,[37] but the possibility of durable remission has led many investigators to favor intensive therapy for patients with FM.

Results according to stage
Stage I–II
A number of recent studies have suggested that about half of patients with stage I–II low grade lymphoma may be curable (Table 2).[38–45] This potential for cure seems highest for those with stage I presentations; in some series, patients with stage II disease have outcomes no different than those with stage III and IV. Most of these reports for stage I–II patients have employed involved field radiation therapy alone. Given the high frequency of occult abdominal disease in clinically staged patients, there have been several trials of more extensive therapy for stage I–II patients. At Stanford University, a

177

Table 2. *Treatment results for stage I–II low grade lymphoma*

Author	Therapy	Number of patients	% Survival 5-yr	% Survival 10-yr	% Failure-free 5-yr	% Failure-free 10-yr
Fuller[38]	XRT	62[a]	65		35	
Gospodarowicz[25]	XRT	190[a]	75	66	55	53
Paryani[39]	XRT	124[a]	84	68	62	54
McLaughlin[40]	XRT	76[a]	74		37	
	CT ± XRT		73		64	
Gomez[41]	XRT	29	75	66	62	55
	CT + XRT					
Monfardini[42]	XRT	26	62		55	
	CT + XRT		93		63	
Lawrence[43]	XRT or CT	54[a]	83	69	60	48
Richards[44]	XRT	57	79		61	
	XRT + CT				94	
McLaughlin[45]	CT + XRT	44	88		74	

[a]includes patients with FLC.

subset of patients who received total lymphoid radiation had a better freedom from relapse rate than those who received involved or extended field radiation.[39] At the MD Anderson Cancer Center, a subset of patients who received chemotherapy with or without radiotherapy had a better relapse-free survival rate than those who received radiotherapy alone.[40] Likewise, at St Bartholomew's Hospital patients who received adjuvant chemotherapy had more durable remissions than those who received XRT alone.[44] However, other trials have noted no apparent increase in the cure rate when chemotherapy was used as an immediate adjunct after XRT.[46] Thus, the use of XRT alone as initial therapy, reserving chemotherapy for use if relapse occurs, remains a common approach.

In a recent prospective trial at MD Anderson of COP-Bleo + XRT for stage I–II LGL, a preliminary analysis shows a 74% failure-free survival at 5 years for the first 44 patients so treated, suggesting that chemotherapy has a favorable impact.[45]

Stages III and IV
Natural history
The majority of patients with LGL have stage III–IV disease at the time of diagnosis. Most experience confirms that they are, in general, responsive to either single agent or combination chemotherapy, and that complete remis-

sion will occur in most cases. However, with the possible exception of patients with follicular mixed lymphoma, the remission obtained is not durable and up to 75% will relapse within four years. Thus, a pattern of response and relapse is observed, with an average median survival of 7 years (range 5–10 years) in most series. The risk for late relapse has been assumed to be indefinite, leading to the conclusion that these patients are incurable.[47] This premise of incurability is the basis for current controversy about the timing and role of initial therapy for these patients.

The failure to cure most patients with conventional therapy has meant that in stage III–IV disease, treatment has become increasingly selective. The policy of minimizing treatment with the hope of maximizing the patient's quality of life has been the aim of several studies. This argument about quality of life may be profoundly influenced by preliminary results from an ongoing NCI study of 'watchful waiting' versus intensive chemotherapy plus radiotherapy.[48] In this NCI study, early reports suggest that patients who receive early intensive therapy enjoy more time in remission off therapy than patients managed expectantly. Longer follow-up on this trial is needed.

The original description of the expectant, 'watch and wait' policy was reported by investigators at Stanford,[49] who have recently reported on their experience with 83 patients,[50] selected from an overall population of 214 patients seen over a 20-year period. The actuarial survival of the 83 patients was 82% at 5 years with a median survival of 11 years. Treatment was eventually required in 60% of the group, in general, for slowly progressive disease. The median time until therapy was required was 3 years and was determined by criteria including disease progression, the development of symptoms of bone marrow failure, or the development of disease in threatening sites. The time to treatment depended on the histology: for patients with FM, the time to treatment was 16.5 months, while it was 48 months for those with FSC, and 72 months for SL. Spontaneous remissions were observed in 19 patients (23%). In 6 patients, this was a complete regression. Two-thirds of the 19 had the FSC subtype.

Thus, in the Stanford experience, deferral of initial therapy was feasible for selected good risk patients. Other investigators have estimated that 60–86% of stage III–IV patients could be candidates for such an approach.[48,51] In the Stanford experience, the survival results for the deferred therapy group were similar to the results for unselected patients who were treated definitively at diagnosis. It should be noted that no survival advantage was seen for this group, despite their selection as prognostically favorable patients without threatening disease. So, while the feasibility of this approach is apparent, the ultimate benefit is uncertain. Hopefully, further information on this issue will be provided by the NCI randomized trial or by careful comparison of 'watch and wait' patients with treated patients with similar prognostic factors.

The 'watch and wait' policy is associated with some risks. Progressive disease can worsen the odds for treatment success for patients with stage III disease, many of whom may have long-term remissions with XRT or combined modality programs.[52-54] For stage IV patients, the development of adverse prognostic features such as bulky adenopathy, elevated serum LDH, or multiple extranodal sites could jeopardize the chance for treatment response. Thus, if the 'watch and wait' policy is taken, close follow-up is mandatory, and criteria for institution of therapy should be carefully defined.

The phenomenon of histological transformation may be another reason to be cautious about the 'watch and wait' approach. Most reports about transformed lymphoma have been based on patients who had received prior therapy; patient outcome in these reports was usually dismal.[55,56] Since de novo large cell lymphoma is potentially curable, DeVita and Hubbard speculated that untreated patients with LGL who transformed might also be potentially curable.[57] However, the management of patients who transform while under observation appears to be difficult, based on their low overall CR rate (43%) in the NCI randomized study.[48] The Stanford experience comparing rebiopsy in untreated and protocol patients showed a transformation rate that was similar (44 and 42%) between the groups, suggesting that treatment is not a factor in the development of transformation.[50] On the other hand, in the NCI randomized trial, transformation was seen in 6 of 41 patients on 'watch and wait', a large number for a study with short follow-up and an apparent contrast with their intensive therapy patients.

The 'watchful waiting' approach accepts that most patients will die of their disease. Currently available treatment approaches do not cure a meaningful fraction of stage IV patients. Controversies on the timing and choice of initial therapy are likely to persist until clinical trials identify potentially curative therapies.

Therapy

Once the decision is made to initiate therapy, there are additional controversies about whether complete remission should be the primary goal of therapy, and about the related issue of whether combination chemotherapy is superior to single alkylating agent therapy. For stage III patients, the role of radiation therapy is another controversial issue.

The impact of complete remission

Several studies have demonstrated a significant survival advantage for patients who achieve remission.[58,59] Most investigators make attainment of CR a primary goal of therapy.[60] While 'good partial remission' or 'probable complete remission' may be tantamount to CR, it is clear that patients who fail to respond represent an adverse group for whom improved therapy is badly needed.

The frequency of CR, like the time to treatment failure, is an important objective parameter on which to base comparisons of treatments. Survival, while obviously of key importance, is influenced by numerous features other than initial therapy. CR rates and TTF data have the merit of being solely attributable to the chosen therapy.

Single agents vs combinations

The range of reported response rates for single agents and combination chemotherapy regimens overlap considerably, with single agents yielding 30–70% CR[61,62] and combinations yielding 55–78% CR.[63,64] Combination chemotherapy regimens typically lead to more rapid attainment of CR than do single alkylators, which can require 3 years or more of continuous therapy to achieve CR.[65] Thus, in the occasional patient for whom a rapid response is needed (obstructive uropathy, etc), combination chemotherapy is indicated. In other cases, the choice is debatable. Single alkylators are certainly well tolerated; but drawbacks include somewhat lower CR rates than combinations, the established inability to cure, and the potential to cause leukemia.[66] In comparison, combinations have more short-term toxicity but are usually not required for a protracted period; they can induce long-term remissions in some cases, but also do not cure the majority of stage IV patients and they too can sometimes, at least for some regimens, cause leukemia.[48]

The role of radiotherapy for stage III disease

Three centers have reported results for patients with stage III LGL employing radiotherapy with or without chemotherapy (Table 3). In 1981, Cox reported on a small group of patients with stage III follicular lymphoma who received total lymphoid irradiation, and he described a 61% relapse-free survival rate at 5 years with a suggestion of a plateau in the RFS curve.[52] Later, Paryani reported long-term remission in about 40% of patients with stage III follicular LGL who received total lymphoid irradiation.[53] At MD Anderson Cancer Center, a combined modality approach using CHOP-Bleo chemotherapy and radiotherapy resulted in a 59% 5-year RFS rate for patients with low grade histologies (FSC and FM).[54] This fraction of patients with long-term remissions is considerably higher than with most reports of chemotherapy alone for stage III–IV disease. Thus, for many patients with stage III disease, combined modality therapy or radiation therapy alone can be effective and potentially important treatment approaches.

Stage III–IV: conventional chemotherapy

Chemotherapy has been the most common approach for patients with stage III–IV LGL. There have been a few reports of radiotherapy for stage IV pateints, either alone or integrated with chemotherapy, without any clear benefit.[65,67,68] As mentioned earlier, it is still debatable whether initial combination chemotherapy is superior to single alkylating agent therapy in terms

P McLaughlin, F Cabanillas and A C Newland

Table 3. *Treatment results for stage III low-grade lymphoma*

Author	Therapy	Number of patients	% Survival 5-yr	% Survival 10-yr	% Failure-free 5-yr	% Failure-free 10-yr
Cox[52]	XRT	29[a]	78		61	
Paryani[53]	XRT	66	78	50	60	40
McLaughlin[54]	CHOP − B + XRT	53	88		59	

[a]includes patients with FLC.

of long-term survival. However, the majority of recent investigations focus on combination chemotherapy, in part because: (a) there is quicker attainment and perhaps higher frequency of response; (b) some subsets of patients, such as those with follicular mixed histology, may have the potential for long term remission; and (c) no one is satisfied with the failure of single agent therapy to cure these patients.

In general, most studies of combination chemotherapy report CR rates of 55–78% (Table 4).[69–74] The median failure-free survival is about 3 years for most reported regimens, with a relapse-free survival at 5 years of 20–30%. There may be the potential for more durable remissions for patients with FSC lymphoma who receive COPP, as recently reported by the Eastern Cooperative Oncology Group, although earlier experience with COPP at the NCI did not suggest this.[69] The role of doxorubicin remains controversial. At MD Anderson Cancer Center, superior CR rates and survival were seen with CHOP compared to a historical group of COP treated patients.[75,76] The Southwest Oncology Group have reported no significant difference between CHOP-Bleo and COP-Bleo.[70] The BNLI noted a higher CR rate with CHOP compared to chlorambucil, but comparable disease-free survival and overall survival.[77] Somewhat higher morbidity was noted with CHOP compared with either COP[76] or chlorambucil.[77]

Once CR has been achieved, the difficulty is to maintain it. Unfortunately, because of the nature of the disease with its slow tempo, any study would need to be large and with prolonged follow-up to detect any significant differences. Two possible approaches are available: the first is to maintain the remission with protracted chemotherapy, or consolidate it with some form of grafting procedure; the second is to utilize modern developments with the biologic response modifiers.

A number of maintenance strategies with chemotherapy have been reported.[72,78] The duration of induction therapy has varied in many of these studies, as has the duration and type of maintenance therapy. However, the general observation with this approach has been a modest prolongation of remission with no ultimate survival advantage.

Table 4. *Treatment results for stage III–IV low-grade lymphoma*

Author	Therapy	Number of patients	% CR	% 5-yr survival	% 5-yr Failure-free of all pts
Anderson[69]	CVP				18 (DSL)
	C-MOPP	91	70	69	17 (FSC)
	BACOP				61 (FM)
Jones[70]	COP-Bleo	77	71	50	29
	CHOP-Bleo	75	72	57	38
Steward[72]	CVP	84	57	60	18
	CVP + Maint.	78	54	46	27
Ezdinli[71]	CP	48	64	62	22
	BCVP	53	64	58	26
	COPP	27	78	70	57
Anderson[73]	MBACOD	18	56	46	22
McLaughlin[74]	CHOP-Bleo + IFN	127	73	67	41

The earliest reports of the use of biological response modifiers were with BCG. At MD Anderson, BCG maintenance therapy was associated with more durable remissions.[79] In early reports from the Southwest Oncology Group, the inclusion of BCG in induction therapy was associated with prolonged survival, while maintenance BCG showed no effect.[70] More recent reports from the SWOG have questioned the earlier impression of prolonged survival with BCG.[80]

Maintenance therapy with alpha-interferon after CHOP-Bleo induction has been employed since 1982 at MD Anderson, and preliminary reports from that study have shown a statistically significant prolongation of remission with this strategy.[74] For all 127 patients on the study, the 5 year failure-free survival was 41% compared to 28% for historical control patients ($P = 0.08$).

The use of high dose cyclophosphamide and total body irradiation (TBI), or high dose combination regimens, are increasingly being investigated in conjunction with bone marrow infusion as consolidation for patients in remission on completion of conventional treatment for relapsed intermediate and high grade lymphoma. Unfortunately, bone marrow involvement is common in the LGL, but several groups have explored the possibility of bone marrow purging to deal with this problem.[81,82] So far, bone marrow transplant approaches have only been reported in the setting of relapsed disease. However, as problems of efficacy and toxicity are clarified, some groups have initiated trials with bone marrow transplantation as a consolidation approach for some patients in first remission. These studies necessarily have to focus on young patients, usually less than 50 years old, whose prognosis has usually been superior to elderly patients. Thus, it may be difficult to make comparisons of transplantation strategies versus standard therapy.

Salvage therapy following relapse

At the time of relapse, repeat biopsy is recommended to rule out the possibility of transformation. If the histology is still low grade, therapy can be withheld until there is disease progression or until there are symptoms. In the St Bartholomew's Hospital study following this policy, retreatment was required on average every 33 months; remission and duration of remission did not differ significantly for the first 3 treatment courses, although there was a predictable trend for shorter remissions following multiple relapses.[29] Others have noted a significantly worse outlook following 2 or more relapses.[83] Still, retreatment with the same single agent or combination regimen can be effective, particularly in patients who responded well to initial induction therapy.

A number of salvage chemotherapy regimens and phase II single agent studies have reported results by cell type. In general, patients with LGL have response rates comparable to those with intermediate grade lymphoma, although a lower proportion of responses are complete. A few agents have appeared to be particularly effective for patients with LGL, including alpha-interferon[84,85] fludarabine,[86] mitoxantrone,[87,88] and the related drug bisantrene.[89]

Future prospects

Using prognostic indicators that have been delineated, including tumor bulk, elevated LDH, and elevated beta-2 microglobulin, coupled with the clinical behavior of the lymphoma, it is possible to identify subsets of patients with different expected prognoses. In the community setting, such stratification could provide some basis for decisions about individualized therapy. In the research setting, it can permit stratification of treatment based on risk, and it can provide a more rational basis to identify clinically comparable patient populations receiving different therapies. Thus, both in the community and in the research setting, a careful staging evaluation is increasingly important.

The older patient

For the asymptomatic older patient with indolent disease, conservative management can sometimes be appropriate. When the lymphoma is aggressive, and when treatment is required at presentation, we should consider whether we should accept the known results and limitations of current conventional therapy or whether we have anything in addition to offer this age-group. In a study of mitoxantrone in combination with chlorambucil and prednisolone, 7 of 8 elderly patients responded and 3 remain in CR at greater than 2 years.[90] The regimen was well tolerated, although there was one early cardiac death in a patient who had previously received maximum doses of doxorubicin.

The younger patient

For the younger patient, the conventional approach is not particularly attractive. If they respond to alkylating agent therapy, they are faced with the long-term risks of prolonged exposure to these agents. Alternatively, if they fail to respond, the prognosis is poor with a median survival of only 2 years. Thus, new approaches are urgently needed.

In theory, the most attractive approach is to achieve a true complete remission and then prevent relapse, with its attendant risks of resistant or transformed disease and bone marrow failure. Neither of these aims is straightforward. As yet, none of the established combination chemotherapy regimens has been proven to achieve more durable remissions than single agent therapy, although the comparison with high grade lymphoma suggests that this may be the case. Alternative approaches include the utilization of current regimens in a modified fashion or the investigation of new combinations.

Bone marrow transplantation (BMT)

High dose therapy and BMT may be curative in relapsed lymphoma, even with advanced disease. Most reports show that the response is better and toxicity less if transplantation occurs in remission. Autologous bone marrow transplantation is the most practical transplant approach for patients with LGL, who are often too old for allogeneic transplant. As mentioned previously, the frequency of bone marrow involvement in LGL has prompted research on purging techniques. The group from the Dana Farber Cancer Institute have recently reported their experience using cyclophosphamide and total body irradiation as a preparative regimen, and using monoclonal antibodies directed against B cell antigens in conjunction with complement in an attempt to lyse residual tumor cells prior to autologous marrow transplantation.[81] Their results have been encouraging with 34 out of 49 stringently selected patients remaining in a complete unmaintained remission at a median follow-up of 11 months, with none of the 17 patients with follow-up greater than 11 months having relapsed. Although most of their patients were high and intermediate grade, some were low grade and these had a particularly encouraging high rate of response. The group from the University of Minnesota treated a less highly selected group of patients, including 3 patients with refractory LGL.[82] Continuous CR has been achieved for 5 of 10 patients transplanted in CR or PR in their series, but none of 7 patients transplanted with refractory disease has had sustained remissions. These results are more in keeping with results in series employing unpurged marrow. Thus, while theoretically appealing and technically feasible with satisfactory engraftment, it remains unproven that there is any benefit from the removal of tumor cells from bone marrow harvest specimens by monoclonal antibody treatment or other techniques.

The results of a number of studies show that transplantation can offer durable remissions in up to 25% of patients with advanced lymphoma. It remains to be seen, however, whether this applies to patients with low grade lymphoma, and whether it confers a survival advantage, with the possibility of cure, if performed at an earlier phase of the disease.

Targeted therapy

Treatment with tumor-specific anti-idiotype monoclonal antibody has been developed, primarily by the group from Stanford, utilizing the idiotype specificity of the unique cell surface immunoglobulin that is present on each B cell lymphoma. Occasional dramatic responses have occurred,[91] although overall results have not been encouraging. There is generally doubt about the efficacy of the treatment for several reasons. Although the mechanism of tumor lysis is not known, it most probably occurs by phagocytosis of antibody coated tumor cells. Continuing response assumes that there is not a finite capacity of the host effector system. There is also often tumor heterogeneity, with additional variable antigen expression, which will leave some of the tumor undetectable by the monoclonal antibody. If there is truly a limited repertoire of idiotypes for the majority of LGL, this problem might be overcome with cocktails of multiple idiotype antibodies.[92] Other targeted therapy approaches have utilized pan-B monoclonal antibodies conjugated to either toxins or radioisotopes.[93-95] Early clinical trials with these agents are promising. Many challenges remain, including optimizing radiation dosimetry for isotopes, and overcoming the theoretical need to deliver toxin to every tumor cell for the toxin conjugates. Other potential problems for both anti-idiotype and monoclonal antibody therapies include antigenic modulation, as is seen in CLL, and the fact that most tumors shed free antigen into the serum, which would act as a blocking antibody, soaking up the infused antibody. Finally, the immunogenicity of the xenogeneic immunoglobulin provokes anti-antibody activity.

Biological response modifiers

Alpha-interferon has been shown to have activity in the low grade lymphomas. In trials using the recombinant product, partial and occasional complete remissions have been seen. There is documented synergy in vitro between alpha-interferon and some chemotherapeutic agents, and clinical trials are currently in progress to assess combinations in vivo.[96,97]

There are a number of other agents that are available and await assessment, including interleukin 2 and the colony stimulating factors. Of these latter,

GM-CSF and G-CSF are particularly interesting as they stimulate normal bone marrow activity, and have been demonstrated to reduce the period of myelosuppression following chemotherapy,[98] thus creating the opportunity for more timely and intensive therapy which should translate into more effective disease control. In addition to this adjunctive role of the colony stimulating factors, it is foreseeable that evolving understanding of B-cell growth factors and their receptors will lead to therapies capable of direct modulation of the growth of these lymphomas.

References

(1) Rappaport H. Tumors of the hematopoietic system. In: *Atlas of tumor pathology.* Section III, Fascicle 8. Armed Forces Institute of Pathology. Washington, DC, 1966: 97–161.

(2) Lennert K, Mohri N. Histopathology and diagnosis of non-Hodgkin's lymphoma. In: Lennert K, ed. *Malignant lymphomas other than Hodgkin's disease: histology–cytology–ultrastructure–immunology.* Berlin: Springer-Verlag, 1978: 302–13.

(3) Lukes RJ, Collins RD. New approaches to the classification of the lymphomata. *Br J Cancer* 1975; 31 (Suppl 2): 1–28.

(4) Non-Hodgkin's Lymphoma Pathologic Classification Project. National Cancer Institute sponsored study of classifications of non-Hodgkin's lymphomas: summary and description of a working formulation for clinical usage. *Cancer* 1982; 2112–35.

(5) Ezdinli EZ, Costello W, Wasser LP et al. Eastern Cooperative Oncology Group experience with the Rappaport classification of non-Hodgkin's lymphomas. *Cancer* 1979; 43: 544–50.

(6) NCI Non-Hodgkin's Classification Project Writing Committee. Classification of non-Hodgkin's lymphomas. *Cancer* 1985; 55: 91–5.

(7) Dvoretsky P, Wood GS, Levy R, Warnke RA. T-lymphocyte subsets in follicular lymphomas compared with those in non-neoplastic lymph nodes and tonsils. *Human Pathol* 1982; 13: 618–25.

(8) Jaffe ES, Braylan RC, Nanba K, Frank MM, Berard CW. Functional markers: a new perspective on malignant lymphomas. *Cancer Treat Rep* 1977; 61: 953–62.

(9) Deegan MJ. Membrane antigen analysis in the diagnosis of lymphoid leukemias and lymphomas: differential diagnosis, prognosis as related to immunophenotype, and recommendations for testing. *Arch Pathol Lab Med* 1989; 113: 606–18.

(10) Bremer K. Cellular renewal kinetics of malignant non-Hodgkin's lymphomas. In: Mathe G, Seligmann M, Tubiana M, eds. *Recent results in cancer research, vol 65.* Berlin: Springer-Verlag, 1978: 5–11.

(11) Ellims PH, Gan TE, Medley G. Clinical relevance of markers of cell proliferation in human lymphoid malignancies: a concise review. *Eur J Cancer Clin Oncol* 1982; 18: 1229–35.

(12) Srigley J, Barlogie B, Butler JJ et al. Heterogeneity of non-Hodgkin's lymphoma probed by nucleic acid cytometry. *Blood* 1985; 65: 1090–6.

(13) Yunis JJ, Oken MM, Kaplan ME, Ensrud KM, Howe RR, Theologides A. Distinctive chromosomal abnormalities in histologic subtypes of non-Hodgkin's lymphoma. *N Eng J Med* 1982; 307: 1231–6.

(14) Tsujimoto Y, Cossman J, Jaffe E, Croce CM. Involvement of the *bcl-2* gene in human follicular lymphoma. *Science* 1985; 228: 1440–4.

(15) Lee MS, Blick MB, Pathak S et al. The gene located at chromosome 18 band q21 is rearranged in uncultured diffuse lymphomas as well as follicular lymphomas. *Blood* 1987; 70: 90–5.

(16) Gahrton G, Juliusson G, Robert K-H. Chromosomal aberrations in chronic lymphocytic leukemia. In: Polliack A, Catovsky D, eds. *Chronic lymphocytic leukemia*. Chur: Harwood Academic Publishers, 1988: 289–304.

(17) Speaks SL, Sanger WG, Linder J et al. Chromosomal abnormalities in indolent lymphoma. *Cancer Genet Cytogenet* 1987; 27: 335–44.

(18) Tsujimoto Y, Yunis J, Onorato-Showe L, Erikson J, Nowell PC, Croce CM. Molecular cloning of the chromosomal breakpoint of B-cell lymphomas and leukemias with the t(11;14) chromosome translocation. *Science* 1984; 224: 1403–6.

(19) Ngan BY, Nourse J, Cleary ML. Detection of chromosomal translocation t(14;18) within the minor cluster region of *bcl-2* by polymerase chain reaction and direct genomic sequencing of the enzymatically amplified DNA in follicular lymphomas. *Blood* 1989; 73: 1759–62.

(20) Chen-Levy Z, Nourse J, Cleary ML. The *bcl-2* candidate proto-oncogene product is a 24-kilodalton integral-membrane protein highly expressed in lymphoid cell lines and lymphomas carrying the t(14;18) translocation. *Mol Cell Biol* 1989; 9: 701–10.

(21) Lee MS, Chang KS, Cabanillas F, Freireich E, Trujillo JM, Stass SA. Detection of minimal residual cells carrying the t(14;18) by DNA sequence amplification. *Science* 1987; 237: 175–8.

(22) Jones SE, Fuks Z, Bull M et al. Non-Hodgkin's lymphomas: IV. Clinicopathologic correlation in 405 cases. *Cancer* 1973; 31: 806–23.

(23) Vianna NJ. The malignant lymphomas: epidemiology and related aspects. *Pathobiol Ann* 1977; 7: 231–55.

(24) Rudders RA, Kaddis M, DeLellis RA, Casey H Jr. Nodular non-Hodgkin's lymphoma (NHL): factors influencing prognosis and indications for aggressive treatment. *Cancer* 1979; 43: 1643–51.

(25) Gospodarowicz MK, Bush RS, Brown TC, Chua T. Prognostic factors in nodular lymphomas: a multivariate analysis based on the Princess Margaret Hospital experience. *Int J Radiat Oncol Biol Phys* 1984; 10: 489–97.

(26) Rosenberg SA. Validity of the Ann Arbor staging classification for the non-Hodgkin's lymphomas. *Cancer Treat Rep* 1977; 61: 1023–7.

(27) Simon R, Durrleman S, Hoppe RT et al. The non-Hodgkin lymphoma pathologic classification project: long-term follow-up of 1153 patients with non-Hodgkin lymphoma. *Ann Intern Med* 1988; 109: 939–45.

(28) Romaguera JE, McLaughlin P, North L et al. Multivariate analysis of prognostic factors in stage IV follicular low-grade lymphoma: a tumor burden model. *J Clin Oncol*, 1991; 9: 762–9.

(29) Gallagher CJ, Gregory WM, Jones AE et al. Follicular lymphoma: prognostic factors for response and survival. *J Clin Oncol* 1986; 4: 1470–80.

(30) Stein RS, Greer JP, Cousar JB et al. Malignant lymphomas of follicular centre cell origin in man. VII. Prognostic features in small cleaved cell lymphoma. *Hematol Oncol* 1989; 7: 381–91.

(31) Litam P, Swan F, Cabanillas F et al. Correlation of serum beta 2 microglobulin with prognosis in low grade lymphoma and its association with other prognostic variables. *Ann Intern Med*, 1991; 114: 855–60.

(32) Ligler FS, Smith RG, Kettman JR et al. Detection of tumor cells in the peripheral blood of nonleukemic patients with B-cell lymphoma: analysis of 'clonal excess'. *Blood* 1980; 55: 792–801.

(33) Smith B, Weinberg DS, Robert NJ et al. Circulating monoclonal B lymphocytes in non-Hodgkin's lymphoma. *N Eng J Med* 1984; 311: 1476–81.

(34) Hu E, Thompson J, Horning S et al. Detection of B-cell lymphoma in peripheral blood by DNA hybridisation. *Lancet* 1985; ii: 1092–5.

(35) Heifetz LJ, Fuller LM, Rodgers RW et al. Laparotomy findings in lymphangiogram-staged I and II non-Hodgkin's lymphomas. *Cancer* 1980; 45: 2778–86.

(36) Longo DL, Young RC, Hubbard SM et al. Prolonged initial remission in patients with nodular mixed lymphoma. *Ann Intern Med* 1984; 100: 651–6.

(37) Glick JH, Barnes JM, Ezdinli EZ, Berard CW, Orlow EL, Bennett JM. Nodular mixed lymphoma: results of a randomized trial failing to confirm prolonged disease-free survival with COPP chemotherapy. *Blood* 1981; 58: 920–5.

(38) Fuller LM, Banker FL, Butler JJ, Gamble JF, Sullivan MP. The natural history of non-Hodgkin's lymphomata stages I and II. *Br J Cancer* 1975; 31 (Suppl 2): 270–85.

(39) Paryani SB, Hoppe RT, Cox RS, Colby TV, Rosenberg SA, Kaplan HS. Analysis of non-Hodgkin's lymphomas with nodular and favorable histologies, stage I and II. *Cancer* 1983; 52: 2300–7.

(40) McLaughlin P, Fuller LM, Velasquez WS, Sullivan-Halley JA, Butler JJ, Cabanillas F. Stage I–II follicular lymphoma. Treatment results for 76 patients. *Cancer* 1986; 58: 1596–602.

(41) Gomez GA, Barcos M, Krishnamsetty RM, Panahon AM, Han T, Henderson ES. Treatment of early stages I and II nodular, poorly differentiated lymphocytic lymphoma. *Am J Clin Oncol* 1986; 9: 40–4.

(42) Monfardini S, Banfi A, Bonadonna G et al. Improved five year survival after combined radiotherapy–chemotherapy for stage I–II non-Hodgkin's lymphoma. *Int J Radiat Oncol Biol Phys* 1980; 6: 125–34.

(43) Lawrence TS, Urba WJ, Steinberg SM et al. Retrospective analysis of stage I and II indolent lymphomas at the National Cancer Institute. *Int J Radiat Oncol Biol Phys* 1988; 14: 417–24.

(44) Richards MA, Gregory WM, Hall PA et al. Management of localized non-Hodgkin's lymphoma: the experience at St Bartholomew's Hospital 1972–1985. *Hematol Oncol* 1989; 7: 1–18.

(45) McLaughlin P, Fuller L, Hagemeister F et al. Combination chemotherapy and radiotherapy for stage I–II low-grade lymphoma. *Ann Oncol*, 1991; 2 (Suppl 2): 137–40.

(46) Jeliffe AM, Vaughan-Hudson G. Multicentre studies and the treatment of lymphoma. In: McElwain TJ, Lister TA, eds. *The lymphomas. Ballière: Clinical haematology*. Philadelphia: W.B. Saunders, 1987: 235–64.

(47) Rosenberg SA. Non-Hodgkin's lymphoma: selection of treatment on the basis of histologic type. *N Eng J Med* 1979; 301: 924–8.

(48) Young RC, Longo DL, Glatstein E, Ihde DC, Jaffe ES, DeVita VT. The treatment of indolent lymphomas: watchful waiting v aggressive combined modality treatment. *Semin Hematol* 1988; 25 (Suppl 2): 11–16.

(49) Portlock CS, Rosenberg SA. No initial therapy for stage III and IV non-Hodgkin's lymphomas of favorable histologic types. *Ann Intern Med* 1979; 90: 10–13.

(50) Horning SJ, Rosenberg SA. The natural history of initially untreated low-grade non-Hodgkin's lymphomas. *N Eng J Med* 1984; 311: 1471–5.

(51) Mead GM, Macbeth FR, Ryall RDH, Williams CJ, Whitehouse JMA. A report on a prospective trial of no initial therapy in patients with asymptomatic favourable prognosis non-Hodgkin's lymphoma. *Hematol Oncol* 1984; 2: 179–88.

(52) Cox JD, Komaki R, Kun LE, Wilson JF, Greenberg M. Stage III nodular lymphoreticular tumors (non-Hodgkin's lymphoma): results of central lymphatic irradiation. *Cancer* 1981; 47: 2247–52.

(53) Paryani SB, Hoppe RT, Cox RS, Colby TV, Kaplan HS. The role of radiation therapy in the management of stage III follicular lymphomas. *J Clin Oncol* 1984; 2: 841–8.

(54) McLaughlin P, Fuller LM, Velasquez WS et al. Stage III follicular lymphoma: durable remissions with a combined chemotherapy–radiotherapy regimen. *J Clin Oncol* 1987; 5: 867–74.

(55) Ostrow SS, Diggs CH, Sutherland JC, Gustafson J, Wiernik PH. Nodular poorly differentiated lymphocytic lymphoma: changes in histology and survival. *Cancer Treat Rep* 1981; 65: 929–33.

(56) Cullen MH, Lister TA, Brearley RL, Shand WS, Stanfeld AG. Histological transformation of non-Hodgkin's lymphoma: a prospective study. *Cancer* 1979; 44: 645–51.

(57) DeVita VT, Hubbard SH. The curative potential of chemotherapy in the treatment of Hodgkin's disease and non-Hodgkin's lymphomas. In: Rosenberg S A, Kaplan H S, eds. *Malignant lymphomas: etiology, immunology, pathology, treatment*. New York: Academic Press, 1982: 379–416.

(58) Diggs CH, Wiernik PH, Ostrow SS. Nodular lymphoma: prolongation of survival by complete remission. *Cancer Clin Trial* 1981; 4: 107–14.

(59) Lister TA, Cullen MH, Beard ME J et al. Comparison of combined and single-agent chemotherapy in non-Hodgkin's lymphoma of favourable histological type. *Br Med J* 1978; 1: 533–7.

(60) Portlock CS. Deferral of initial therapy for advanced indolent lymphomas. *Cancer Treat Rep* 1982; 66: 417–19.

(61) Hoogstraten B, Owens AH, Lenhard RE et al. Combination chemotherapy in lymphosarcoma and reticulum cell sarcoma. *Blood* 1969; 33: 370–8.

(62) Jones SE, Rosenberg SA, Kaplan HS, Kadin ME, Dorfman RF. Non-Hodgkin's lymphomas: II. Single agent chemotherapy. *Cancer* 1972; 30: 31–8.

(63) Kennedy BJ, Bloomfield CD, Kiang DT, Vosika G, Peterson BA, Theologides

A. Combination versus successive single agent chemotherapy in lymphocytic lymphoma. *Cancer* 1978; 41: 23–8.

(64) Luce JK, Gamble JF, Wilson HE et al. Combined cyclophosphamide, vincristine, and prednisone therapy of malignant lymphoma. *Cancer* 1971; 28: 306–17.

(65) Hoppe RT, Kushlan P, Kaplan HS, Rosenberg SA, Brown BW. The treatment advanced stage favorable histology non-Hodgkin's lymphoma: a preliminary report of a randomized trial comparing single agent chemotherapy, combination chemotherapy, and whole body irradiation. *Blood* 1981; 58: 592–8.

(66) Pedersen-Bjergaard J, Ersboll J, Sorensen HM et al. Risk of acute nonlymphocytic leukemia and preleukemia in patients treated with cyclophosphamide for non-Hodgkin's lymphomas. *Ann Intern Med* 1985; 103: 195–200.

(67) Brereton HD, Young RC, Longo DL et al. A comparison between combination chemotherapy and total body irradiation plus combination chemotherapy in non-Hodgkin's lymphoma. *Cancer* 1979; 43: 2227–31.

(68) Mendenhall NP, Noyes WD, Million RR. Total body irradiation for stage II–IV non-Hodgkin's lymphoma: ten-year follow-up. *J Clin Oncol* 1989; 7: 67–74.

(69) Anderson T, Bender RA, Fisher RI et al. Combination chemotherapy in non-Hodgkin's lymphoma: results of long-term followup. *Cancer Treat Rep* 1977; 61: 1057–66.

(70) Jones SE, Grozea PN, Metz EN. Improved complete remission rates and survival for patients with large cell lymphoma treated with chemoimmunotherapy. A Southwest Oncology Group Study. *Cancer* 1983; 51: 1083–90.

(71) Ezdinli EZ, Anderson JR, Melvin F, Glick JH, Davis TE, O'Connell J. Moderate versus aggressive chemotherapy of nodular lymphocytic poorly differentiated lymphoma. *J Clin Oncol* 1985; 3: 769–75.

(72) Steward WP, Crowther D, McWilliam LJ et al. Maintenance chlorambucil after CVP in the management of advanced stage, low-grade histologic type non-Hodgkin's lymphoma: a randomized prospective study with an assessment of prognostic factors. *Cancer* 1988; 61: 441–7.

(73) Anderson KC, Skarin AT, Rosenthal DS et al. Combination chemotherapy for advanced non-Hodgkin's lymphomas other than diffuse histiocytic or undifferentiated histologies. *Cancer Treat Rep* 1984; 68: 1343–50.

(74) McLaughlin P, Cabanillas F, Hagemeister F et al. Alpha-interferon prolongs remission in stage IV low grade lymphoma [Abstract]. *Proc ASCO* 1990; 9: 267.

(75) Cabanillas F, Smith T, Bodey GP, Gutterman JU, Freireich EJ. Nodular malignant lymphomas: factors affecting complete response rate and survival. *Cancer* 1979; 44: 1983–9.

(76) Kalter S, Holmes L, Cabanillas F. Long-term results of treatment of patients with follicular lymphomas. *Hematol Oncol* 1987; 5: 127–38.

(77) Vaughan-Hudson G. BNLI trial of CHOP vs chlorambucil in aggressive low grade stage III–IV non-Hodgkin's lymphoma: a preliminary report. *Br J Haematol* 1990; 74 (Suppl 1): 13.

(78) Ezdinli EZ, Harrington DP, Kucuk O, Silverstein MW, Anderson J, O'Connell MJ. The effect of intensive intermittent maintenance therapy in advanced low-grade non-Hodgkin's lymphoma. *Cancer* 1987; 60: 156–60.

(79) Cabanillas F, Freireich EJ. Intensive treatment of nodular non-Hodgkin's lymphoma. In: Wiernik PH, ed. *Controversies in oncology*. New York: John Wiley & Sons, 1982: 31–43.

(80) Jones SE, Grozea PH, Miller TP et al. Chemotherapy with cyclophosphamide, doxorubicin, vincristine, and prednisone alone or with levamisole or with levamisole plus BCG for malignant lymphoma: a Southwest Oncology Group Study. *J Clin Oncol* 1985; 3: 1318–24. 82.

(81) Takvorian T, Canellos GP, Ritz J et al. Prolonged disease-free survival after autologous bone marrow transplantation in patients with non-Hodgkin's lymphoma with a poor prognosis. *N Eng J Med* 1987; 316: 1499–505.

(82) Hurd DD, LeBien TW, Lasky LC et al. Autologous bone marrow transplantation in non-Hodgkin's lymphoma: monoclonal antibodies plus complement for ex vivo marrow treatment. *Amer J Med* 1988; 85: 829–34.

(83) Spinolo J, McLaughlin P, Hagemeister FB et al. Factors associated with response, survival and transformation in recurrent low grade follicular lymphomas [Abstract]. *Proceedings of the Third Intl Conference on Malignant Lymphoma* – Lugano, Switzerland, 1987: 57.

(84) Wagstaff J, Loynds P, Crowther D. A phase II study of human rDNA alpha-2 interferon in patients with low grade non-Hodgkin's lymphoma. *Cancer Chemother Pharmacol* 1986; 18: 54–8.

(85) Foon KA, Roth MS, Bunn PA. Interferon therapy of non-Hodgkin's lymphoma. *Cancer* 1987; 59: 601–4.

(86) Redman J, Cabanillas F, McLaughlin P, Hagemeister F, Velasquez W, Swan F, Rodriguez M, Plunkett W, Keating M. Fludarabine phosphate: a new agent with major activity in low grade lymphoma [Abstract]. *Proc AACR* 1988; 29: 211.

(87) Gams RA, Bryan S, Dukart G et al. Mitoxantrone in malignant lymphomas. *Invest New Drugs* 1985; 3: 219–22.

(88) Coltman CA Jr, McDaniel TM, Balcerzak SP, Morrison FS, Von Hoff DD. Mitoxantrone hydrochloride in lymphoma. A Southwest Oncology Group Study. *Invest New Drugs* 1983; 1: 65–70.

(89) McLaughlin P, Cabanillas F, Hagemeister FB, Velasquez W. Activity of bisantrene in refractory lymphoma. *Cancer Treat Rep* 1987; 71: 631–3.

(90) Jones L, Cotter FE, Lord D, Newland AC. Phase 2 study of mitozantrone in combination with chlorambucil and prednisolone for relapsed and refractory non-Hodgkin's lymphoma. *Hematol Oncol* 1990; 8: 41–5.

(91) Miller RA, Maloney DG, Warnke R, Levy R. Treatment of a B cell lymphoma with monoclonal anti-idiotype antibody. *N Eng J Med* 1982; 306: 517–22.

(92) Miller RA, Hart S, Samoszuk M et al. Shared idiotypes expressed by human B-cell lymphomas. *N Eng J Med* 1989; 321: 851–7.

(93) Press OW, Eary JF, Badger CC et al. High-dose radioimmunotherapy of B cell lymphomas. In: Vaeth J M, Meyer J L, eds. *The present and future role of monoclonal antibodies in the management of cancer*. Front Radiat Ther Oncol. Basel, Karger, 1990; 24: 204–13.

(94) DeNardo SJ, DeNardo GL, O'Grady LF et al. Pilot studies of radioimmunotherapy of B cell lymphoma and leukemia using I-131 Lym-1 monoclonal antibody. *Antibody, Immunocon and Radiopharm* 1988; 1: 17–33.

(95) Nadler L, Schlossman SF. Treatment of B-cell non-Hodgkin's lymphomas with immunotoxins [Abstract]. *Proceedings of the Fourth Intl Conference on Malignant Lymphoma* – Lugano, Switzerland, 1990: 60.

(96) Rohatiner AZS, Richards MA, Barnett MJ, Stansfeld AG, Lister TA. Chlorambucil and interferon for low grade non-Hodgkin's lymphoma. *Br J Cancer* 1987; 55: 225–6.

(97) Ozer H, Anderson JR, Peterson BA et al. Combination trial of subcutaneous interferon alfa-2b and oral cyclophosphamide in favorable histology, non-Hodgkin's lymphoma. *Invest New Drugs* 1987; 5: 27–33.

(98) Yoshida T, Nakamura S, Ohtake S et al. Effect of granulocyte colony-stimulating factor on neutropenia due to chemotherapy for non-Hodgkin's lymphoma. *Cancer* 1990; 66: 1904–9.

The management of high grade non-Hodgkin's lymphomas

J M VOSE and J O ARMITAGE

Introduction: management of the high grade lymphomas

The working formulation for classification of the non-Hodgkin's lymphomas divides the high grade non-Hodgkin's lymphomas into three major categories: malignant lymphoma – large cell immunoblastic, malignant lymphoma – lymphoblastic, and malignant lymphoma – small noncleaved cell.[1] Overall, this category represents approximately 12–18% of all the non-Hodgkin's lymphomas.[1] Many of these high grade lymphomas present in young patients with almost half of childhood non-Hodgkin's lymphomas (NHL) in this category.[1] Although the total number of high grade lymphomas is small, because they often affect young patients, the economic and personal impact of these lymphomas is often great.

The category of malignant lymphoma – large cell immunoblastic would be considered diffuse 'histiocytic' lymphoma in the Rappaport classification system. Because of a small but significant difference in survival and certain morphologic distinctions, these cases were separated from the diffuse large cell type in the working formulation. However, the remarkable variations in the proportion of immunoblastic lymphomas seen in different series suggests that the distinction between the two groups is difficult and inconsistent (Table 1). Other analyses have failed to demonstrate a statistical difference.[6] Furthermore, because the large cell and large cell immunoblastic categories are clinically similar, the inclusion of immunoblastic lymphomas in the high grade category has been controversial. Because of the clinical similarities, many oncologists would evaluate and treat immunoblastic NHL in a manner similar to diffuse large cell NHL. However, certain subsets of what would normally be considered intermediate lymphomas often behave in an aggressive clinical manner and could, in effect, be considered high grade lymphomas. An important example would be advanced stage peripheral T-cell

All correspondence to: Dr J M Vose, The University of Nebraska Medical Center, Department of Internal Medicine, Section of Oncology/Hematology, 600 South 42nd Street, Omaha, NE 68198-3330, USA

Cambridge Medical Reviews: Haematological Oncology Volume 1

Table 1. *Diagnosis of DLC vs immunoblastic NHL*

Reference	Study	Patients	DLC	IBL
2	LNH–84	438	63%	37%
3	CAP–BOP	137	53%	47%
4	m/M–BACOD	121	100%	0%
5	MACOP–B	114	67%	33%

DLC = Diffuse large cell lymphoma.
IBL = Immunoblastic lymphoma.

lymphoma which could be included in one of several different histological subtypes including diffuse mixed small and large cell, diffuse large cell, or diffuse large cell – immunoblastic. Each of these subtypes of high grade non-Hodgkin's lymphomas will now be considered individually with respect to clinical presentation, diagnosis and treatment.

Lymphoblastic non-Hodgkin's lymphoma

This histological category was originally included in the diffuse poorly differentiated lymphocytic lymphomas of the Rappaport classification; however, based on clinical and pathological grounds, it is clearly a distinct entity. In 1975, Barcos and Lukes used the term 'convoluted lymphocytic lymphoma' to describe the distinct clinical presentation of this lymphoma.[7] Nathwani et al[8] subsequently recognized both convoluted and non-convoluted cell types in these lymphomas and classified them as lymphoblastic lymphomas.

The clinical presentation of lymphoblastic lymphoma is often very distinctive with 60–75% of the patients presenting with a large mediastinal mass.[9] Often complications resulting from the mediastinal mass such as superior vena cava syndrome or tracheal compression brings the patient to medical attention. Males are more frequently affected than females (2 : 1), and the peak incidence is during the second decade.[9] Although lymphoblastic lymphoma sometimes appears to be localized at diagnosis, it evolves rapidly to disseminated systemic lymphoma. Bone marrow involvement is present at diagnosis in approximately 30% of the cases; however, as the disease progresses or at relapse, 80% of the cases develop bone marrow and eventually peripheral blood involvement.[10] The central nervous system (CNS) is also involved with lymphoblastic lymphoma in approximately 30% of the cases at diagnosis. As the disease disseminates, and also through peripheral blood contamination, the percentage of cases with CNS lymphoma increases. This fact directs special detail to the clinical evaluation and treatment of the CNS in these patients.

Because this lymphoma is usually of T-cell origin, and often involves the bone marrow and peripheral blood, it is frequently difficult to separate from

T-cell acute lymphoblastic leukemia. The St Jude Children's Hospital staging system for childhood non-Hodgkin's lymphoma includes patients in the lymphoblastic lymphoma category if they meet the other clinical characteristics and have less than 25% lymphoblasts in the bone marrow.[11] However, other systems use a lower cutoff such as 10%.[12] In addition to the usual T-cell cases, there have also been rare cases of lymphoblastic lymphoma reported to be of pre-B,[13] or natural killer cell (NK)[14,15] phenotype. The cases involving the NK cells are unusual in that they are reported much more frequently in female than male patients.[15]

As with all malignancies, a rapid and accurate histological diagnosis is the first step toward the proper therapy for the patient. After this initial pathological diagnosis, staging procedures should be carried out including computerized axial tomography (CT) scans of the chest, abdomen and pelvis, a bone marrow biopsy, and a spinal tap for CNS cell count and cytology. These studies should be completed rapidly. Because of the aggressiveness of this tumor, treatment should not be delayed for an extended period of time to complete these staging procedures. Lymphoblastic lymphomas, when treated with conventional chemotherapy regimens used for other aggressive non-Hodgkin's lymphomas, often demonstrate excellent initial responses. However, many patients relapse and eventually die of progressive disease that is unresponsive to salvage therapy at conventional doses. Because of these discouraging results, therapeutic trials were designed specifically for the treatment of lymphoblastic lymphoma. Several series have now evaluated ALL-type regimens in patients with lymphoblastic lymphoma. The LSA2-L2 protocol was found to be significantly more effective than the more traditional non-Hodgkin's lymphoma protocol COMP for the treatment of childhood lymphoblastic lymphoma in 1 trial. In that trial, children with lymphoblastic lymphoma had a 76% two-year disease-free survival when treated with LSA2-L2 protocol compared to only 26% for the COMP treated patients.[16]

The treatment of lymphoblastic lymphoma in adults is less well defined in the literature. One study by Levine et al[10] described 15 adult patients who were treated with a modified LSA2-L2 protocol for lymphoblastic lymphoma. This study resulted in a 73% complete remission rate and an actuarial survival rate at 5 years of 40%. Another evaluation of the treatment of adults with lymphoblastic lymphoma was done by Coleman et al[17] who treated 13 patients with an intensive chemotherapy protocol combined with CNS prophylaxis. This study reported a 100% complete remission rate and a 3-year actuarial disease-free survival rate of 56%.

With several trials demonstrating that patients could have long-term survival after receiving treatment for lymphoblastic lymphoma, the evaluation of prognostic factors was pursued in order to identify patients who would possibly benefit from alternative therapy. Coleman et al,[18] in a subsequent evaluation, divided their patients into good and poor prognostic groups based on several patient characteristics. Poor prognosis patients were defined as having bone marrow involvement, CNS involvement, or a lactic dehydrogenase (LDH) greater than 300 IU/ml (ie normal value). These poor prognosis patients had a 5-year freedom from relapse of 19% compared to the good prognosis group without these characteristics who had a 5-year freedom from relapse of 94% (Table 2). Other studies have also agreed with these factors as denoting poor prognosis,[19,20] while at least one study did not show that bone marrow/peripheral blood tumor burden was consistent with a poor prognosis.[21]

Based on the results in these poor prognosis patients, several preliminary trials have now been conducted evaluating the use of high dose therapy with allogeneic or autologous bone marrow transplantation for hematopoietic rescue. Twenty-six consecutive patients in 5 different French Centers were transplanted during first complete response (CR) for poor prognosis lymphoblastic lymphoma between October 1982 and October 1987. Thirteen of these patients received an allogeneic bone marrow transplant from an HLA identical sibling with the remaining patients receiving an autologous transplant. The conditioning regimens used in this trial consisted of high dose chemotherapy with either cyclophosphamide (120 mg/kg) or high dose melphalan (140 mg/m^2) followed by either single exposure 10 Gy or fractionated 12 Gy TBI. At the time of publication, the median observation time was 22 months (range 1 to 69). Eighteen patients remained alive in first CCR from 9 to 69 months after BMT with a median follow-up time of 25 months. The actuarial 4-year disease-free survival (DFS) was 70% with the last relapse reported at 10 months post-transplant. Nine out of 13 autografted patients and 8 out of 13 allografted patients were in CCR at the time of publication (Table 3). The major reason for failure was disease relapse. Six patients relapsed between 1 and 10 months after BMT. The mediastinum was the initial site of relapse in each case. Two patients died after allogeneic BMT, 1 with severe acute graft-versus-host disease (GVHD) and 1 of unexplained sudden death. No toxic death occurred after autologous BMT, and all surviving patients had a Karnofsky score of 90 to 100%.[22] Although this study is somewhat heterogenous with respect to conditioning regimens and hematopoietic stem cell source, it appears that these results represent a marked improvement over the previous results of conventional therapy in these poor prognosis patients. One other trial at the City of Hope National Medical Center evaluated 5 patients with poor prognosis lymphoblastic lymphoma who were treated with high dose cyclophosphamide and total body irradiation followed by an allogeneic bone marrow transplant in first complete remission.[23] At the time of publication, 4 of the patients were alive in complete remission at 8, 14, 21, and 47 months post-transplant. One patient died of recurrent lymphoma 17 months post-transplant. This trial also produced encouraging results in poor prognosis patients with bone marrow, CNS,

Table 2. *Prognostic characteristics for lymphoblastic lymphoma*

	Good prognosis	Poor prognosis
Bone marrow involvement	Negative	Positive
CNS involvement	Negative	Positive
LDH	≤300 IU/ml	≥300 IU/ml
5 year freedom for relapse when treated with ALL-like regimen	94%	19%

Table 3. *Bone marrow transplantation for poor prognosis in lymphoblastic lymphoma in first complete response*

	Autologous	Allogeneic	Total
Patients	13	13	26
Age (years)	16–39	15–43	16–43
Median age (years)	23	22	23
Male : Female	11 : 2	9 : 4	20 : 6
Patients in CCR at time of publication	9 (69%)	8 (61%)	17 (65%)

and/or skin involvement. Another study from Europe evaluated 12 patients who underwent high dose cyclophosphamide and total body irradiation while in first complete remission from induction therapy with LSA$_2$-L$_2$ for lymphoblastic lymphoma. At the time of publication, 9 patients were alive and well following autologous BMT. Larger scale randomized trials will be needed to answer the important question concerning the proper management of patients with lymphoblastic lymphoma. The best timing for the transplant, the most effective conditioning regimen, and the most useful hematopoietic stem cell source – autologous (bone marrow vs. peripheral stem cell) or allogeneic have yet to be defined.

Small non-cleaved lymphomas
The small non-cleaved cell lymphomas (SNCL) of the working formulation were formerly known as undifferentiated lymphomas in the Rappaport scheme. Small non-cleaved cell lymphomas can be divided, histologically, into Burkitt's and non-Burkitt's lymphomas, but the distinction between the two is subjective and depends primarily upon the degree of cellular pleomorphism and the proportion of cells with a single large nucleolus. This distinction is not usually clinically significant since both subtypes behave in a similar aggressive manner.[25]

The chromosomal translocations identified in SNCL include t(8;14) (70%), t(8;22) (20%), t(2;8) (10%).[26] The c-*myc* oncogene located on chromosome 8 is involved in all of these translocations and is juxtaposed with the gene from one of the immunoglobulin loci. The immunoglobulin heavy chain locus is located on chromosome 14, while the immunoglobulin kappa and lambda light chains are located on chromosomes 2 and 22, respectively. There are also a small number of patients with tumors with both t(8;14) and t(14;18) translocations which most likely represents the development of a small non-cleaved cell lymphoma in a pre-existing follicular lymphoma.[26]

The role of Epstein–Barr virus (EBV) in the pathogenesis of SNCL may occur when the infection is latent in B lymphocytes which are targets for a transformational event, thus increasing the possibility that 'random chromosomal breaks' will generate the specific translocation in a single cell clone. The cases of 'endemic' SNCL in Africa are associated with significantly elevated antibody titers to a variety of EBV antigens, and between 80–90% of the tumors contain multiple copies of EBV DNA genome.[27,28] The association of EBV in 'sporadic' cases of SNCL in the United States is approximately 15–20%.[29]

The clinical presentation of the majority of patients with SNCL in the United States and Europe is that of an abdominal tumor, although other presentations may involve the lymphatic system, CNS, testis, or skeleton.[30] Most patients with African SNCL present with jaw tumors, particularly patients less than age 5.[31] Bone marrow involvement is rare in both endemic and sporadic SNCL at presentation, 20% and 8% respectively.[32] However, at the time of relapse, the percentage of patients with marrow involvement is approximately 50–60%. Central nervous system disease can present as meningeal infiltration, cranial nerve involvement, intracerebral disease, or as a paraspinal mass causing spinal cord compression.[33] Central nervous system presentations occur in approximately 5–15% of the cases; however, as with bone marrow involvement, this percentage rises at relapse.

Due to problems with a large tumor burden, patients with SNCL can experience tumor lysis syndrome with treatment. Therefore, prior to treatment, patients should have allopurinol administered with hydration and diuresis in an attempt to minimize this response. Dialysis is also sometimes needed due to renal failure with subsequent electrolyte abnormalities. Although a percentage of patients present with localized SNCL, local therapy such as radiation is not curative.[34] However, several different combination chemotherapy regimens have now been shown to be efficacious.

Most therapeutic trials for the treatment of SNCL have been carried out in a pediatric population, with few large trials in adults available for comparison. There have been a few reported cases of African Burkitt's lymphoma that have been cured with a single dose of cyclophosphamide.[35] Several multiagent chemotherapy protocols have now been studied in this patient population. Most of the protocols utilize cyclophosphamide along with several other agents such as doxorubicin, cytarabine, methotrexate, or additional agents. The importance of CNS prophylaxis has now been documented in several trials with a significant decrease in CNS relapse in those patients treated with prophylaxis.[36]

Protocols such as the LSA2-L2 regimen that were designed for lymphoblastic lymphoma seem to be inferior to protocols specifically designed for SNCL. This was confirmed in a children's cancer study group trial (CCSG) in which patients were treated either with a modified LSA2-L2 protocol or the COMP protocol (cyclophosphamide, oncovin, methotrexate, and prednisone). In this analysis, children with stage III or IV SNCL had a 24-month failure-free survival rate of 57% for the 38 patients treated with COMP and 28% for the 33 patients treated with LSA2-L2.[37] However, children with localized stage I or II SNCL responded well to both multi-agent chemotherapy regimens. This report demonstrated a 24-month failure-free survival rate of 89% for 28 patients with localized SNCL treated with COMP, and an 84% failure-free survival for 32 patients treated with LSA2-L2.[37] As is the case with lymphoblastic NHL, the serum LDH level can be predictive of patient outcome[38] (Fig. 1). Patients with limited disease, such as localized or completely resectable abdominal disease, have an excellent prognosis and may be able to receive less extensive disease. For example, one study demonstrated that patients with SNCL and localized disease had similar results when treated with a truncated 6 month protocol as when treated with a more complex 18 month protocol.[39]

There have been few reports on the treatment of SNCL strictly in adults. One study from Stanford reported 18 adult patients with SNCL who were treated with cyclophosphamide, doxorubicin, vincristine, prednisone, systemic and intrathecal methotrexate, as well as radiation therapy to unresectable masses >10 cm.[40] In this analysis the patients with poor prognostic factors including unresected tumor bulk >10 cm, pretreatment LDH of >500 IU/l, or involvement of the CNS or bone marrow had a significantly worse prognosis with a projected relapse-free survival of 28.6% compared with 100% for those patients without those features.[40] This and other analyses of the treatment of patients with SNCL have identified several subgroups of patients which may benefit from more aggressive therapy such as bone marrow transplantation.

One of the original reports of patients with relapsed or resistant Burkitt's lymphoma treated with high dose chemotherapy and autologous bone marrow transplantation was by Appelbaum in 1978. This article described 14 patients who were treated with BACT (carmustine, cytosine arabinoside, cyclophosphamide, 6-thioguanine) high-dose therapy followed by autologous bone marrow transplantation.[41] This first publication reported 3 of the 14 patients alive 9+, 19+, and 29+ months post-transplant.[41] Another large

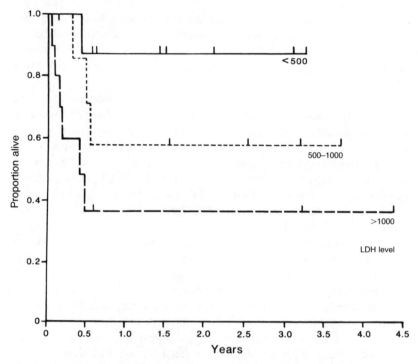

Fig. 1. Lactic dehydrogenase (LDH) as a measure of tumor burden versus proportion of patients alive and disease-free following treatment with the St Jude total therapy B protocol for SNCL (*J Clin Oncol* 1986; 4:1732–9).

experience of high-dose chemotherapy and autologous bone marrow transplantation for SNCL has been reported by Philip et al.[42] A report of their 5-year experience evaluated 28 patients transplanted using the BACT or BEAM protocol as high dose therapy followed by autologous bone marrow transplantation. The overall disease-free survival at the time of publication was 46% with a median observation time post ABMT of 22 months. This also included 5 out of 10 long-term survivors who had previous CNS disease. It should be pointed out that these results would have been difficult to achieve with conventional chemotherapy in a similar patient population. With the identification of the poor prognostic variables as outlined above, the indications for transplantations have changed for patients with SNCL. Many oncologists would now advocate high-dose chemotherapy and transplantation for patients with these poor prognostic characteristics in first complete remission or, at best, response in order to improve on the historical results.

Because of a fairly high percentage of patients who may have occult tumor cells in their bone marrow with poor prognosis or relapsed SNCL, the use of purged marrow or allogeneic marrow has been advocated by some transplant centers. Explosive leukemia-like regrowth of SNCL has been reported following high-dose chemotherapy and autologous bone marrow transplantation in several studies.[42,43] Furthermore, Burkitt's lymphoma cells can grow in an in vitro culture system from histologically negative bone marrow.[44,45] A trial utilizing purged bone marrow from Baumgartner et al[46] evaluated 5 patients transplanted for SNCL. Four of the patients who were in first CR at the time of transplant were free of tumor at a median observation time of 19 months post-transplant; however, the patient who was transplanted in second partial remission died on day 48 after ABMT from generalized relapse.[47] One example of an allogeneic study was reported by O'Leary et al.[47] There were 6 patients with SNCL who received high-dose chemotherapy followed by allogeneic bone marrow transplantation in this analysis. One patient died early in the transplant course of the remaining 5 patients, 3 were alive in remission at the time of publication.[47] Further clinical trials will be needed in order to define the exact role of high-dose therapy with transplantation in the treatment of patients with SNCL. Also, the most appropriate source of hematopoietic stem cells needs further study.

Peripheral T-cell lymphoma

Some series would also include peripheral T-cell lymphomas (PTCL) in the category of high-grade NHL. Although several series have found that the immunophenotype of a NHL does not predict the outcome of treatment,[48-50] several large studies utilizing uniform treatment have found that T-cell NHL patients do not have as good a long-term disease-free survival as their B-cell counterparts.[51,52] A recent analysis from our institution evaluated 110 uniformly treated patients with diffuse mixed, diffuse large cell or immunoblastic NHL of whom 91 (83%) had a B-cell NHL and 19 (17%) had a T-cell NHL. The patients with stage I–III had similar complete remission rates (B-cell 82% vs. T-cell 91%, p = NS), as well as similar 3 year overall survivals (B-cell 58% vs. T-cell 73%, p = NS). However, the stage IV B-cell patients had a higher CR rate than their stage IV T-cell counterparts (67% vs. 0%, p = 0.002), as well as a much improved overall survival at 3 years (44% vs. 0%, p = 0.002).[51] Based on that information, we now recommend early autologous bone marrow transplantation for patients with high risk (ie high stage or large tumor bulk) PTCL.

Conclusions

The advent of modern combination chemotherapy for the treatment of the non-Hodgkin's lymphomas has been one of the great advances in oncology in the past decades. However, not every patient suffering from an aggressive lymphoma can yet be cured. The use of specific chemotherapy regimens has improved the results in some subgroups. Furthermore, the recognition that groups with a poor prognosis can be identified who need more intensive therapy has led to trials of high-dose therapy and transplantation. Many more clinical trials will be needed to answer the important remaining clinical questions regarding high-grade non-Hodgkin's lymphomas.

References

(1) Summary and description of a working formulation for clinical usage. The non-Hodgkin's lymphoma pathologic classification project. NCI Sponsored Study of Classification of lymphoblastic lymphomas. *Cancer* 1982; 49: 2112–35.

(2) Coiffier B, Gisselbrecht C, Herbrecht R et al. LNH-84 regimen: a multicenter study of intensive chemotherapy in 737 patients with aggressive malignant lymphoma. *J Clin Oncol* 1989; 7: 1018–26.

(3) Vose JM, Armitage JO, Weisenburger DD et al. The importance of age in survival of patients treated with chemotherapy for aggressive non-Hodgkin's lymphoma. *J Clin Oncol* 1988; 6: 1838–44.

(4) Shipp MA, Harrington DP, Khatt MM et al. Identification of major prognostic subgroups of patients with large-cell lymphoma treated with m-BACOD or M-BACOD. *Ann Intern Med* 1986; 104: 757–65.

(5) Connors J M, Klimo P. Updated clinical experience with MACOP-B. *Semin Hematol* 1987; 24: 26–34.

(6) Fisher RI, Hubbard SM, DeVita VT et al. Factors predicting long-term survival in diffuse mixed, histiocytic, or undifferentiated lymphoma. *Blood* 1981; 58: 45–51.

(7) Barcos MP, Lukes RJ. Malignant lymphoma of convoluted lymphocytes – a new entity of possible T-cell type. In: Sinks L F, Godden J O, eds. *Conflicts in childhood cancer. An evaluation of current management*, vol 4, New York: Liss, 1975: 147.

(8) Nathwani BN, Kim H, Rappaport H. Malignant lymphoma, lymphoblastic. *Cancer* 1976; 38: 964–83.

(9) Rosen PJ, Feinstein DI, Pattengale PK et al. Convoluted lymphocytic lymphoma in adults: a clinicopathologic entity. *Ann Intern Med* 1978; 89: 319–24.

(10) Levine AM, Forman SJ, Meyer PR et al. Successful therapy of convoluted T-lymphoblastic lymphoma in adults. *Blood* 1983; 61: 92–8.

(11) Murphy SB. Childhood non-Hodgkin's lymphoma. *N Eng J Med* 1978; 299: 1446–8.

(12) Weinstein MJ, Cassidy JR, Levey R. Long term results of the APO protocol (vincristine, doxorubicin [adriamycin], and prednisone) for the treatment of mediastinal lymphoblastic lymphoma. *J Clin Oncol* 1983; 1: 537–41.

(13) Cossman J, Chused TM, Fisher RI et al. Diversity of immunologic phenotypes of lymphoblastic lymphoma. *Cancer Res* 1983; 43: 4486–90.

(14) Swerdlow SH, Habeshaw JA, Richards MA et al. T lymphoblastic lymphoma with Leu-7 positive phenotype and unusual clinical course: a multiparameter study. *Leukemia Res* 1985; 9: 167–73.

(15) Sheibani K, Nathwani BN, Winberg CD et al. Antigenically defined subgroups of lymphoblastic lymphoma: relationship to clinical presentation and biologic behavior. *Cancer* 1987; 60: 183–90.

(16) Wollner N, Wachtel AE, Exelby PR et al. Improved prognosis in children with

intraabdominal lymphoblastic lymphoma following LSA$_2$-L$_2$ protocol chemotherapy. *Cancer* 1980; 45: 3034–9.

(17) Coleman LN, Cohen JR, Burke JS et al. Lymphoblastic lymphoma in adults: results of a pilot protocol. *Blood* 1981; 57: 679–84.

(18) Coleman LN, Picozzi VJ, Cox RS et al. Treatment of lymphoblastic lymphoma in adults. *J Clin Oncol* 1986; 4: 1628–37.

(19) Steuli RA, Kaneko Y, Variakojis D et al. Lymphoblastic lymphoma in adults. *Cancer* 1981; 47: 2510–16.

(20) Magrath IT, Janus C, Edwards BK et al. An effective therapy for both undifferentiated (including Burkitt's) lymphoma and lymphoblastic lymphomas in children and young adults. *Blood* 1984; 63: 1102–11.

(21) Slater DE, Mertelsmann R, Loziner B et al. Lymphoblastic lymphoma in adults. *J Clin Oncol* 1986; 4: 57–67.

(22) Milpied N, Ifrah N, Kuentz M et al. Bone marrow transplantation for adult poor prognosis lymphoblastic lymphoma. In: Dicke KA, Spitzer G et al, eds. *Proc IVth International Autologous Bone Marrow Transplantation*. Houston, TX 1989: 247–52.

(23) Nademanee AP, Forman SJ, Schmidt GM et al. Allogeneic bone marrow transplantation for high risk lymphoblastic lymphoma during first complete remission. *Blut* 1987; 55: 11–16.

(24) Santini G, Coser P, Chisesi T et al. Autologous bone marrow transplantation for advanced stage adult lymphoblastic lymphoma in first complete remission. A pilot study of the lymphoblastic lymphoma co-operative study group (NHLCSG). *Bone Marrow Transplantation* 1989; 4: 399–404.

(25) Hutchison RE, Murphy SB, Fairclough DC et al. Diffuse small noncleaved cell lymphoma in children, Burkitt's versus non-Burkitt's types. *Cancer* 1989; 64: 23–8.

(26) The fifth international workshop on chromosomes in leukemia-lymphoma: Correlation of chromosome abnormalities with histologic and immunologic characteristics in lymphoblastic lymphoma and adult T-cell leukemia-lymphoma. *Blood* 1987; 70: 1554–64.

(27) Lindahl T, Klein G, Reedman BM et al. Relationship between Epstein–Barr virus (EBV) DNA and the EVB-determined nuclear antigen (EBNA) in Burkitt's lymphoma biopsies and other lymphoproliferative malignancies. *Int J Cancer* 1974; 13: 764–9.

(28) Henle G, Henle W, Clifford P et al. Antibodies to Epstein–Barr virus in Burkitt's lymphoma and control groups. *J Natl Cancer Inst* 1969; 43: 1147–52.

(29) Magrath IT. Burkitt's lymphoma: clinical aspects and treatment. In: Newlander D W, ed. *Diseases of the lymphatic system: diagnosis and therapy*. New York: Springer-Verlag, 1983: 103–9.

(30) Levine PH, Kamaraja LS, Connelly RR et al. The American Burkitt's lymphoma registry: eight years experience. *Cancer* 1982; 49: 1016–22.

(31) Burkitt OP. General features and facial tumors. In: Burkitt DP, Wright DH, eds. *Burkitt's Lymphoma*, London: E&S Livingstone, 1970: 6–15.

(32) Magrath IT, Ziegle JL. Bone marrow involvement in Burkitt's lymphoma and its relationship to acute B-cell leukemia. *Leukemia Res* 1980; 4: 33–59.

(33) Ziegler JL, Bluming AZ, Morrow RH et al. Central nervous system involvement in Burkitt's lymphoma. *Blood* 1970; 36: 718–28.

(34) Jenkin RDT, Sonley MJ, Stephens CA et al. Primary gastro-intestinal tract lymphoma in childhood. *Radiology* 1969; 92: 763–7.

(35) Arseneau JC, Canellos GP, Banks PA et al. American Burkitt's lymphoma: a clinicopathologic study of 30 cases. I. Clinical factors relating to prolonged survival. *Am J Med* 1975; 58: 314–21.

(36) Sullivan MP, Ramirez I. Curability of Burkitt's lymphoma with high-dose cyclophosphamide high-dose methotrexate therapy and intrathecal chemoprophylaxis. *J Clin Oncol* 1985; 3: 627–36.

(37) Anderson JR, Wilson JF, Jenkin DT et al. Childhood non-Hodgkin's lymphoma. The results of a randomized therapeutic trial comparing a 4-drug regimen (COMP) with a 10-drug regimen (LSA$_2$-L$_2$). *N Eng J Med* 1983; 308: 559–65.

(38) Murphy SB, Bowman WP, Abromowitch M et al. Results of treatment of advanced stage Burkitt's lymphoma and B-cell (SIG+) acute lymphoblastic lymphoma with high-dose fractionated cyclophosphamide and coordinated high-dose methotrexate and cytarabine. *J Clin Oncol* 1986; 4: 1732–9.

(39) Siegel S, Chilcote R, Coccia P et al. A decade of progress in childhood non-Hodgkin's lymphoma (NHL): the children's cancer study group (CCSG) experience. Third International Conference on Malignant Lymphoma, Lugano, Switzerland, 1987: 44.

(40) Bernstein JI, Coleman N, Strickler JG et al. Combined modality therapy for adults with small noncleaved cell lymphoma (Burkitt's and non-Burkitt's type). *J Clin Oncol* 1986; 4: 847–58.

(41) Appelbaum FR, Deisseroth AB, Graw RG et al. Prolonged complete remission following high dose chemotherapy of Burkitt's lymphoma in relapse. *Cancer* 1978; 41: 1059–63.

(42) Philip T, Biron P, Philip I et al. Massive therapy and autologous bone marrow transplantation in pediatric and young adult Burkitt lymphoma (30 courses in 28 patients in 5 year experience). *Eur J Cancer Clin Oncol* 1986; 22: 1015–19.

(43) Vaughan WP, Weisenberger DD, Sanger W et al. Early leukemic recurrence of non-Hodgkin's lymphoma after high dose antineoplastic therapy with autologous bone marrow rescue. In: *Progress in bone marrow transplantation*, Alan R Liss Inc, 1987: 787–96.

(44) Joshi SS, Kessinger A, Mann SL et al. Detection of malignant cells in histologically normal bone marrow using culture techniques. *Bone Marrow Transpl* 1978; 1: 303–10.

(45) Philip I, Philip T, Favrot M et al. Establishment of lymphomatous cell lines from bone marrow samples from patients with Burkitt's lymphoma. *J Nat Cancer Inst* 1984; 73: 835–7.

(46) Baumgartner C, Delaleu B, Imbach P et al. Autologous bone marrow transplantation for Burkitt's lymphoma: marrow purging with anti-Y 29/55 monoclonal antibody and complement. *IARC Sci Publications* 1985; 60: 435–9.

(47) O'Leary M, Ramsay NK, Nesbit ME et al. Bone marrow transplantation for lymphoblastic lymphoma in children and young adults. *Am J Med* 1983; 74: 497–501.

(48) Levine AM, Taylor CR, Schneider DR et al. Immunoblastic sarcoma of T-cell versus B-cell origin: I. Clinical Features. *Blood* 1981; 58: 52–61.

(49) Lippman SM, Miller TP, Spier CM et al. The prognostic significance of immunophenotype in diffuse large cell lymphoma: a comparative study of the T-cell and B-cell phenotype. *Blood* 1988; 72: 436–41.

(50) Horning SJ, Weiss CM, Crabtree CG et al. Clinical and phenotypic diversity of T-cell lymphomas. *Blood* 1986; 67: 1578–82.

(51) Armitage JO, Vose JM, Linder J et al. Clinical significance of immunophenotype in diffuse aggressive non-Hodgkin's lymphoma. *J Clin Oncol* 1989; 7: 1783–90.

(52) Coiffier B, Berger F, Bryon P-A et al. T-cell lymphomas: immunologic, histologic, clinical, and therapeutic analysis of 63 cases. *J Clin Oncol* 1988; 6: 1584–9.

CNS prophylaxis – who and how?

O B EDEN

Introduction

Since the 1960s, remarkable progress has been made in the management of childhood lymphoblastic leukaemia so that, in most published series, at least 50% of presenting patients are expected to be alive and disease-free 5 years later. Real cure is now considered feasible. The use of 'prophylactic' central nervous system (CNS) treatment has been considered a prerequisite for such long-term disease-free survival since, before its introduction, at least 50% of children developed overt CNS leukaemia whilst still in systemic remission.[1,2,3] Few such patients eventually survived. Most quite rapidly developed bone marrow relapse but deaths from neurological dysfunction were rare even in the presence of multiple CNS recurrences.[4] Remission duration following overt CNS relapse was short in these early series and, even in a recent review of primary CNS relapses in the Medical Research Council (MRC) UKALL Trials between 1977 and 1987, only 23 out of 116 children with such relapses remain without subsequent events. Remission duration prior to the overt CNS event determined chance of survival.[5] More worrying is the fact that over 50% of the survivors in this series are severely limited, either neurologically, educationally or both. Prevention of overt CNS disease in the maximum number of patients must be attempted. However, so-called prophylactic CNS treatment has been increasingly associated with long-term neurological sequelae. When Pinkel and his group[6,7] at St Jude Children's Research Hospital first pioneered presymptomatic CNS irradiation, overall survival was the preoccupation of clinicians. Increasingly, quality of survival has also become an important consideration.

More recently, doubt was cast even as to whether meningeal relapse truly influenced total survival or duration of haematological remission in at least one series of standard risk patients.[8] In many ALL treatment protocols the 'gold standard' of cranial irradiation and intrathecal methotrexate is being abandoned in favour of high dose systemic chemotherapy and/or intrathecal

All correspondence to: Department of Haematology, Royal Hospital for Sick Children, 17 Millerfield Place, Edinburgh EH9 1LF, UK.

Cambridge Medical Reviews: Haematological Oncology Volume 1
© Cambridge University Press 1991

therapy only. Some such efforts to reduce toxicity have been associated with a significant increase in actual CNS disease.

In acute nonlymphoblastic leukaemia (ANLL) where survival has been prolonged, a similar incidence of overt extramedullary relapse as seen in ALL has been evident. However, there is even less consensus as to optimal preventative therapy for such patients. For the lymphomas, lymphoblastic tumours with high CNS relapse risk can be considered with ALL but localized non-lymphoblastic, and abdominal histiocytic disease may not require 'prophylaxis'.

It would therefore appear opportune to consider the pathogenesis of CNS leukaemia; who is especially at risk?; what the evidence is for toxicity and data on alternative methods of control.

Pathogenesis
Most of what we know about CNS disease comes from studies of ALL. As leukaemic cells circulate, microhaemorrhages deposit them within tissues. Within the CNS, the initial process in the development of CNS disease in ALL and ANLL is the migration of blasts from the walls of superficial arachnoid veins into the surrounding adventitia.[9] As the size of any such deposit increases, the arachnoid trabeculae are destroyed with subsequent penetration of cerebrospinal fluid (CSF) channels over the surface of the brain. Further growth will lead to impingement on grey and white matter, disruption of the pia–glial membrane and hence direct infiltration of neural tissues. Leukaemic blasts do not apparently penetrate the parenchymal capillaries directly, but reach the parenchyma after arachnoid disruption. Since the 1960s, it has been assumed that all children with lymphoblastic leukaemia at least have cells in the walls of the arachnoid veins or in the adventitia. Only a small minority have discernible cells within the CSF and even fewer any overt neurological signs. The term CNS prophylaxis is a misnomer if we are assuming that cells are actually present at the time of diagnosis, and a better term would be CNS minimal disease therapy.

Actual parenchymal disease is rarely seen these days except after multiple relapses. Even more rarely isolated nodular disease can be seen, but its pathogenesis has never been adequately defined. Isolated peripheral or cranial nerve lesions are somewhat more common especially in acute non-lymphoblastic leukaemia (ANLL). Lumbar puncture is essential at diagnosis to define the extent of disease and does not carry a risk of seeding the CSF.[10] The increased incidence of CNS relapse paralleled the overall improvement in disease-free survival for acute lymphoblastic leukaemia (ALL) and, as median duration of survival has improved for other acute leukaemias and high risk lymphomas, so the CNS relapse rate has increased in these conditions also. Control of systemic disease with longer haematological remissions was achieved in the late 1960s without drugs being given in high enough concentration to reach the sites of minimal disease around the arachnoid vessels. These cells would proliferate and eventually lead to significant disease.

In the lymphomas, direct extension of the tumour from erosion of the base of the skull, paranasal sinuses or orbit have all been described. The unusual enigma of primary CNS lymphoma is most often a solitary lesion at presentation whilst secondary dissemination can lead to 'meningeal'-type disease as in ALL or multiple small, often ill-defined, masses. They tend to occur in periventricular sites involving basal ganglia, corpus callosum, thalamus or septum pellucidum.[11]

Incidence, relative risk and timing
Acute lymphoblastic leukaemia
For ALL, prior to the introduction of CNS specific therapy, the median time from diagnosis to CNS relapse was 9 months and the incidence was between 50 and 70% of those diagnosed. In most published modern series the risk is now less than 10% overall with some more at risk than others. Historically, up to 5% of newly diagnosed patients were reported to have overt CNS disease at diagnosis.[12] In more recent series, such as the MRC UKALL VIII Study and Trial, 2.8% of entrants had CSF blasts at diagnosis, half with <5 cells/mm^3 and half with >5/mm^3.[13] Factors which increase the risk of CNS disease at diagnosis appear to include age under 1 year, a white cell count in excess of $100 \times 10^9/l$ and both T and B cell phenotype (possibly not independent of WBC).

CNS relapse can occur in all forms of leukaemia and appears to increase with improving survival. Without attempts at prevention the rate of CNS relapse in ALL has been estimated to be 4% per month for 2 years and thereafter 1% per month. With CNS therapy reported risk factors have included:

(1) Infants under 2 years and maybe those over 10 years at diagnosis.
(2) Those with an initial high white cell count ($>50 \times 10^9/l$).
(3) Those with marked organomegaly and lymphadenopathy.
(4) T cell and B cell ALL.
(5) Low initial platelet count.[14]

It is easy to explain the reasons for at least some of these factors. Extravasation of blood carrying blasts is more likely to occur with low platelet counts, and greater blast spillage will occur in those with high initial white cell counts. Patients with high initial white cell counts have earlier CNS relapses often on therapy. Most patients under 1 year and those with T and B cell disease have high white cell counts and the phenotype and age itself may not be independent prognostic indicators for overt CNS disease. Although these features predict for higher risk of CNS relapse, to date, no group of leukaemia

Table 1. *MRC UKALL VIII study and trial isolated CNS relapses*

Patient category	'Low'	'Average'	'High'
Girls	2.8% (2/71)	7.7% (17/221)	9.1% (6/66)
Boys	6.4% (8/125)	7.0% (17/244)	12.5% (8/64)

% (Number of relapses/Number in category).
'Low'   = aged 3–6 years, initial WBC $< 10 \times 10^9/1$.
'Average' = all patients with WBC 0–$50 \times 10^9/1$ except 'Low' group.
'High'   = all with WBC $> 50 \times 10^9 1$.

patients has been shown to be completely free of risk. Table 1 shows the relative risk by low, average and high risk grouping for patients in the MRC UKALL VIII Study and Trial. Even amongst girls aged 3 to 6 years with white cell counts under $10 \times 10^9/1$ at diagnosis, there were 2 CNS relapses. The dividing line for increased risk by white cell count in this series was at 50 $\times 10^9/1$. There did not appear to be a significant sex difference in incidence.[13]

These results were obtained with standard induction therapy using vincristine, prednisolone, asparaginase with or without daunorubicin (no difference in CNS relapse rate whether daunorubicin was given or not) and 18 Gy cranial irradiation plus 6 intrathecal injections of methotrexate (age determined dosage). Consideration has been given to the early incorporation of high dose systemic chemotherapy, especially methotrexate, first to supplement cranial irradiation and intrathecal medication and latterly to replace it. To be effective, any prophylaxis must take place when cell numbers in and around arachnoid veins are minimal.[14,15] Even for those with low risk, if only intrathecal therapy is used, it must start at once before any seeded cells advance into the adventitia. If not eradicated, early blast cells are beyond the reach of intrathecally injected drugs and are protected from cytocidal concentrations of systemic chemotherapy by the blood–CSF barrier.[15] Indeed, low concentrations of anti-leukaemic drugs in the CSF and, more important, in the adventitia may predispose to the development of resistance in this blast cell population.

Nesbit et al[8] reported that 81% of CNS relapses in the Children Cancer Group (CCG) protocols 101 and 143 occurred by 36 months from diagnosis. In the MRC UKALL VIII series, only 3 out of 59 isolated CNS relapses occurred more than 6 months after stopping treatment.[13]

Acute non-lymphoblastic leukaemia

CNS relapse can occur in all forms of leukaemia[16] including acute myeloblastic (AML), acute myelomonocytic (AMML), acute monocytic (AMoL) and chronic myeloid leukaemia (CML)[17] but with lower incidence probably as a result of inferior survival.[18] If duration at risk is considered,

CNS relapse in AML is as frequent as in ALL. In ANLL, there would appear to be a higher incidence of isolated nerve lesions especially seventh cranial nerve palsies.

Non-Hodgkin's lymphoma

CNS involvement is reported both at presentation (13%) and at relapse in Burkitt's lymphoma.[11] Incidence has recently declined when high dose systemic methotrexate and cytosine arabinoside have been included in treatment programmes.

There is a lower incidence of CNS disease at diagnosis in lymphoblastic lymphoma, but it is found in T cell disease especially with bone marrow infiltration. Either at diagnosis or in relapse, the most common presentation is with cranial nerve palsies or meningeal infiltration, but intracerebral disease is more common than in leukaemia. This is seen as a direct extension of primary tumours in the head and neck and also with failure of eradication of meningeal disease.

The risk of CNS disease in patients who have small non-cleaved non-Burkitt's lymphomas with resected localized abdominal lymphomas appears to be very small and many advocate no 'prophylaxis' for them. Currently, all other lymphomas do receive some form of CNS treatment although most do not have irradiation.

Development of the gold standard therapy in ALL

The initial use of craniospinal irradiation, although quite effective, was associated with excessive myelosuppression from the spinal component. The 'optimum' therapy developed by Pinkel and his group consisted of 24 Gy cranial irradiation in 14 or 15 fractions over 17–18 days and 5 intrathecal injections of methotrexate (12 mg/m^2) every 3–4 days. The total radiotherapy dosage was reduced to 20 Gy for 1 year-olds and 15 Gy for those under 1 year. Reduced numbers of higher dose fractions increased the relapse rate from 5 to 8% in one series.[19] Monthly, or even longer gap-pulsed radiotherapy, and intrathecal methotrexate has not proven more efficacious or noticeably less toxic.[20]

Modifications which do appear to have been worthwhile are the adjustment of methotrexate dosage by age which appears to correlate better with CSF volume than surface area (12.5 mg for all over 3 years, 10 mg for those 2–3 years, 7.5 mg for those 1–2 years and 5 mg for those under 1 year) and using weekly rather than twice weekly lumbar punctures (no loss of efficacy and reduced morbidity). The Children's Cancer Study Group have also demonstrated that 18 Gy (10 fractions over 12–14 days) is as efficacious as 24 Gy for those with an initial white cell count under $50 \times 10^9/1$.[21] For those with a high tumour burden there was a trend for lower CNS relapse with 24 Gy compared with 18 Gy, but the difference was of borderline statistical significance. In the

Table 2. *Randomized studies using high dose methotrexate in childhood ALL*

Study	Patient No.	HDMTX	Control	Outcome MTX:R/T
(1) CALGB 7611	506	500 mg/M² over 24 h +I/T MTX Q 10 wk	24 Gy cranial	Higher CNS relapses Lower testic relapses Lower haem relapses in standard risk patients
(2) CCG/NCI 191 7701	180 Ave+ high risk	33.6 g/M² over 24 h ×4 Q 6 monthly	24 Gy cranial + 5 I/T MTX	No difference CNS, testic or haem relapses In high risk excess CNS relapses in both arms
CCG/NCI 144 84A	166 Ave risk		I/T MTX	In progress
(3) St Jude	309 Low + Ave	1 g/M² over 24 h ×15 I/T MTX +Standard maintenance	18 Gy cranial + I/T MTX +Rotating maintenance	Haem + testic relapses lower overall DFS better CNS relapses no difference but high in Int risk group.

Modified from Bleyer W A. High dose methotrexate in childhood ALL.
In: *Proceedings of workshop. The role of clinical pharmacology*, Prague 1989: 19–31.

1. Data from Freeman A I, Weinberg V, Brecker L et al. Comparison of intermediate dose methotrexate with cranial irradiation for the post-induction treatment of acute lymphoblastic leukæmia in children. *New Eng J Med* 1983; 308: 477–84.
2. Data from Poplack et al.[42]
3. Data from Abromowitch et al.[38]

MRC UKALL VIII Study, 24 Gy was retained for those with an initial white cell count over $100 \times 10^9/1$, but CNS relapses were still at an unacceptable rate of nearly 20% in this group of patients. For these high risk patients standard irradiation and intrathecal therapy is clearly inadequate.

Two problems have emerged in the last decade:

(1) Standard therapy is inadequate for some patients, most specifically those with an initial high white cell count in the peripheral blood.
(2) Standard therapy is associated with unacceptable toxicity for low-risk patients with an otherwise high chance of long-term disease-free survival.

Toxicity of standard CNS treatment
CNS irradiation alone
Acute toxicity Acute neurological problems are rarely seen, and are usually transient and not severe. Intermittent vomiting, anorexia, headache and even some drowsiness can occur during cranial irradiation. It usually lasts only 1–2 days and is not associated with neurological signs. Very rarely, in the presence of previous severe neurological deficit or marked CNS disease, signs and symptoms of raised intracranial pressure can be detected. Lymphopenia and consequential risks of infection, especially with atypical organisms such as *Pneumocystis* are greatest during, and soon after, cranial irradiation.

Subacute toxicity Between 5 and 10 weeks post-cranial irradiation, even with total dosages of only 18 Gy, at least 50% of patients may experience a period of somnolence lasting anywhere from 7–30 days. During this 'somnolence syndrome' most patients feel drowsy, lethargic and generally unwell. They may be nauseated, but total anorexia, fever, dysphasia, ataxia, transient papilloedema and worsening of inherent neurological deficit have all been reported.[22] Transient electro-encephalograph (EEG) changes (diffuse slow waves) increases in CSF protein[23] and in procoagulant activity have all been reported.[24] Younger children, under 3 years, may have a more severe illness. There appears to be a temporary inhibition of myelin synthesis but recovery appears to be complete, and there does not appear to be any correlation with late neurological sequelae. The presence or absence of somnolence does not appear to correlate with tumour load or risk of subsequent CNS relapse. Concomitant use of steroids appears to minimize or prevent the syndrome and can be used to treat it when it develops.[22]

Late toxicity Cerebral atrophy, calcification and necrosis can occur as late sequelae of whole brain irradiation. Necrosis is very rare with irradiation dosages under 50 Gy but both atrophic changes and calcification are recorded with dosages in the usual leukaemia range of 18–24 Gy and, quite frequently, with retreatment following CNS relapse. Calcification is most frequently seen in the basal ganglia and in subcortical areas. Computerized tomography (CT) scanning may not be a fine enough tool to detect subclinical damage[24] but magnetic resonance imaging is proving superior.[25]

Intrathecal medication
Methotrexate This can induce an acute arachnoiditis with headache, pain at the site of lumbar puncture, nausea and vomiting, fever and even raised intracranial pressure. This appears to be rare in childhood occurring in less than 5% of cases, although mild symptoms are not too infrequent following lumbar punctures. Occasionally, a picture very similar to bacterial meningitis can be seen.

Subacute toxicity in the form of myelopathy or encephalopathy can occur after repeated intrathecal medication, especially when included as part of maintenance therapy (incidence between 3 and 10%).[26]

Late toxicity from intrathecal methotrexate alone is rare. Bleyer has reported very minimal abnormalities in 3 out of 8 children treated with intrathecal methotrexate alone and all 8 had normal CT scans.[27]

Intrathecal cytosine arabinoside and triple therapy (cytosine, hydrocortisone and methotrexate)

The addition of steroids appears to decrease acute toxicity although seizures have been reported following the use of intrathecal cytosine with or without hydrocortisone.[28] Although for all intrathecal therapy, the drug preparations used, presence of preservatives within the fluid injected, the concentration of the drug, and the method of administration, may all influence the incidence of reactions.

Triple therapy may be associated with a slightly higher incidence or even more severe late toxicity including necrotizing leukoencephalopathy and ascending paralysis (thought to be an effect of the cytosine arabinoside).[29]

Combined therapy of CNS irradiation and intrathecal methotrexate

The vast majority of leukaemia patients have been treated with combined modality therapy over the last 2 decades.

Acute encephalopathies have been described with onset within a few hours of commencement of irradiation and the first intrathecal injection. Such are rare but can prove fatal and are thought to occur more frequently where there is a high initial intracranial tumour load.

It is essentially the late sequelae which have been worrying and led to the moves to drop irradiation from minimal CNS disease treatment schedules. The literature is full of conflicting papers on the subject but those given 24 Gy cranial irradiation and 5–6 intrathecal injections are now generally accepted to have some degree of deterioration in performance IQ in the range of 15–25 points with relative preservation of verbal IQ skills. The global IQ score may be relatively preserved because of this, although most series do show a fall in mean IQ of 10–15 points.[30,31] Those under 3 years at treatment appear to have greatest deficit.[32] Bleyer's group have also reported that patients receiving spinal irradiation, rather than intrathecal medication, have significantly higher performance IQs confirming the suspicion that the methotrexate is additive to the radiation causing these sequelae. Preliminary reports do not suggest that the reduction of cranial irradiation dosages from 24 Gy to 18 Gy actually reduces the impact on performance.[33]

There is less agreement about the incidence of CT scan and nuclear magnetic resonance imaging (MRI) image abnormalities, but changes are more frequently reported on both forms of scan when combined modality therapy has been used than with either radiation or intrathecal medication alone. Risk factors for the development of CT changes include those under 3 years at diagnosis, girls, and if there has been a previous overt CNS relapse. The changes seen are periventricular hypodensities which can decrease with time and calcifications which conversely may take many years to develop.

Other toxicities Partial or complete growth hormone deficiency and premature onset of puberty are now recognized sequelae of standard CNS therapy secondary, it is thought, to an impact on the hypothalamus. With radiotherapy dosages of 18–24 Gy it appears that the release of growth hormone releasing hormone rather than that of growth hormone itself is the principal cause of the problem, although all the factors associated with premature onset of puberty are not yet recognized.

Can we manage with less or no irradiation? From a multitude of studies, late toxicity appears to be more likely and of greater degree whenever cranial irradiation is included and least with intrathecal methotrexate alone. However, in the CCG 101 study[34] which compared craniospinal irradiation with extended sanctuary irradiation (liver, spleen, gonads), craniospinal irradiation only and intrathecal methotrexate only, an excess of CNS relapses was seen with the latter and patients required recall for delayed irradiation. In more recent studies, where more selected patients with low-risk features (white cell count $<10 \times 10^9/1$ have been given intrathecal methotrexate only, no excess of CNS relapses has been seen, but, unlike in their earlier study, the CCG in study 161, have continued methotrexate during maintenance chemotherapy. The paediatric oncology group (POG) AlinC 11 protocol incorporate triple intrathecal chemotherapy both during induction and on into maintenance with a resulting 5% relapse rate equi-efficacious with those receiving cranial radiotherapy and 5 intrathecal injection only in previous studies, provided the patients did not have high initial tumour load or lymphoma/leukaemia-type presentation with bulk disease.[35] The interesting finding from the CCG 101 study is that, to date, despite higher CNS relapses in the intrathecal methotrexate and delayed radiotherapy arm, overall and haematological relapse-free survival is not significantly worse than for the arms which included initial irradiation.[36] The CCG 143 study used a cranial radiotherapy dose of 18 Gy (10 fractions over 12–14 days) and no excess of CNS relapses was seen except in those with initial white cell counts $>50 \times 10^9/1$. From previous studies using 24 Gy irradiation, there appeared to be a marginal benefit for the higher dose of irradiation for the high WBC patients but the incidence difference was of marginal statistical significance. The CCG also showed that cranial irradiation with intrathecal therapy appeared to be superior in terms of CNS control to craniospinal irradiation.[21] There has been a uniform reduction in radiotherapy dosages following these findings, but

217

preliminary results do not suggest that this will be associated with a significant reduction in late neurotoxicity.[33]

Green et al[37] retrospectively reviewed a number of studies comparing those given standard therapy with radiation and intrathecal methotrexate with those receiving prolonged courses of triple intrathecal chemotherapy only, and with those receiving intermediate dose systemic methotrexate plus intrathecal methotrexate. The lowest CNS relapse rates (reaching significance) were recorded for those given irradiation in both standard ($p<0.05$) and high-risk patient ($p<0.001$) categories but the lowest haematological relapse rate for standard risk patients was achieved with systemic intermediate dose methotrexate (500 mg/M^2). In high risk patients, the best relapse free and total survival was obtained with cranial irradiation. Where there was a high CNS relapse rate, total survival was poorest, but, where it was lowest, it did not necessarily predict for overall good survival. The most important point appeared to be to achieve the best overall leukaemia cell kill. This review was, of course, of a series of studies and not a randomized comparative study. In addition, the systemic methotrexate dosages used in these studies were low compared with current practice.

In ALL there is increasing evidence that systemic methotrexate can be utilized to replace cranial irradiation, at least for standard risk patients. Abromowitch et al[38] compared: (a) methotrexate systemically injected in a dose of 1 g/M^2 along with intrathecal methotrexate during the early phase and first 18 months of maintenance with (b) cranial irradiation (18 Gy) and intrathecal methotrexate during induction and the first 18 months of maintenance included in an otherwise standard chemotherapy protocol for non-T non-B ALL patients with initial white cell count under 100×10^9/l. Patients with neurological signs at diagnosis or any CSF blasts were excluded. Overall CNS relapse rates were comparable ($p = 0.17$) between the 2 arms at an aproximate level of 10%, but overall remission duration and disease-free survival was superior in the patients given systemic methotrexate (4 year remission-free survival 67% compared with 56%). Moe et al had achieved very similar results with 74% 5 year disease-free survival for standard risk and 50% for high white count patients using 500 mg/M^2 of systemic methotrexate. The CNS relapse rate in their series was also 10%.[39]

Methotrexate has limited lipid solubility which limits its ability to cross into the cerebro-spinal fluid and, as a consequence historically, it was injected directly into the CSF (either at lumbar or ventricular level). When injected into the ventricles there is a highly variable half-life (range 3.9–20 hours) whilst lumbar injection leads to less than 10% of the drug reaching the ventricles. In contrast, when injected systemically methotrexate has a uniform distribution throughout the different CNS compartments.[40] The CSF–serum ratio (1–5%) depends on dose, duration of infusion and serum concentration reached. Borsi et al demonstrated that at 500 mg/M^2 30% and even at $1 g/M^2$ 22% of patients did not achieve CSF levels of $10^{-6} M$ which is considered to be essential for therapeutic effect. Once methotrexate dosages were escalated to the range $6–8 g/M^2$ cytocidal concentrations were uniformly achieved.[41] Younger children (under 4 years) appear to need higher dosages to achieve adequate CSF concentration due to more rapid clearance.

Escalation of dosages of methotrexate to more than $33 g/M^2$ have been attempted. In a joint study between the Children's Cancer Study Group (CCSG) and the National Cancer Institute (NCI) in America randomization between cranial irradiation (24 Gy) plus 5 intrathecal methotrexate injections and these very high dose methotrexate dosages showed no differences in CNS relapse rate between the 2 arms.[42] This protocol was for intermediate and poor risk patients only. Of particular interest was the difference in recorded toxicity. Those receiving conventional radiotherapy and intrathecal methotrexate were shown to have the well-recognized fall in full-scale IQ and underachieved in reading, spelling and arithmetic tests. Unlike the other studies, they also had some deterioration in verbal IQ. In contrast, those receiving systemic high dose methotrexate had no fall in full-scale IQ, had a small rise in verbal IQ and just a modest fall in arithmetic skills.[43] These are preliminary findings and the patients require much longer term follow-up to be clear about the differential toxicity.

Such toxicity studies are crucial if we are to uniformly abandon what is known to be effective therapy, at least for standard and low-risk patients. The incidence of neurological sequelae with high dose methotrexate has been reported as being between 5 and 15%, but most are transient in nature.[44] Preliminary results suggest a much lower incidence of learning difficulties than with irradiation. The great advantages of the high dose systemic methotrexate is that it is distributed throughout the body, including the pharmacological sanctuaries such as the CNS, that it may overcome cell resistance mechanisms by a sheer concentration effect and also prevent emergence of drug-resistant clones. Clearly, this agent has the advantage of a potential rescue in the form of folinic acid. When given after the CSF, methotrexate concentration falls below the concentration cytotoxic to leukaemic cells, folinic acid rescues normal cells and possibly some lymphoblasts outwith the CNS, but none within the CNS. Given $6–8 g/M^2$ of methotrexate intravenously (1/10 of the dose as an initial first hour prime and the rest over 23 hours) the CSF concentration falls below $10^{-6}M$ at about 36 hours post-initiation of the 24-hour infusion. This is when folinic acid should be started. With dosages of methotrexate as high as $33 g/M^2$ the addition of intrathecal therapy may not be needed.[45]

For ALL and the lymphoblastic lymphomas, it would seem very reasonable to avoid irradiation and use systemic high dose methotrexate to provide CNS and systemic treatment. It is legitimate to attempt to ask whether there are low risk patients who do not need to receive such therapy which is clearly expensive, time-consuming and associated with some non-neurological acute sequelae (for example, hepatopathy, nephropathy and mucositis). By randomized trial it is worth trying to identify those who can be managed by intrathecal therapy only (induction phase plus during continuing therapy) as the Paediatric Oncology Group have been using for some time (using triple therapy). The United States Children's Cancer Study Group (CCG 161) and the MRC are testing this hypothesis using intrathecal methotrexate only. So far, there is not uniform agreement as to which risk categories this therapy is applicable. For patients with high initial white cell counts (especially >100 × $10^9/l$), standard cranial radiotherapy at 18 or 24 Gy has failed to adequately control CNS disease in up to 20% of patients and, since overall disease-free survival is still disappointing in this group of patients, the higher dosages of systemic methotrexate which we can now deliver safely offer a promise of benefit. There is clearly an extra advantage of high dose methotrexate in its lack of significant marrow suppression and both the LMB[46] group and United Kingdom Children Cancer Study Group[47] have interposed high dose methotrexate at the nadir of counts following myelosuppressive therapy when treating advanced B cell lymphomas.

Cytosine forms the mainstay, albeit at somewhat reduced dosage compared with these lymphoma protocols, in the ANLL protocols. Using longer courses of cytosine, and incorporating intrathecal injections thereof, has not been associated with a dramatic rise in CNS relapses as one might expect with improved survival in ANLL. Mild tremor or nystagmus are seen quite frequently with the use of high dose cytosine, but cerebellar encephalopathy, which may prove fatal, appears much more common in adults than in children.

Conclusions

There is a risk of overt CNS relapse developing in acute leukaemias and in non-Hodgkin's lymphoma of childhood. Historically, this risk has been reduced by the universal application of cranial irradiation (18–24 Gy) and intrathecal medication, usually methotrexate. Long-term sequelae, most notably learning difficulties, in young children have generated studies using either intrathecal therapy only or high dose systemic methotrexate. For low-risk patients certainly (white cell count <10 × $10^9/l$), and maybe average or standard risk patients (white cell count 10–50 × $10^9/l$), intrathecal methotrexate or triple therapy may be adequate if it is continued intermittently during the first 18–24 months of treatment, and not just given for 5–6 injections early in therapy. Further confirmation is required for whom this is adequate therapy. For high risk patients, systemic methotrexate offers the unique opportunity to give systemic and CNS high dose therapy (ie total body attack) at the same time.

Very careful monitoring of sequelae long term is essential to ensure that efficacy and safety are at least equal, if not considerably less, with systemic methotrexate than with irradiation. Monitoring must include checks for acute neurological toxicity, liver and renal dysfunction, growth disturbance, endocrinopathy, learning difficulties, global IQ scale and, of course, secondary neoplasia. There is very good evidence that neurotoxicity in leukaemia after CNS treatment is proportional to the number of modalities used. The safest, to date, appears to be the use of systemic high dose methotrexate. If combined modality therapy is used, the sequencing must be very carefully planned. Although intrathecal methotrexate can be given before, during and after, cranial irradiation, there is a risk that post-radiotherapy intrathecal methotrexate may increase neurotoxicity. If systemic methotrexate is given, it must be given prior to radiotherapy. If given after, there is very high risk of leukoencephalopathy developing.

References

(1) Evans AE. Central nervous system involvements in children with acute leukaemia. A study of 921 patients. *Cancer* 1964; 17: 256–8.

(2) Hyman CB, Bogle JM, Brubaker CA, Williams SK, Hammond D. CNS involvement by leukaemia in children. Relationship to systemic leukaemia and description of clinical and laboratory manifestations. *Blood* 1965; 25: 1–12.

(3) Hardisty RM, Norman PM. Meningeal leukaemia. *Arch Dis Child* 1967; 42: 441–7.

(4) Ortega JA, Nesbit ME, Sather HN et al. Long term evaluation of a CNS prophylactic trial – treatment comparison and outcome after CNS relapse in childhood ALL. A report of the Children's Cancer Study Group. *J Clin Oncol* 1987; 5: 1646–54.

(5) Darbyshire PJ, Eden OB, Richards S. *Analysis of primary CNS relapse occurring in children on MRC trials between 1977–1987.* Personal communication 1990.

(6) Aur RJA, Simone JV, Hustu HO et al. CNS therapy and combination chemotherapy of childhood lymphocytic leukaemia. *Blood* 1971; 37: 272–81.

(7) Hustu HO, Aur RJA, Verzosa MS et al. Prevention of CNS leukaemia by irradiation. *Cancer* 1973; 32: 585–97.

(8) Nesbit ME, D'Angio GJ, Sather HN et al. Effect of isolated CNS leukaemia on bone marrow remission and survival in childhood ALL. *Lancet* 1981; i: 1386–9.

(9) Thomas LB. Pathology of leukaemia in brain and meninges. P.M. Studies of patients with acute leukaemia and of mice given inoculations of L1210 leukaemia. *Cancer Res* 1965; 25: 1555–71.

(10) Miller DR. Acute lymphoblastic leukaemia. *Paediatric Clinics of North America* 1980; 27: 269–91.

(11) Magrath IT. *The non Hodgkin's lymphomas: clinical features and staging.* London: Edward Arnold, ed, 1990: 180–99.

(12) Sullivan MP, Vietti TJ, Fernack DJ et al. Clinical investigations in the treatment of meningeal leukaemia: radiation therapy regimens versus conventional intrathecal methotrexate. *Blood* 1969; 34: 301–19.

(13) Eden OB, Lilleyman JS, Shaw MP, Richards S, Peto J. *Results of Medical Research Council Childhood Leukaemia Trial UKALL VIII. Br J Haematol* 1991: in press.

(14) West RJ, Graham-Pole J, Hardisty RM, Pike MC. Factors in pathogenesis of central nervous system leukaemia. *Br Med J* 1972; 3: 311–14.

(15) Rall DP, Zubrod CG. Mechanisms of drug absorption and excretion. *Ann Rev Pharmacol & Toxicol* 1962; 2: 109.

(16) Hunt WE, Bournoncle BA, Meagher JN. Neurological complications of leukaemia and lymphomas. *J Neurosur* 1959; 16: 135.

(17) Kwaan HC, Pierre RV, Long DL. Meningeal involvement as first manifestation of acute myeloblastic transformation in CGL. *Blood* 1969; 33: 348–52.

(18) Evans A, Gilbert ES, Zandstra R. The increasing incidence of central nervous system leukaemia in children. *Cancer* 1970; 26: 404–9.

(19) Medical Research Council Working Party on Leukaemia in Childhood. Report on UKALL V: An attempt to reduce the immunosuppressive effects of therapy in childhood acute lymphoblastic leukaemia. *J Clin Oncol* 1986; 4: 1758–64.

(20) Mastrangelo R, Romanini A, Cellini N et al. Intermittent intrathecal methotrexate and fractional radiation (M-IMFRA) plus chemotherapy in childhood leukaemia. *TUMORI* 1978; 64: 607–11.

(21) Nesbit ME, Sather HM, Robinson LL et al. Presymptomatic central nervous system therapy in previously untreated childhood acute lymphoblastic leukaemia: comparison of 1800 rads and 2400 rads. A report from Children's Cancer Study Group. *Lancet* 1981; i: 461–6.

(22) Pizzo PA, Poplack DG, Bleyer WA. Neurotoxicities of current leukaemia therapy. *Am J Pedia Hematol & Oncol* 1979; 1: 127–40.

(23) Parker D, Malpas JS, Sandland R, Sheaff PC, Freeman JE, Paxton A. Outlook following 'somnolence syndrome' after prophylactic cranial irradiation. *Br Med J* 1978; 1: 554.

(24) O'Hare AE, Eden OB, Simpson RM, Donaldson A, Sainsbury CPQ. Cranial computerised tomography and cerebrospinal fluid procoagulant activity in childhood acute lymphoblastic leukaemia. *Pedia Hematol & Oncol* 1988; 5: 103–13.

(25) Packer RJ, Zimmerman RA, Bilaniuk LT. Magnetic resonance imaging in the evaluation of treatment related central nervous system damage. *Cancer* 1986; 58: 635–40.

(26) Ochs J, Bowman WP, Pui CH et al. Seizures in childhood lymphoblastic leukaemia patients. *Lancet* 1983; i: 793–8.

(27) Bleyer WA. Neurological sequelae of methotrexate and ionising radiation: a new classification. *Cancer Treat Rep* 1981; 61: 89–98.

(28) Eden OB, Wood T, Goldie W, Etcubanas E. Seizures following intrathecal cytosine arabinoside in young children with acute lymphoblastic leukaemia. *Cancer* 1978; 42: 53–8.

(29) Price RA. Therapy related central nervous system diseases in children with acute lymphoblastic leukaemia. In: Mastrangelo R, Poplack DG, Roccardo R, eds. *Central nervous system leukaemia*. Boston: Martinus Nijhoff, 1983: 71–82.

(30) Eiser C. Intellectual abilities among survivors of childhood leukaemia as a function of CNS irradiation. *Arch Dis Child* 1978; 53: 391–5.

(31) Moss HA, Nannis ED, Poplack DG. The effects of prophylactic treatment of the central nervous system on the intellectual functioning of children with acute lymphocytic leukaemia. *Am J Med* 1981; 71: 47–52.

(32) Jannoun L. Are cognitive and educational development affected by age at which prophylactic therapy is given in acute lymphoblastic leukaemia? *Arch Dis in Child* 1983; 58: 953–8.

(33) Chessells JM, Cox T, Cavanagh N et al. Methotrexate, cranial irradiation and neurotoxicity in childhood acute lymphoblastic leukaemia. *Proc Internat Soc Paediat Oncol* 1987; 16: 102–3.

(34) Nesbit ME, Sather H, Robinson LL et al. Sanctuary therapy: A randomised trial of 724 children with previously untreated acute lymphoblastic leukaemia. A report of the Children's Cancer Study Group. *Cancer Res* 1982; 42: 674–80.

(35) Sullivan MP, Chen T, Dyment PK et al. Equivalence of intrathecal chemotherapy and radiotherapy as central nervous system prophylaxis in children with acute lymphatic leukaemia. A Pediatric Oncology Group Study. *Blood* 1982; 60: 948–58.

(36) Ortega JA, Nesbit ME, Sather HN et al. Long term evaluation of a CNS prophylaxis trial – treatment comparisons and outcome after CNS relapse in childhood ALL. A report from the Children's Cancer Study Group. *J Clin Oncol* 1987; 5: 1646–54.

(37) Green DM, Freeman AL, Sather HN et al. Comparison of three methods of central nervous system prophylaxis in childhood acute lymphoblastic leukaemia. *Lancet* 1980; i: 1398–403.

(38) Abromowitch M, Ochs J, Pui CH et al. High dose methotrexate improved clinical outcome in children with acute lymphoblastic leukaemia. St Jude Total Therapy Study X. *Med & Pediat Oncol* 1988; 16: 297–303.

(39) More PJ, Seip M, Finne PH. Intermediate dose methotrexate in childhood acute lymphocytic leukaemia in Norway. *Haematologia* 1981; 14: 257–63.

(40) Shapiro WR, Young DF, Mehta BM. Methotrexate distribution in cerebrospinal fluid after intravenous ventricular and lumbar injection. *New Eng J Med* 1975; 293: 161–6.

(41) Borsi JD, Moe PJ. A comparative study on the pharmacokinetics of methotrexate in a close range of 0.5 g to 33.6 g/M^2 in children with acute lymphocytic leukaemia. *Cancer* 1987; 60: 5–13.

(42) Poplack DG, Reaman G, Bleyer WA et al. Central nervous system preventative therapy with high dose methotrexate in ALL. *Proc Am Soc Clin Oncol* 1984; 3: 294.

(43) Brouwers P, Moss H, Reaman G et al. Central nervous system preventative therapy with systemic high dose methotrexate versus cranial radiation and intrathecal methotrexate. Longitudinal comparison of effects of treatment on intellectual function of children with ALL. *Proc Am Soc Clin Oncol* 1987; 6: 158.

(44) Jaffe N, Takaue Y, Anzai et al. Transient neurologic disturbance induced by high dose methotrexate treatment. *Cancer* 1985; 56: 1356–60.

(45) Bleyer WA. High dose methotrexate in childhood acute lymphoblastic leukaemia. How high should the dose be? *Proc Internat Soc Paediat Oncology Workshop*. The role of clinical pharmocology. Borsi JD, ed. 1989: 19–31.

(46) Patte C, Philip T, Rodary C et al. Improved survival rate in children with Stage III & IV B cell NHL and leukaemia using multiagent chemotherapy: results of a study of 114 children from the French Paediatric Oncology Society. *J Clin Oncol* 1986; 8: 1219–26.

(47) Hann IM, Eden OB, Pinkerton R, Barnes J. 'Macho' chemotherapy for Stage IB B cell lymphoma and B cell ALL. *Br J Haematol* 1990, in press.

Multiple myeloma: host–tumour and tumour–host interactions

D E JOSHUA

Introduction

The development of an antigen specific immunoglobulin, the final product of the normal humoral immune response, is one of the most tightly regulated phenomena in immunology. Antigen specificity is achieved by a number of processes. Immunoglobulin gene rearrangements provide a large pre-existing repertoire of B-lymphocytes, while additional extensive qualitative changes occur in antibody structure during an affinity maturation process involving somatic mutation of heavy and light chain variable regions.[1,2] Concurrently, but independently of somatic mutation, isotype switch recombination results in the replacement of antibody constant regions.[2,4]

It is therefore not surprising that, in lymphoproliferative disorders characterized by antibody production such as myeloma, there exist active regulatory control mechanisms which reflect the mechanisms required for production and expression of normal immunoglobulin. The network theory of Jerne[5] proposes such regulatory processes occur as a result of an autoimmune response to idiotypes developed during the humoral immune response. Thus abnormalities of the normal immune response (hypogammaglobulinaemia and impaired immune responsiveness) as well as immunoregulatory attempts to control tumour proliferation are represented.

Malignancies of the B-cell lineage can occur in populations of cells which vary in their ability to undergo somatic mutation and isotype switch. Very little somatic mutation is seen in chronic lymphatic leukaemia, small lymphocytic lymphoma and acute lymphocytic leukaemia.[6–8] In contrast, malignancies of the immune system occurring at stages after somatic mutation and isotype switch overwhelmingly involve IgG or IgA immunoglobulin expression and are associated with the presence of extensive mutations including point mutations.[9–11] The presence of somatic mutations in such

All correspondence to: Haematology Department, Royal Prince Alfred Hospital, Camperdown NSW 2050, Australia.

Cambridge Medical Reviews: Haematological Oncology Volume 1

malignancies, of which multiple myeloma is the classic example, argues against the clonogenic cell being a primitive or pre-B B-cell, as has been suggested by many authors.[12-15] In order to fulfil the requirements of antigen dependence, somatic cell mutation, isotype class switch and idiotypic immunoglobulin production which is characteristic of myeloma, we have argued that the proliferative cell is of germinal centre origin.[16]

Multiple myeloma is characterized by the excessive malignant production of an idiotypic protein. Yet, even in this pathological process, there is evidence that immunoregulatory control mechanisms are active and play a role in the pathogenesis of the disease. This review will discuss the unique nature of the immune deficiency associated with myeloma (tumour–host interaction) and, using evidence both from the murine plasmacytoma model and from human myeloma, will argue that the host is able to influence the state of proliferation of the malignant clone. This phenomenon is especially seen with respect to the maintenance of the plateau phase of myeloma.

Plateau phase is a hypoproliferative state and it is postulated that, in myeloma immunoregulatory control mechanisms actively inhibit the stage of B-cell proliferation and mutation that normally occurs within the germinal centre. This inhibition may in part be light chain specific.

Humoral immunodeficiency associated with myeloma
Clinical studies
Recurrent infections, usually involving highly pathogenic organisms, are a predominant clinical feature and a cause of both morbidity and mortality in myeloma.[17] It is not known precisely which subpopulations of myeloma patients are most at risk, to which type of infection they are most vulnerable or at what stage during the course of the disease the risk of infection is greatest. Early data suggested a high incidence of pneumococcal bacterial pneumonia,[18,19] and this has remained the classical dogma in most reviews.[20] In the 1970s and 1980s, reports of gram negative infections were increasing.[21] Some studies have demonstrated a biphasic pattern of infections occurs, with encapsulated organisms predominating early in the course of the disease and gram-negative organisms terminally,[22] but this is not supported by other studies.[23]

Patients with myeloma have low levels of circulating antibodies to Staphylococcal alpha-toxin and streptolysin 0.[24] In addition, they demonstrate reduced levels of agglutinins to E. coli, sheep red blood cells and type specific agglutinins for human A and B erythrocytes.[25,26] Patients with myeloma have also been shown to have impaired responses to pneumococcal polysaccharide I and II which results in the failure of protection by pneumococcal vaccines.[27] The recent availability of intravenous gammaglobulin preparations has renewed interest in the prophylactic use of immunoglobulin in myeloma. A large trial to investigate this question is currently in progress by the MRC Myeloma Trials group.

To differentiate between true primary and secondary responses, Cone and Uhr[28] studied the response to the bacteriophage ∅X174 in patients with myeloma and chronic lymphatic leukaemia. This was regarded as a true primary stimulus. The secondary response to diphtheria toxin was also studied. In chronic lymphatic leukaemia, both primary and secondary responses were impaired, while in patients with myeloma there was an impaired primary response but a normal secondary response. This defect was not related to paraprotein isotypes. Harris and co-workers[29] studying the humoral immune response to keyhole limpet haemocyanin in myeloma observed a prolonged induction time for IgM production and reduced titres of antibody. Patients with benign paraproteinaemias also had a decreased primary immune response and a normal secondary response.[30] Weits et al studied the primary and secondary antibody responses to *Helix pomatia* haemocyanin in a group of patients with paraproteins. These patients had been followed for at least 3 years before the study and were documented as having non-progressive disease. Primary responses were impaired, but, in contrast, the responses to previously encountered antigens, tetanus and diphtheria toxoid, were normal. This fact suggests the impaired humoral immune status seen in such patients is a manifestation of immune regulation per se, rather than due to the malignant process.

The aetiology of immune deficiency state is complex and will be discussed below, but it involves both hypogammaglobulinaemia and an impaired primary immune response to both T-dependent and T-independent antigens. Immunosuppression occurs at low tumour loads and is a specific effect of the malignancy. It is unlike the immunosuppression associated with viral infections or cancer in general.

Cellular immunity associated with myeloma

In general, patients with myeloma are able to mount delayed hypersensitivity reactions to common antigens. They can also be sensitized to new antigens such as 2, 4-dinitro-1-fluorobenzene and keyhole limpet haemocyanin.[29] The clinical correlate of these findings is the lack of fungal and viral infections as predominant clinical problems in myeloma, with the exception of those patients receiving high dose corticosteroids in new chemotherapy regimens and those patients undergoing bone marrow transplantation.[31,32] In vitro studies show that peripheral blood lymphocytes from myeloma patients have a normal response to stimulation by PHA and pokeweed mitogen, but a marginally reduced response in an antigen induced proliferation assay.[33]

Other investigators have shown defective cytotoxic T-lymphocyte generation and a deficiency in the ability to generate lymphokine activated killer activity,[34] together with abnormal T-cell clonogenic potential in patients with myeloma.[35] These data demonstrate both T- and B-cell defects in myeloma.

The mechanism of immunodeficiency
Murine plasmacytoma model
Transplantable plasma cell tumours of Balb/c mice have many of the characteristics of human myeloma. They elaborate monoclonal paraproteins and the host animals develop hypogammaglobulinaemia.[36] In addition, mice bearing these tumours have the immune defect typical of human myeloma, that is, a depressed primary immune response with normal secondary responses and a marginally deficient cellular immunity.[37,28]

The mechanism of this immune defect has been extensively investigated. It has been postulated on the basis of in vitro evidence that the myeloma induces 'suppressor' monoctyes or macrophages. The development of these suppressor macrophages is believed to be due to a plasmacytoma secreted product called 'PC factor' which has no immunosuppressive properties per se but induces macrophages to secrete a soluble factor 'plasmacytoma induced macrophage substance' (PIMS), which suppresses antibody production and B-cell proliferation. The relationship of this substance to the known interleukins is not known.[39–42] Other investigators, using in vivo transfer experiments, have failed to demonstrate that macrophages, even from the very suppressive plasmacytoma TEPC-183, are immunosuppressive.[38] In addition, supraoptimal numbers of normal[43] or heat-killed macrophages[44] are very effective inhibitors of the primary response in vitro. These factors, together with the demonstration of an increase in red pulp macrophages induced by the murine plasmacytoma TEPC-183,[45] have led us to postulate that the defect in murine plasmacytomas is an antigen sequestration phenomenon. A similar defect is caused by systemic murine *Mycobacterium lepraemurium* and in murine malarial infection.[47] Thus we have postulated that lack of antigen binding by the appropriate antigen presenting cells, ie interfollicular dendritic cells, and uptake by tumour infiltrating macrophages may cause the reduced primary immune response in the mouse model. The fact that the primary defect can be abrogated by the use of Freund's adjuvant or by increasing antigen load supports this theory.[38]

In addition to the macrophage-associated defect detectable in the murine plasmacytoma, other workers have demonstrated T-cells with immunosuppressive properties. Studies with IgA secreting plasmacytomas show mice bearing these tumours have increased numbers of T-cells carrying Fc receptors specific for the isotype of the paraprotein.[48,49] These cells appear to be suppressor cells and inhibit immunoglobulin production. The exact role these cells play in causing immune suppression is not clear.

Human myeloma

A reduction in polyclonal immunoglobulin occurs in almost all patients with myeloma. Studies on IgG myeloma have demonstrated hypercatabolism of the residual normal IgG to a level almost twice that seen in control subjects. IgG is, however, the only class of immunoglobulin that exhibits a direct concentration–hypercatabolism relationship. Thus patients with IgA myeloma and reduced IgG levels have a normal catabolism of IgG; IgA catabolism in contrast is independent of its serum concentration and the depressed values of immunoglobulins in IgA myeloma predominantly reflect reduced synthesis.[50]

Studies of the immune defect in human myeloma have produced data both in agreement with, and in conflict to, the concepts postulated from the murine plasmacytoma model. Hence a circulating suppressor phagocytic cell has been described in myeloma by some but not all authors.[51–53] Data on T-cell numbers are conflicting. Several reports have described a reduction in CD4 positive T-cells in myeloma, whereas other studies do not confirm these data.[54,55] Similarly, T-cells with Fc receptors specific for the myeloma protein, and which suppress immunoglobulin secretion, have abnormalities in T-helper and suppressor function.[56,57] Petersen and his colleagues in a recent study failed to show any significant abnormalities in T-cell function and point out that chemotherapy may be responsible for the previously described abnormalities.[53] A CD5 positive B-cell present in the blood and spleen of patients with myeloma has been shown to mediate immunosuppression.[58] Recently, a plasma cell line with immunosuppressive properties was isolated. The cell line secreted a 10–15 kD substance capable of suppressing, by more than 50%, the production of immunoglobulin by pokeweed mitogen-stimulated normal human peripheral blood cells.[59] The cell line did not have the classical phenotype of plasma cells, being CD5 positive, and the role of such cells in myeloma-induced immunosuppression remains unclear.

Pilarski and her colleagues in a detailed series of papers have shown a marked deficiency of mature B-cells in myeloma. They have demonstrated that memory specificities for certain recall antigens remain, consistent with the finding of relatively unimpaired secondary responses in myeloma.[60–62] Pilarski regards the defect of myeloma as being a block in B-cell maturation with an accumulation of precursor cells. This concept is consistent with animal data showing that B-cells from plasmacytoma bearing mice are functionally capable of mounting antibody responses when transferred to normal mice.[38] Pilarski has postulated that the immune deficiency results from auto-immune reactivity against immunoglobulin and immunoglobulin-related epitopes, generated as a result of high levels of monoclonal immunoglobulin present and so is consistent with the network theory of Jerne.[5]

An as yet unexplained phenomenon is that of light chain isotype suppression. Non-malignant rectal mucosal plasma cells show a decreased expression of the light chain isotype concordant with the malignant paraprotein.[63,64] The mechanism of light chain isotype suppression is not known, but it cannot be the full explanation of hypogammaglobulinaemia in myeloma since complete suppression of isotype-specific light chain would only be able to reduce immunoglobulin levels to 30% of normal. The appreciation that the presence of light chain isotype suppression in the blood is a marker of stable disease has led to concepts of host–tumour interactions playing a role in the maintenance of the plateau phase state in myeloma.[65]

Host-mediated effects on tumour growth
Murine plasmacytoma
In addition to the effect of the tumour has on the host immune system, there is evidence that the host immunological mechanisms can modulate tumour growth. Thus early studies with the murine plasmacytomas MOPC 315 and MOPC 460 showed that idiotype specific tumour rejection can be elicited by immunizing with myeloma proteins.[66] Of great interest is the fact that the immunogenic portion of the paraprotein is the variable portion of the light chain, the heavy chain being ineffective. For example, in the murine plasmacytoma MOPC 315, idiotypic reactive T-cells are stimulated by whole 315 immunoglobulin and 315 light chain but not by purified 315 heavy chain.[67] Similar results suggesting that it is the light chain that is involved in immunoregulatory processes have been found in the plasmacytoma T15[68] and in studies using human myeloma cell lines.[69] The role of light chains in B-cell immunoregulation will be discussed further below. In addition to immunization studies with myeloma proteins, antigens in tolerogenic form,[70] antigen–antibody complexes,[71] carrier-specific helper and suppressor T-cells,[72] idiotype specific T-cells[73] and allo reactive T-cells[74] have all been shown to be capable of modulating plasmacytoma growth and function.

Multiple myeloma
Unlike remission in acute leukaemia, plateau phase in myeloma is not characterized by the complete morphological disappearance of the tumour, but represents a state in which tumour progression does not occur despite persistence of a significant bone marrow plasma cell infiltrate and an elevated but stable paraprotein level. Plateau phase can be achieved in approximately 50% of patients with myeloma. Haematological remission with complete disappearance of measurable disease is only rarely obtained with standard melphalan therapy, although its frequency is increased with the newer intensive regimens such as high dose melphalan or intensive multiagent therapy plus alpha-interferon.[79,80] There is no relationship between initial percentage fall in paraprotein level and duration of plateau (Joshua et al, in press).

Plateau phase is characterized by a low labelling index of bone marrow plasma cells,[77] a lack of response to standard chemotherapy,[78] the presence of light chain isotype suppression,[64] and the absence of elevated numbers of CD10 positive and CD38 positive lymphocytes circulating in the peripheral blood.[79,80]

Although light chain isotype suppression of B-cells in the peripheral blood of patients with myeloma had been noted by previous authors,[81,82] its significance and clinical associations was not addressed. We reported that light chain isotype suppression in the peripheral blood of patients with myeloma was associated with plateau phase or stable disease.[64] Our studies have also demonstrated that light chain isotype suppression is a marker of stable disease at presentation.[83] In addition, longitudinal monitoring of patients demonstrates that the establishment and subsequent loss of light chain isotype suppression heralds disease progression and is a valuable monitor of disease activity.[84] Loss of suppression is not always due to malignant cells being present in the peripheral blood and can occur without monotypic heavy chain gene rearrangements being detected.[85]

The existence of plateau phase implies that the differentiation of myeloma precursor cells into the plasma cell pool is being balanced by plasma cell death. Plasma cell life span in humans has not been well studied, but experimental studies point to short-lived plasma cells being produced after interaction with extrafollicular digitating cells, and long-lived plasma cells being produced as a result of interaction with follicular dendritic cells within the lymphoid follicle.[86] These long-lived plasma cells home to the bone marrow and are the putative cells of origin of myeloma.

The possibility that plateau phase results from increased plasma cell death and therefore increased cellular turnover is not supported by kinetic studies. In addition, low levels of serum thymidine kinase, a marker of cellular proliferation, are correlated with plateau phase and light chain isotype suppression.[87] This is consistent with the theory that plateau phase is a state of hypoproliferation of both plasma cells[77] and plasma cell precursors. The lack of correlation between the duration of plateau phase and the direct effect of chemotherapy (as measured by the percentage fall in paraprotein) further reinforces the concept of maintenance of plateau phase being under immunological control.

Evidence that light chains play a regulatory role in B-cell immunoregulation

The mechanism of light chain isotype suppression is unknown. Recent data, however, point to light chains playing a role in regulatory control of B-cell proliferation and clonal expansion of B-cells which is unrelated to their antigen binding role.

Light chains also appear to play an essential role in immunoglobulin secretion, as documented from observations on myeloma mutants. In contrast to the spontaneous loss of heavy chain synthesis in plasma cell mutants, it is extremely rare for such mutants to lose the capacity to secrete light chain.[88] In the murine plasmacytoma models, there is further evidence that free light chains may have a significant clonal regulatory function. As mentioned previously, in the plasmacytoma M315, idiotype reactive T-cells are stimulated by whole 315 immunoglobulin and 315 light chain, but not by purified 315 heavy chain.[67,68]

Surplus free light chain unassociated with heavy chain is secreted throughout B-cell maturation.[89] Mitogen-activated normal mononuclear cells in addition secrete significant amounts of light chain unassociated with heavy chain.[90] Furthermore, malignant kappa plasma cells in myeloma, in some cases at least, bear free kappa light chains on their plasma membrane, as do human plasmacytoma lines.[91,92]

In myeloma, an excess of light chain is produced. The idiotypic epitopes expressed on this light chain present a continuum of specificity from public idiotypes to private idiotypes. A sharing of idiotypes on myeloma proteins and normal light chains together with feedback inhibition may account for light chain isotype suppression and tumour inhibition.

Precursor cell dynamics in myeloma

Studies on the kinetics of plasma cells in myeloma have suggested that a precursor compartment of proliferating cells is present, feeding the predominantly non-proliferating plasma cell pool.[16] We have reported data using levels of serum thymidine kinase as a monitor of the proliferative state of a tumour cell population which supports the view that tumour stability and plateau phase in myeloma is due to inhibition of proliferation of the precursor cell.[87]

There has been considerable debate regarding the maturity of the cells undergoing malignant transformation in myeloma. A number of investigators favour the concept that the proliferative or precursor cell in myeloma is of stem cell origin. In contrast, we have argued that this cell must arise late in B-cell ontogeny and is of germinal centre origin for the following reasons: (1) the neoplastic proliferation occurs in a cell that is committed to the production of idiotypic proteins and has stable heavy and light chain gene rearrangements, (2) there is a critical requirement for antigen exposure in the development of mineral oil-induced murine plasmacytomas, (3) the overwhelming predominance of IgG and IgA paraproteins in myeloma place the final malignant event as following isotype switch, (4) cells of germinal centre phenotype, ie CD10 and CD38 positive, frequently circulate in the peripheral blood of myeloma patients and their occurrence correlates with progressive disease and loss of light chain isotype suppression.[16] The putative precursor cell retains two crucial properties of germinal centre cells; the ability to participate in the hypermutation process of the germinal centre and the ability to home to the bone marrow and to differentiate into an antibody-producing plasma cell.

Somatic mutation as a marker of B-cell ontogeny with reference to myeloma

There is considerable evidence that somatic mutation does not take place during the initial stages of the immune response, but is a phenomenon of the reaction occurring in the germinal centre.[86] Somatic mutation occurs both before and after isotype switch at a rate close to 10^{-3} per cell per generation.[93] Somatic mutation is thought to occur together with cell division and such remarkable frequencies of mutation imply that the rate of B-cell division is extremely high. High rates of B-cell proliferation only occur during primary B-lymphopoiesis or following antigen activation. These rates of mutation are considerably higher than those normally observed in animal or bacterial cells (normally $10^{-5} - 10^{-8}$/cell/generation). Weitzman[94] has shown such rates are obtained in mouse myeloma cells where mutant progeny were generated at 10^{-2}/cell/generation. Mutations usually result in the loss of ability to synthesize heavy chains. Since myeloma progenitor cells retain the capacity for somatic mutation, both in animals and humans, then myeloma is separated clearly from malignancies of B-cells which are pre-germinal centre in origin, eg the mu-positive, delta-positive cell of chronic lymphatic leukaemia and small lymphocytic lymphoma in which somatic mutation is not found. This is in marked contrast to follicular non-Hodgkin's lymphoma in which somatic mutation is common.[6,7] Other B-cell tumours also lack somatic mutation. Bird and colleagues[8] have demonstrated that somatic mutation does not occur in childhood acute lymphoblastic leukaemia, but immunoglobulin heavy chain genes continue to rearrange de novo within neoplastic B-cell precursor populations.

Further evidence against the precursor cell of myeloma being a pre-B-cell comes from studies utilizing molecular biological techniques. There is, for example, no preferential use of the VH(V) family gene. This recently described immunoglobulin V_H family is close to the D_H and J_H genes and is preferentially rearranged in immature B cell tumours. In a recent study only 1 patient out of 28 with myeloma had rearrangements of this gene. This is in contrast to B-chronic lymphocytic leukaemia (B-CLL) or acute lymphoblastic leukaemia (ALL) where rearrangements are seen in one third of patients.[95] Thus the postulate that the clonogenic B-cell in myeloma is an early or pre-B-cell is not supported by these studies, which firmly place the site of origin of this cell after the somatic mutation phase of the germinal centre reaction.

Site of host–tumour interaction in myeloma

We have recently published a proposed mechanism for antigen-driven selection in germinal centres and postulated that unselected mutants die from apoptosis. Germinal centre cells were isolated from human tonsil by negative selection of IgD and CD39 positive lymphocytes. Such isolated cells have the morphology and phenotype of germinal centre centrocytes and rapidly die in culture by apoptosis unless stimulated by phorbol ester or anti-IgM.[96] Cells which have been rescued from apoptosis have the phenotype of myeloma precursor cells and develop plasmablast cell morphology.[16] As apoptosis is not a feature of myeloma (unlike Burkitt's lymphoma), it is possible that inhibition is being exhibited on B-cell division (and therefore mutation) in a cell that has been antigen selected initially in the germinal centre, but whose subsequent malignant proliferation is independent of antigen. The relationship between proliferation and somatic mutation would explain the high levels of mutations in myeloma proteins seen in progressive disease. For example, in a number of cases, the transition from benign to malignant gammopathy has been accompanied by proliferation of variant new clones with idiotypic determinants shared by the original clone.[97,98] Other cases have been documented where new clones develop on the transition from plateau induced by chemotherapy to active relapse.[99]

Thus, although the site of host inhibition of B-cell proliferation remains unknown, a position at the germinal centre would account for both the immune deficit in myeloma, since antibody affinity maturation would not occur, and the inhibitory effect on tumour proliferation.

Conclusion

In human myeloma, the tumour has profound effects on the host's immune responses. The immune deficit is of major clinical importance and results in significant morbidity and mortality. It is unlike the immune deficit caused by viral infections or by cancer in general and appears to be a specific immunoregulatory phenomenon. As well as interference with the immune mechanisms of the host, it seems likely that the host immune mechanisms are activated in response to the presence of the tumour. This is seen especially in plateau phase disease which is a hypoproliferative state due to inhibition of myeloma precursor activity.

We have postulated that the myeloma precursor cell is of germinal centre origin, able to participate in the process of somatic mutation and home to the bone marrow. It seems possible that inhibition of proliferation, together with a reduction in somatic mutation, occurs under the influence of immunomodulatory control mechanisms. This may be, in part, light chain specific and is supported by the evolution of increased somatic mutants, associated with increased precursor cell proliferation as the disease progresses.

References

(1) Berek C, Griffiths GM. Molecular events during maturation of the immune response to oxazolone. *Nature* 1985; 316: 412–16.

(2) Wysocki L, Manser T, Fefter ML. Somatic evolution of variable region structures during an immune response. *Proc Natl Acad Sci USA* 1986; 83: 1847–51.

(3) Cebra JJ, Komisar JL, Schweitzer PA. C_H isotype 'switching' during normal B-lymphocyte development. *Ann Rev Immunol* 1984; 2: 493–7.

(4) Gilmore GL, Yang JQ, Marcu KB, Birshtein BK. Absence of somatic mutation in the variable region of MPC 11 variants expressing a different heavy chain isotype. *J Immunol* 1987; 139: 619–24.

(5) Jerne NK. Towards a network theory of the immune system. *Ann Immunol* (Paris) 1974; 125C: 373–89.

(6) Pratt LF, Rassenti L, Larrick J, Robbins B, Banks PM, Kipps TJ. IgV region gene expression in small lymphocyte lymphoma with little or not somatic hypermutation. *J Immunol* 1989; 143: 699–707.

(7) Kipps TJ, Fong S, Tomhave E, Chen PP, Goldfien RD, Carson DA. High-frequency expression of a conserved kappa light chain variable region gene in chronic lymphocytic leukaemia. *Proc Natl Acad Sci USA* 1987; 84: 2916–20.

(8) Bird J, Galili N, Link M, Stites D, Sklar J. Continuing rearrangement but absence of somatic hypermutation in immunoglobulin gene of human B cell precursor leukaemia. *J Exp Med* 1988; 168: 229–45.

(9) Hobbs JB. Monitoring myelomatosis. *Arch of Int Med* 1975; 135: 125–30.

(10) Cognse M, Bakhshi A, Korsmeyer SJ, Guglielmi P. Gene mutations and alternate RNA splicing result in truncated IgL chains in human gamma II chain disease. *J Immunol* 1988; 141: 1738–44.

(11) Davidson A, Preud'homme JL, Solomon A, Chang MD, Beede S, Diamond B. Idiotypic analysis of myeloma proteins: anti-DNA activity of monoclonal immunoglobulins bearing an SLE idiotype is more common in IgG than IgM antibodies. *J Immunol* 1987; 138: 1515–18.

(12) Barlogie B, Epstein J, Selvanayagam P, Alexanian R. Plasma cell myeloma – new biological insights and advances in therapy. *Blood* 1989; 73: 865–75.

(13) Epstein J, Barlogie B, Katzmann J, Alexanian R. Phenotypic heterogeneity in aneuploid multiple myeloma indicates pre-B-cell involvement. *Blood* 1988; 71: 861–5.

(14) Grogan TM, Durie BGM, Spier CM, Richter L, Vela E. Myelomonocytic antigen positive multiple myeloma. *Blood* 1989; 73: 763–9.

(15) Bergsagel D. Plasma cell neoplasma and acute leukaemia. *Clin in Haematol* 1982; 11: 221–34.

(16) Warburton P, Joshua DE, Gibson J, Brown RD. CD10-(CALLA)-positive lymphocytes in myeloma: evidence that they are a malignant precursor population and are of germinal centre origin. *Leukemia and Lymphoma* 1989; 1: 11–20.

(17) Kyle RA. Multiple myeloma: review of 869 cases. *Mayo Clinic Proceedings* 1975; 50: 29–40.

(18) Zinneman HH, Hall WH. Recurrent pneumonia in multiple myeloma and some observations on immunologic response. *Ann Int Med* 1954; 41: 1152–63.

(19) Fahey JL, Scoggins R, Utz J, Szwed C. Infections, antibody response and

gammaglobulin components in multiple myeloma and macroglobulinanaemias. *Am J Med* 1963; 35: 690–707.

(20) Durie B, Salmon S. The current status and future prospects of treatment for multiple myeloma. *Clin in Haematol* 1982; 11: 181.

(21) Meyers BRN, Hirshman SL. Axelrod IA. Current patterns of infection in multiple myeloma. *Am J Med* 1972; 52: 87–92.

(22) Savage DG, Lindenbaum J, Garrett TJ. Biphasic pattern of bacterial infection in multiple myeloma. *Ann Int Med* 1982; 96: 47–50.

(23) Epersen F, Birgens H, Hertz J, Drivsholm A. Current patterns of bacterial infection in myelomatosis. *Scand J Infect Dis* 1984; 16: 169–73.

(24) Marks J. Antibody formation in myelomatosis. *J Clin Pathol* 1953; 6: 62–3.

(25) Lawson HA, Stuart CA, Paull AM et al. Observations on the antibody content of the blood in patients with multiple myeloma. *N Eng J Med* 1955; 252: 13–18.

(26) Linton AL, Dunnigan MG, Thomson JA. Immune responses in myeloma. *Br Med J* 1963; 2: 86–9.

(27) Birgins HS, Espersen F, Hertz JG, Pederson FK, Drivsholm A. Antibody response to pneumococcal vaccination in patients with myelomatosis. *Scand J Haematol* 1983; 30: 324–30.

(28) Cone L, Uhr JW. Immunological deficiency disorders associated with chronic lymphatic leukaemia and multiple myeloma. *J Clin Invest* 1964; 43: 2241–8.

(29) Harris JE, Alexanian R, Hersh EM, Migliore P. Abnormal immune response to keyhold limpet haemocyanin with multiple myeloma. *Ann Int Med* 1969; 70: 1084.

(30) Weits J, de Gast GC, The TH, Marrink J, Mandema E. Immune response in asymptomatic paraproteinemia 1. Primary and secondary antibody response to Helix pomatia haemocyanin. *Scand J Immunol* 1976; 5: 1163–9.

(31) Barlogie G, Smith L, Alexanian R. Effective treatment of advanced multiple myeloma refractory to alkylating agents. *N Eng J Med* 1984; 310: 1353–6.

(32) Barlogie B, Hall R, Zander A, Dickie K, Alexanian R. High dose melphalan with autologous bone marrow transplantation for multiple myeloma. *Blood* 1986; 67: 1293–301.

(33) Paglieroni T, MacKenzie MR. Studies on the pathogenesis of an immune defect in multiple myeloma. *J Clin Invest* 1977; 59: 1120–3.

(34) Massaia M, Bianchi A, Dianzani C, Attisano C, Boccadora M, Pileri A. Defective cell mediated immunity in monoclonal gammopathies. In: Barlogie B, Alexanian R, eds. *Proceedings of the Second International Workshop in Myeloma.* Houston: University of Texas, 1989: 5.

(35) Pilarski LM, Mant MJ, Ruether BA et al. Abnormal clonogenic potential of T-cells from multiple myeloma patients. *Blood* 1985; 66: 1266–71.

(36) Fenton MR, Havas HF. The effect of plasmacytomas on serum immunoglobulin levels of Balb/c mice. *J Immunol* 1975; 114: 793–801.

(37) Jacobson DR, Zolla-Pazner S. Immunosuppression and infection in multiple myeloma. *Seminars in Oncol* 1986; 13: 282–90.

(38) Joshua DE, Brown G, MacLennan ICM. Immune suppression in Balb/c mice bearing the plasmacytoma TEPC-183: evidence for normal lymphocyte but defective macrophage function. *Int J Cancer* 1979; 23: 663–72.

(39) Kolb J-P, Arrian S, Zolla-Pazner S. Suppression of the humoral immune

response by plasmacytomas: mediation by adherent mononuclear cells. *J Immunol* 1977; 118: 702–9.

(40) Kennard J, Zolla-Pazner S. Origin and function of suppressor macrophages in myeloma. *J Immunol* 1980; 124: 268–73.

(41) Katzmann JA. Myeloma-induced immunosuppression: a multistep mechanism. *J Immunol* 1978; 121: 1405–9.

(42) Ullich S, Zolla-Pazner S. Immunoregulatory circuits in myeloma. *Clin in Haematol* 1982; 11: 87–111.

(43) Ptak W, Gersham R. Immunosuppression effected by macrophage surfaces. *J Immunol* 1975; 115: 1346–50.

(44) Ptak W, Naidorf R, Gershon R. Interface with the transmission of T cell-derived messages by macrophage membranes. *J Immunol* 1977; 119: 444–9.

(45) Joshua DE, Humphrey JH, Grennan Deirdre, Brown G. Immunosuppression in Balb/c mice bearing the plasmacytoma TEPC-183: massive increase in red pulp macrophages induced by the tumour. *Immunology* 1980; 40: 223–8.

(46) Watson SR, Suivic VS, Brown IN. Defect of macrophage functions in the antibody response to sheep erythrocytes in systemic Mycobacterium lepraemurium infection. *Nature* 1975; 256: 206–8.

(47) Warren HS, Weidarz WD. Malarial immunodepression in vitro: adherent spleen cells are functionally defective as accessory cells in the response to horse erythrocytes. *Eur J Immunol* 1976; 6: 816–19.

(48) Hoover RG, Dieckgraefe BK, Lake J et al. Lymphocyte surface membrane immunoglobulin in myeloma. III. IgA plasmacytomas induce large numbers of circulating, adult-thymectomy-sensitive theta+, Lyt-1⁻ 2+ lymphocytes with IgA-Fc receptors. *J Immunol* 1982; 129: 2329–31.

(49) Hoover RG, Lynch RG. Isotype-specific suppression of IgA: suppression of IgA responses in BALB/c mice by T alpha cells. *J Immunol* 1982; 130: 521–3.

(50) Waldmann TA, Strober W. Metabolism of immunoglobulins. *Prog Allergy* 1969; 13: 1–110.

(51) Broder S, Humphrey R, Durm M et al. Impaired synthesis of polyclonal (non-paraprotein) immunoglobulins by circulating lymphocytes from patients with multiple myeloma: role of suppressor cells. *N Eng J Med* 1975; 293–87.

(52) Twomey JJ, Laughter AH, Rice L, Ford RJ. Suppression of lymphocyte responses by monocytes with untreated and treated multiple myeloma. *Blood* 1982; 60: 316–32.

(53) Petersen J, Drivsholm A, Brandt M, Ambjørnsen A, Dickmeiss E. B lymphocyte function in multiple myeloma: analysis of T-cell and monocyte-dependent antibody production. *Eur J Haematol* 1989; 42: 193–201.

(54) Mellstedt H, Holm G, Pettersson D et al. T-cells in monoclonal gammopathies. *Scand J Haematol* 1982; 29: 57–62.

(55) Wahlin A, Roos G, Holm J. T-cell subsets in multiple myeloma. Impact of cytostatic treatment. *Blut* 1985; 51: 291–6.

(56) Hoover RG, Hickman S, Gebel HM et al. Expansion of Fc receptor bearing T lymphocytes in patients with immunoglobulin G and immunoglobulin A myeloma. *J Clin Invest* 1981; 67: 308–11.

(57) Oken MM, Kay NE. T-cell subpopulations in multiple myeloma: correlation with clinical disease status. *Br J Haematol* 1981; 49: 629–34.

(58) Mackenzie MR, Paglieroni TG, Warner NL. Multiple Myeloma IV. The EA rosette-forming cell is a Leu-1 positive immunoregulatory B cell. *J Immunol* 1987; 139: 24–8.

(59) Mackenzie MR, Scibienski R, Paglieroni TG. Characterization of an immunosuppressive human plasma cell line. In: Barlogie B, Alexanian R, eds. *Proceedings of the Second International Workshop in Myeloma.* Houston: University of Texas, 1989: 4.

(60) Pilarski LM, Andrews EJ, Mant MJ, Reuther BA. Humoral immune deficiency in multiple myeloma patients due to compromised B-cell function. *J Clin Immunol* 1986; 6: 491–6.

(61) Pilarski LM, Mant MJ, Reuther BA. Pre-B cells in peripheral blood of multiple myeloma patients. *Blood* 1985; 66: 416–22.

(62) Pilarski LM, Reuther BA, Mant MJ. Abnormal function of B lymphocytes from peripheral blood of multiple myeloma patients. *J Clin Invest* 1985; 75: 2024–9.

(63) Leonard RCF, MacLennan CM, Smart Y et al. Light chain isotype associated suppression of normal plasma cell number in patients with multiple myeloma. *Int J Cancer* 1979; 24: 385–93.

(64) Wearne A, Joshua DE, Kronenberg H. Light chain isotype associated suppression of surface immunoglobulin expression on peripheral blood lymphocytes in myeloma during plateau phase. *Br J Haematol* 1984; 58: 563–8.

(65) Joshua DE, Wearne A, Kronenberg H. Indication for therapy in multiple myeloma. Should it be stage or stability? *Lancet* 1985; ii: 210.

(66) Rohrer JW, Lynch RG. Immunoregulation of localised and disseminated murine myeloma: antigen-specific regulation of MOPC-315 stem cell proliferation and secretory cell differentiation. *J Immunol* 1979; 123: 1083–7.

(67) Jorgensen T, Hannestad K. T helper lymphocytes recognised the V_1 domain of the isologous mouse myeloma protein 315. *Scand J Immunol* 1979; 10: 317–23.

(68) McNamara M, Kohler H. Regulatory idiotype-recognising helper T-cells by free light chains and heavy chains. *J Exp Med* 1984; 159: 623–8.

(69) Ioannidis RA, Joshua DE, Warburton T et al. Multiple myeloma: evidence that light chains play an immunoregulatory role in B cell regulation. *Hematol Pathol* 1989; 3: 169–75.

(70) Abbas AK, Claus CGB. Inhibition of antibody production in mouse plasmacytoma cells by antigens. *Eur J Immunol* 1977; 7: 667–73.

(71) Antigen-antibody complexes suppress antibody production by mouse plasmacytoma cells in vitro. *Eur J Immunol* 1978; 8: 217–21.

(72) Rohrer JW, Lynch TG. Specific immunologic regulation of differentiation of immunoglobulin expression in MOPC 315 cells during in vivo growth in diffusion chambers. *J Immunol* 1977; 119: 2045–53.

(73) Abbas AK, Perry LL, Bach BA, Greene MI. Idiotype specific T-cells immunity. I. Generation of effector and suppressor T-lymphocytes reactive with myeloma idiotype determinants. *J Immunol* 1980; 124: 1160–6.

(74) Abbas AK. T lymphocyte-mediated suppression of myeloma function in vitro. I. Suppression by allogeneically activated T lymphocytes. *J Immunol* 1979; 123: 2100–206.

(75) Selby PF, McElwain TJ, Nandi AC et al. Multiple myeloma treated with high dose intravenous melphalan. *Br J Haematol* 1987; 66: 55–8.

(76) Oken MM, Kyle RA, Greipp PR, Kay NE, Tsiatis A, O'Connell MJ. Alternating cycles of VBMCP with interferon (rIFN-alpha 2) in the treatment of multiple myeloma. *Proc Soc Clin Oncol* 1988; 7: 868A.

(77) Greipp PR, Kyle RA. Clinical morphological and cell kinetic differences among multiple myeloma, monoclonal gammopathy of undetermined significance, and smoldering multiple myeloma. *Blood* 1983; 62: 166–72.

(78) Durie BGM, Russell DH, Salmon SE. Reappraisal of plateau phase in myeloma. *Lancet* 1980; ii: 65.

(79) Wearne A, Joshua DE, Brown RD, Kronenberg H. Multiple myeloma: the relationship between CALLA (CD10) positive lymphocytes in the peripheral blood and light chain isotype suppression. *Br J Haematol* 1987; 67: 39–44.

(80) Joshua DE, Ioannidis R, Brown R, Francis SE, Gibson J, Kronenberg H. Multiple myeloma: relationship between light chain isotype suppression, labelling index of plasma cells, and CD38 expression on peripheral blood lymphocytes. *Am J Haematol* 1988; 29: 5–11.

(81) Van Kemp B, Reynaert PH, Broodtaerts L. Studies on the origin of the precursor cell in multiple myeloma Waldenstrom's macroglobulinaemia and benign monoclonal gammopathy. *Clin Exp Immunol* 1982; 44: 82–6.

(82) Nicholls M, Vincent P, Repka E, Saunders J, Gunz F. Isotypic discordance of paraproteins and lymphocyte surface immunoglobulins in myeloma. *Blood* 1981; 57: 192–5.

(83) Wearne A, Joshua DE, Young GAR, Kronenberg H. Multiple myeloma: light chain isotype suppression – a marker of stable disease at presentation. *Eur J Haematol* 1987; 38: 43–9.

(84) Wearne A, Joshua DE, Kronenberg H. Monitoring myeloma – light chain isotype suppression a new parameter. *Aust NZ J Med* 1985; 15: 629–33.

(85) Joshua DE. Biology of multiple myeloma – host–tumour interactions and immune regulation of disease activity. *Hematol Oncol* 1988; 6: 83–8.

(86) MacLennan CM, Gray D. Antigen-driven selection of virgin and memory B cells. *Immunol Rev* 1986; 91: 61–85.

(87) Brown RD, Ioannidis RA, Joshua DE, Kronenberg H. Serum thymidine kinase as a marker of disease activity in patients with multiple myeloma. *Aust NZ J Med* 1989; 19: 226–32.

(88) Kohler G, Potash M, Lehrach H, Shulman M. Deletions in immunoglobulin mu chains. *EMBO J* 1982; 1: 555–63.

(89) Gordon J. Molecular aspects of immunoglobulin expression by human B cell leukaemias and lymphomas. *Ad Cancer Res* 1984; 41: 71–154.

(90) Hopper JE, Papagiannes E. Evidence by radioimmunoassay that mitogen activated human blood mononuclear cells secrete significant amounts of light chain Ig unassociated with heavy chain. *Cell Immunol* 1986; 101: 122–31.

(91) Diaz-Espada F, Milstein C, Secher D. The regulation of membrane-bound and secreted immunoglobulins in the human lymphoid cell line LICR-LON and human hybridomas. *Mol Immunol* 1987; 24: 595–603.

(92) Boux HA, Raison RL, Walker KZ, Hayden G, Basten A. A tumour associated

antigen specific for human kappa myeloma cells. *J Exp Med* 1983; 158: 1769–74.

(93) Allen D, Cumano A, Dildrop R, Kocks C et al. Timing, genetic requirements and functional consequences of somatic hypermutation during B-cell development. *Immunol Rev* 1987; 96: 5–22.

(94) Weitzman S, Margueles DH, Sharff MD. Mutations in mouse myeloma cells: implications for human multiple myeloma and the production of immunoglobulins. *Ann Intern Med* 1976; 85: 110–16.

(95) Clofent G, Brockly F, Commes T, Lefranc MP, Bataille R, Klein B. No preferential use of the VH(V) family in human myeloma. *Br J Haematol* 1989; 73: 490.

(96) Liu YJ, Joshua DE, Williams GT, Smith CA, Gordon J, MacLennan CM. Mechanism of antigen-driven selection in germinal centres. *Nature* 1989; 342: 929–31.

(97) Carter A, Spira G, Manaster J, Tatarsky I. Spontaneous immunoglobulin changes in human plasma-cell dyscrasia. *Scand J Haematol* 1981; 27: 111–18.

(98) Bartoloni C, Fiamini G, Genthoni N et al. Immunochemical and ultrastructural study of multiple myeloma with a heavy chain protein in the serum. *J Clin Pathol* 1980; 33: 936–45.

(99) Preud'homme JL, Morel-Maroger L, Brouet JC, Mihaesco E, Mery JP, Seligmann M. Synthesis of abnormal heavy and light chains in multiple myeloma with visceral deposition of monoclonal immunoglobulin. *Clin Exp Immunol* 1980; 42: 545–53.

Index

Abelson murine leukaemia virus (Ab-MuLV)
    79–81
abl oncogene 79–81
actinomycin D, and mutant PGP 32
AIDS-related lymphadenopathy, gene
    rearrangements 150, 152
alpha interferon *see* interferon alpha
angioimmunoblastic lymphadenopathy, gene
    rearrangements 150
anti-CD5 immunotoxin, *see* ricin A chain
    H65-RTA
anti-CD19 antibody-blocked ricin
    immunotoxin, in B cell
    malignancies 56–7

B cell lymphoma, anti-CD22 monoclonal
    antibody RTA immunotoxin 58–9
B cell malignancies
    anti-CD19 antibody-blocked ricin
        immunotoxin 56–8
    side effects 58
    gene rearrangements 145, 149–54
BCG therapy, in low-grade lymphomas
    183
bcr gene, and Ph translocation 85
bcr-abl gene
    and acute leukaemias 89–91
    and chronic myelogenous leukaemia 88–9
biological response modifiers in low-grade
    lymphoma 183
    following relapse 186–7
bone marrow transplantation, in AML
    remission
    allogeneic, prognosis 121
        timing 121–2
    autologous (autograft) 122–34
        age factor 122–3
        clinical experience 126–8
        clinical trial assessment 131–4
        factors influencing outcome 128–9
        and graft-versus-host disease 123–4
        purging 124–6; clinical results 129–30
        in second remission 130–11
    classification of AML 114
bone marrow transplantation, and graft-

versus-host disease, use of
    immunotoxins 54–5, 56
bone marrow transplantation, in low-grade
    lymphomas 183
    following relapse 185–6
bone marrow transplantation, in small non-
    cleaved lymphomas 202
breast cancer, positive PGP staining 35–6
Burkitt's/non–Burkitt's lymphoma 199, 200
    see also non-Hodgkin's lymphomas high
        grade
busulphan, during AML remission 131, 133

CAM *see* cellular adhesion molecules
Castleman's disease, gene rearrangements 150
CD structures
    in AML remission 115
    CD5, immunotoxin, *see* ricin A chain
        H65-RTA
    marker, immunotoxin cytotoxicity 55
    CD19, immunotoxin, and B cell
        malignancies 56–8
    CD22, monoclonal antibody, and B cell
        lymphoma 58–9
    RTA immunotoxins targeting leucocyte
        cell surface structures 53, 54
cellular adhesion molecules, effect of GM-
    CSF 11
cellular immunity associated with myeloma
    227–8
central nervous system, prophylaxis 209–23
    leukaemia, acute lymphoblastic, incidence,
        relative risk and timing 211–12
    acute non-lymphoblastic 212–13
    pathogenesis 210–11
    non-Hodgkin's lymphoma 213
    acute lymphoblastic: cytosine
        arabinoside and triple therapy 216;
        gold standard therapy 213–20;
        methotrexate 213–14, 215–16
    irradiation 215–20; combined with
        chemotherapy 217–20; IQ ratings
        219; less or no irradiation 217–20;
        other toxicities 217
    toxicity 215–20

Index

chemotherapy
  in acute lymphoblastic leukaemia 213–20
    with CNS irradiation 217–20
    in low-grade lymphohomas 181–4
    following relapse 184–5, 186
chloroxyadenosine, in hairy cell leukaemia 68
chromosome abnormalities
  in AML prognosis 114
  localization of HGFs 2–4
  Philadelphia *see* Philadelphia chromosome
  translocations, in small non-cleaved
    lymphoma 200
  9, Ph chromosome, distinguishing from
    other anomalies at 9q34, 97–8
  22, Ph chromosome, distinguishing from
    other anomalies at 22qll, 97–8
  see also Philadelphia chromosome
chronic renal failure, use of HGFs 16
colony stimulating factor
  identification 2
  see also granulocyte-CSF: granuloctye
    macrophage-CSF: macrophage-CSF
Condyloma acuminata, interferon alpha 64
CSF *see* colony stimulating factor
cyclophosphamide, during AML remission
  131, 133
cytokines, in minimal residual disease 160
cytomegalovirus pneumonitis, in BMT for
  AML remission 117–19
cytosine arabinoside, in ALL 216, 220

deoxycoformycin, in hairy cell leukaemia
  68–9
digital image microscopy, in minimal residual
  disease 158
dimethyl sulphoxide, and P-glycoprotein
  expression 30
DMSO *see* dimethyl sulphoxide

eosinophils, effects of HGFs 10–11
Epstein–Barr virus, in small non-cleaved
  lymphoma 200
erythropoietin
  clinical use 16
  production 5
  signal transduction 14

G protein activity, erythropoietin, GM-CSF,
  and IL-3, 12
G-CSF *see* granulocyte-CSF
gene rearrangements in lymphoproliferative

disorders 149–54
  B-cell malignancies 149
  Hodgkin's disease 149–50
  Ig and TCR genes, clinical applications,
    152–3
  mixed lineage 150
  non-neoplastic gene rearrangements 150
  T-cell malignancies 149
  translocation involving antigen receptor
    genes 150–2
  translocation (t(14:18)) in lymphomas
    153–4
glucose-6-phosphate dehydrogenase, in AML
  remission 116
glutathione
  depletion and multi-drug resistance 43
  transferases and multi-drug resistance 41–3
  expression 42
  transfection studies 42
GM-CSF *see* granuloctye macrophage-CSF
graft-versus-host disease
  BMT in AML remission 117, 118
  autologous BMT 123–4
  prevention 119–20
  immunotoxins 54
  H65-RTA 55–6
graft-versus-leukaemia, effect after BMT
  116–17, 123
granulocyte-CSF
  biological activity 9–11
  characteristics 7
  clinical use 16–17
  production 4–6
  receptors 6–9
  signal transduction 11–14
granulocyte macrophage-CSF
  biological activity 2
  chromosome location 2–4
  cloning 2–4
  and chromosomal localization 3–4
growth factors
  and haemopoietic regulation 1–28
  see also haemopoietic growth factors
GST *see* glutathione transferases

haematological malignancies
  MDR significance 35–6
  multi-drug resistance 35–6
haemopoiesis
  negative regulators 14–16
  clinical use 17

haemopoietic cells, origin 1–2
haemopoietic growth factors 1–28
  biochemistry 2
  biological activity 2, 9–11
  characteristics 7
  chromosomal localization 2–3
  clinical use 16–17
  cloning 2–4
  molecular size 3
  production 4–6
  receptors 6–9
  signal transduction 11–14
haemopoietic regulation by growth factors
    1–28
  see also haemopoietic growth factors
hairy cell leukaemia
  chloroxyadenosine 68
  deoxycoformycin 68–9
  interferon alpha 64, 68
    mechanism of action 69
HILDA see leukaemia inhibitory factor
HLA identical MLC non-reactive sibling for
    BMT 117
Hodgkin's disease
  gene rearrangements 149
  interferon alpha 72
humoral immunodeficiency associated with
    myeloma 226–7
hypoxanthine phosphoribosyl transferase, in
    AML remission 116

immunodeficiency syndromes, gene
    rearrangements 150
immunoglobulin
  gene, in minimal residual disease 160–1
  gene studies, clinical applications 152–3
  normal rearrangement 146–9
    detection 147–9
immunophenotyping
  in AML 114–15
  in minimal residual disease 158
immunotoxins in haematological oncology
    49–62
  clinical studies 53–9
  conjugated to antibodies 53
  design 50–3
  endocytosis 49–50
  H65-RTA 55–6
  ricin 50–3
  ricin A chain 53
interferon

cell proliferation and differentiation 66
definition 63
effects on cell function 66
gene products 66
gene regulation 65
immune system 66
in low-grade lymphomas 186
in minimal residual disease 160
molecular characteristics 64
molecular level 65–6
receptors 65
signal transduction 65
types 63–5
interferon alpha 63–78
  anti-viral activity 63–4, 66
  in chronic granulocytic leukaemia 70–1
    mechanism of action 71
  in chronic lymphatic leukaemia 72–3
  in essential thrombocythaemia 73
  in hairy cell leukaemia 68
    mechanism of action 69
  in lymphoma 72
  measurement of activity 66–7
  in myelodysplasia 73
  in myelofibrosis 73
  in myeloma 72
  pharmacology 67
  therapeutically available 64
  versus other treatment modalities 68–9
interleukin-1
  biological activity 10
  clinical use 16
  receptors 6, 7, 8
interleukin-2
  in low-grade lymphomas 186
  in minimal residual disease 160
  receptors 6, 8, 7
interleukin-3
  biological activity 2, 9–11
  characteristics 7
  clinical use 16–17
  cloning and chromosomal localization 2–4
  production 4–6
  receptors 6–9
  signal transduction 12, 13
interleukin-4
  clinical use 16
  receptors 6, 8
interleukin-5
  cloning and chromosomal localization 3–4
  production 4

Index

interleukin-6
  biological activity 2, 10
  characteristics 7
  cloning and chromosomal localization 3
  production 4
  receptors 6
interleukin-7
  receptors 6, 8
intron, indications for use 64

kaposi sarcoma, interferon alpha 64
  AIDS-related 64

LAK *see* lymphokine-activated killer cells
leukaemia
  acute lymphoblastic
    childhood, CNS prophylaxis, *see* central
      nervous system, prophylaxis
    with chromosome anomalies at 22qll
      97–8; distinguishing Ph
      translocation 97–8
    clinical features 84–5; Ph+ 89–91
    minimal residual disease 35, 159–60
    and P-glycoprotein 33
  acute myelogenous (myeloid)
    with 9q34 chromosome anomalies 97;
      distinguishing Ph translocation 97
    clinical features 84–5; Ph+ 89–91
    MDR 35
    remission, treatment options 111–43; bone
      marrow transplantation 116–17,
      121–34; *see also* bone marrow
      transplantation in AML remission;
      chemotherapy 113, 116, 131, 132–3;
      classification of AML 114; graft-
      versus-host disease, prevention
      119–21; immunophenotyping
      114–15; nature of remission 115–16;
      options for post-remission treatment
      112; pneumonitis 117–19: CMV
      status 117–19; prevention 118–19;
      seronegative patient 119; prognostic
      factors 114–15; quality of remission
      111–12
  acute non-lymphoblastic, CNS
    prophylaxis, *see* central nervous system,
      prophylaxis
  chronic granulocytic, interferon alpha 64,
    70–1
  chronic lymphatic, interferon alpha 72–3
  chronic myelogenous

and *bcr–abl* gene 88–9
blast crisis, Ph+ 91–4
clinical features, Ph+ chromosome 83–4
Ph negative 94–6, *bcr*+ 94–5; *bcr*– 95–6
hairy cell, *see* hairy cell leukaemia
inhibitory factor, synergistic activity 10
Philadelphia chromosome-positive 81–5
  clinical findings 82–5
  cytogenetic findings 81–2
  variant translocations 81–2
polymerase chain reaction technique 98
lung cancer, and multi-drug resistance 34
lymphoid malignancies, gene rearrangements
  145, 149–54
lymphokine-activated killer cells, hairy cell
  resistance 69
lymphoma
  interferon alpha 72
  low-grade 173–93
    clinical presentation 176
    etiology 175–6
    incidence 175–6
    results of treatment 176–8: stage I–II
      176–8; stage III and, IV 178–80
    staging 176
    therapy controversies, BCG maintenance
      therapy 183; biological response
      modifiers 183: following relapse
      186–7
    bone marrow transplantation 183:
      following relapse 185–6
    combinations, complete remission rates
      182
  conventional chemotherapy stage III–IV
    181–4
  impact of complete remission 180–1
  maintenance of remission 182
  radiotherapy for stage III 181
  salvage therapy following relapse 184:
    future prospects 184; older patients
      184–5; radiotherapy 184; targeted
      therapy 186; younger patients 185
  single agents v. combinations 181
  watch and wait approach 179–80
  non-Hodgkin's *see* non-Hodgkin's
    lymphomas
  positive PGP staining 35–6
  translocation (t(14:18)) 153–4
  see also B cell lymphoma: T cell lymphoma
lymphoproliferative disorders 145–72
  gene rearrangements 145, 149–54

see also gene rearrangements
minimal residual disease 154–61
    see also minimal residual disease
M-CSF *see* macrophage-CSF
macrophage-CSF
  biological activity 2, 9–11
  characteristics 7
  cloning and chromosomal localization 2–4
  production 4–6
  receptors 6–9
  signal transduction 11–14
melphalan, during AML remission 132
methotrexate, in acute lymphoblastic
  leukaemia 213–14
  combined 216
  combined with CNS irradiation 217–20
  intrathecal 215–16
minimal residual disease, in lymphoid
  malignancies 159–61
    clinical perspectives 159–61
    experimental techniques 160–1
    maintenance chemotherapy 159
    phenotypic markers 159
  in lymphoproliferative disorders 154–61
    clinical perspectives 159
    methods to detect 156–8
monoclonal antibodies, in minimal residual
  disease 160
multi-drug resistance, mechanisms 29–48
  chromosomal location 30
  clinical significance 34–5
  genetic studies 30
  genomic organization 30
  glutathione transferases 41–3
    see also glutathione transferases
  haematological malignancies 35–6
  molecular studies 30
  mutation of MDRI gene 32
  P-glycoprotein expression 29–30
    tissue distribution 33
  protein modification 31–2
  regulation 30–3
    summary 33
  reversal 36–7
  RNA stabilization 32
  topoisomerase II 37–41
    see also topoisomerase II
  tumour expression 34–5
multiple myeloma, immune regulation 225–40
  associated cellular immunity 227–8
  associated humoral immunodeficiency
    226–7

B-cell ontogeny, somatic mutation as
  marker 233
B-cell, role of light chains 231–2
host-mediated effects on tumour growth
  230–1
  multiple myeloma 230–1
  plasmacytoma, murine 230
immunodeficiency mechanism 228–301
  human 229–30
  plasmacytoma, murine, in
    immunodeficiency mechanism 228,
    230
precursor cell dynamics 232–3
site of host–tumour interaction 234
murine leukaemia, and oncogenes 79–81
mycosis fungoides, interferon alpha 72
myelodysplasia, interferon alpha 73
myelofibrosis, interferon alpha 73
myeloma
  interferon alpha 72
  multiple, *see* multiple myeloma
  positive PGP staining 35–6

natural killer cells, hairy cell resistance
  69
neutropaenia, use of HGFs 16
neutrophils, effects of HGFs 10–11, 13–14
NK *see* natural killer cells
non-Hodgkin's lymphoma
  CNS prophylaxis 213
  gene rearrangements 150
non-Hodgkin's lymphomas, high-grade
  195–207
  classification 195–6
  lymphoblastic, clinical presentation 196
    diagnosis methods 197
    management 196–9
    prognostic factors 197–8
    treatment 197–9
  peripheral T-cell lymphoma 203
  small non-cleaved 199–203
    bone marrow transplantation 202
    Burkitt's/non-Burkitt's 199
    chemotherapy 201–2
    chromosomal translocations 200
    clinical presentation 200
    Epstein–Barr virus 200
    relapsed, therapy 201–2
    therapeutic trials 200–1
    tumour lysis syndrome 200
non-neoplastic gene rearrangements 150

Index

P-glycoprotein
  in breast cancer 35
  clinical significance tumours 34–5
  homologies 29–30
  in lymphoma 35
  and MDR regulation 30
  and MDR reversal 36–7
  modification 31–2
  molecular and genetic studies 30
  in myeloma 35
  tissue distribution 33
PCR *see* polymerase chain reaction
PGP *see* P-glycoprotein
Ph chromosome, in AML prognosis 114
Philadelphia chromosome, genetics 79–110
  ABL gene 86–7
  BCR gene 85–6
  BCR–ABL gene 88–9
  conclusions 98–100
  essential thrombocythaemia 96–7
  leukaemias, Ph chromosome positive 81–5,
    97–8
  murine leukaemia and oncogenes 79–81
  polymerase chain reaction 98
  translocation, distinguished from other
    anomalies at 22qll and 9q34 97
  Ph, molecular genetics 85–96
phorbol myrisate acetate (PMA)
  and GM-CSF 13–14
  and IL-3 13
Pityriasis lichenoides et varioliformis acuta,
  gene rearrangements 150
PKC *see* protein kinase C
plasmacytoma, murine, and
  immunodeficiency mechanism in myeloma
    228, 238
platelet-derived growth factor receptor 12
pneumonitis and BMT for AML remission
  117–19
  CMV status, patient and recipient 117–19
  prevention 118
  seronegative 119
  seropositive patient 118
polymerase chain reaction
  in immunoglobulin gene rearrangement
    147–9
  in minimal residual disease 156–8
  in TCR gene rearrangement 147
  technique in leukaemia 98
  to analyse MDRI RNA levels 34–5
post-cardiac transplantation, gene

rearrangements 150
protein kinase C, and IL-3 13

renal cell cancer, interferon alpha 64
ricin 50–3
  conjugation to antibody 52
    monoclonal, M-T151 52
  cytotoxicity 52
  isolation 50–1
  structure 51
  toxin entry 51–2
ricin A chain (RTA) immunotoxins 53
  H65-RTA, in graft-versus-host disease 55
  in T cell lymphoma 56
  targeting human leucocyte cell surface
    structures 53, 54
RNA, rapid, transcript sequence analysis of
  clonal TCR, in minimal residual disease
    156
roferon, indications for use 64
RTA *see* ricin A chain

saccharomyces cerevisiae 30, 37
Sjögren's disease, gene rearrangements 150
sodium butyrate, and P-glycoprotein
  expression 30
Southern analysis
  in immunoglobulin gene rearrangement
    147–9
  in minimal residual disease 158
  in TCR gene rearrangement 147–9

T-cell(s)
  lymphoma, immunotoxin H65-RTA 56
  malignancies, gene rearrangements 145,
    149–54
  receptor, clonal, RNA transcript sequence
    in minimal residual disease 156
  receptor gene, in minimal residual disease
    160–1
    normal rearrangement 146–9; detection
      147–9
    studies, clinical applications 152–3
  removal from BMT in AML remission
    119–21
taxol, and mutant PGP 32
TGF alpha or beta, *see* transforming growth
  factor alpha or beta
thrombocythaemia, essential, Ph chromosome
  96–7

thrombocytopaenia, essential, interferon
    alpha 73
topoisomerase I, up regulation 40
topoisomerase II (topo II) 37–41
    abnormally functioning 39–40
    action 37–8
    clinical implications 41
    and drug resistance 39
    as a drug target 38
    glucose deprivation 40
    hypoxia 40
    methylation 40
    point mutations 39–40
    regulation 38–9
    switch to novel form 40–1
    tissue distribution 41

total body irradiation, during AML remission
    133
transforming growth factor alpha, interferon
    inhibition 16
transforming growth factor beta, negative
    regulation 15–16
translocations in lymphoid neoplasia 150–2,
    153–4
    involving antigen receptor genes 150–2
    in lymphomas 153–4
tumours, solid, MDR significance 34–5
tyrosine kinase activity, M-CSF 11–12

vincristin, and mutant PGP 32

wellferon, indications for use 64